The Collected Works of D. W. Winnicott

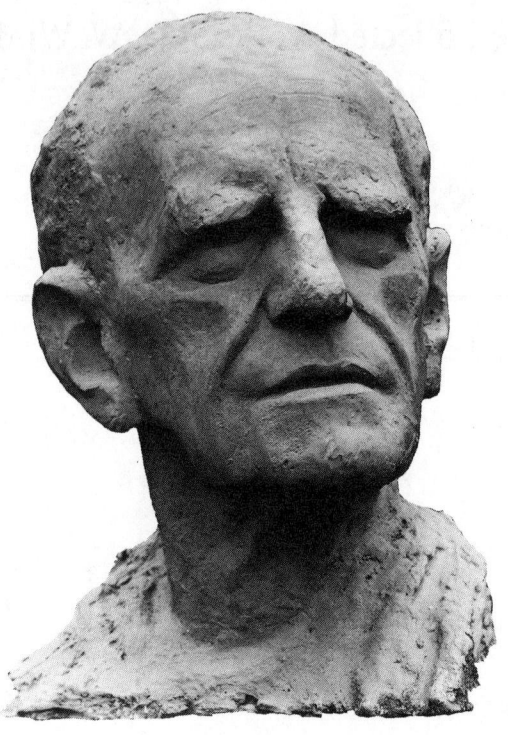

Oscar Nemon's bust of D. W. Winnicott, plaster cast, 1971

Reproduced courtesy of the Oscar Nemon Estate

The Collected Works of D. W. Winnicott

Volume 3, 1946–1951

General Editors
Lesley Caldwell and Helen Taylor Robinson

Assistant Editor
Robert Adès

Managing Editor
Amal Treacher Kabesh

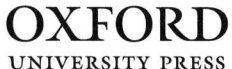

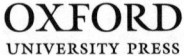
OXFORD
UNIVERSITY PRESS

Oxford University Press is a department of the University of Oxford. It furthers
the University's objective of excellence in research, scholarship, and education
by publishing worldwide. Oxford is a registered trade mark of Oxford University
Press in the UK and certain other countries.

Published in the United States of America by Oxford University Press
198 Madison Avenue, New York, NY 10016, United States of America.

© Oxford University Press 2017

All rights reserved. No part of this publication may be reproduced, stored in
a retrieval system, or transmitted, in any form or by any means, without the
prior permission in writing of Oxford University Press, or as expressly permitted
by law, by license, or under terms agreed with the appropriate reproduction
rights organization. Inquiries concerning reproduction outside the scope of the
above should be sent to the Rights Department, Oxford University Press, at the
address above.

You must not circulate this work in any other form
and you must impose this same condition on any acquirer.

Library of Congress Cataloging-in-Publication Data
Names: Winnicott, D. W. (Donald Woods), 1896–1971, author. |
Caldwell, Lesley, editor. | Taylor Robinson, Helen, editor.
Title: The collected works of D. W. Winnicott / edited by Lesley Caldwell
and Helen Taylor Robinson.
Description: Oxford ; New York : Oxford University Press, [2017] | Includes
bibliographical references and index.
Identifiers: LCCN 2016026458 (print) | LCCN 2016039667 (ebook) |
ISBN 9780199399338 (set) | ISBN 9780190271336 (v. 1) | ISBN 9780190271343 (v. 2) |
ISBN 9780190271350 (v. 3) | ISBN 9780190271367 (v. 4) | ISBN 9780190271374 (v. 5) |
ISBN 9780190271381 (v. 6) | ISBN 9780190271398 (v. 7) | ISBN 9780190271404 (v. 8) |
ISBN 9780190271411 (v. 9) | ISBN 9780190271428 (v. 10) | ISBN 9780190271435 (v. 11) |
ISBN 9780190271442 (v. 12)
Subjects: LCSH: Child psychiatry. | Child psychology. | Psychoanalysis. | Psychotherapy.
Classification: LCC RJ499 .W479 2017 (print) | LCC RJ499 (ebook) | DDC 618.92/8914—dc23
LC record available at https://lccn.loc.gov/2016026458

1 3 5 7 9 8 6 4 2

Printed by Sheridan Books, Inc., United States of America

COMPLETE CONTENTS OF
THE *COLLECTED WORKS OF D. W. WINNICOTT*

VOLUME 1: 1911–1938

Foreword by Christopher Bollas	xlvii
Acknowledgements	li
Editors' Note	lv
General Introduction to the *Collected Works*	lvii
LESLEY CALDWELL AND HELEN TAYLOR ROBINSON	
Introduction to Volume 1	3
KEN ROBINSON	

PART 1 **School to Medical Training, 1911–1920s**

1. Letter to His Mother, Elizabeth, ca. 2 September 1911–1913	27
2. Letter to Stanley Ede, ca. 1912–1913	29
3. Smith, 1913	31
4. Letter to His Family, 3 November 1913	35
5. Letter to His Family, ca. 23 December 1913	37
6. The Night Attack, 1914	39
7. Letter to His Family, 9 May 1914	43
8. The Best Remedy, 1914	45
9. Letter to His Mother, Elizabeth, n.d., late 1916	49
10. Letter to His Family, 9 December 1916	51
11. Letter to His Sister, Violet, 15 November 1919	53
12. A Shropshire Surgeon, 1920	57
13. St Bartholomew's Hospital Amateur Dramatic Club, 1920	59
14. A Reminder to the Binder, 1921	63

15. The Snag, 1921 — 65
16. What Is Worthwhile in Medicine, ca. 1917–1923 — 67

PART 2 First Contributions to Medicine, 1926–1930

1. Varicella Encephalitis and Vaccinia Encephalitis, with Nancy Gibbs, 1926 — 75
2. Case for Diagnosis (? Poliomyelitis with Some Spasticity), 1926 — 91
3. Case for Diagnosis (? Infantile Hemiplegia), 1926 — 93
4. Two Cases of Post-Encephalitic Hypernoea, 1926 — 95
5. Case of Stunted Growth, 1927 — 99
6. The Only Child, 1928 — 101
7. Facial Nerve Paralysis, 1928 — 111
8. Facial Nerve Paralysis, Associated with Fits, 1928 — 113
9. Encephalitis After Measles and Chicken-pox, 1928 — 115
10. Muscle Weakness, Altered Gait and Absent Deep Reflexes after Measles, 1928 — 117
11. Abscess in Frontal Lobe: Post-Mortem Findings in a Case Shown at a Previous Meeting of the Section, with Elisabeth O'Flynn, 1928 — 119
12. Rheumatism in Children, 1929 — 123
13. Hemiplegia Noticed After Diphtheria, 1929 — 127
14. Measles Encephalitis, 1930 — 129
15. Symptoms Suggesting Post-Encephalitis, 1929 — 131
16. The Diagnosis of Chorea, 1929 — 133
17. Enuresis (abstract), 1929 — 141
18. Short Communication on Enuresis, 1930 — 143
19. Pathological Sleeping, 1930 — 149
20. Hæmoptysis: Case for Diagnosis, 1931 — 151
21. Pre-systolic Murmur, Possibly Not Due to Mitral Stenosis, 1931 — 153

22. A Clinical Example of Symptomatology Following
    the Birth of a Sibling, ca. 1931   155

23. Child Psychiatry: The Body as Affected by Psychological
    Factors, ca. 1931   159

24. On In-Patient Treatment for Rheumatic Fever
    and Chorea, ca. 1923–1931   161

PART 3 *Clinical Notes on Disorders of Childhood*, 1931

    Preface   167
    Introduction   169

1. History-Taking   173
2. Physical Examination   187
3. A Note on Temperature and the Importance of Charts   195
4. The Nose and Throat   203
5. The Heart, with Special Reference to Rheumatic Carditis   207
6. Rheumatic Fever   219
7. The Rheumatic Clinic   225
8. Active Heart Disease   229
9. Growing Pains   235
10. Arthritis Associated with Emotional Disturbance   239
11. Fidgetiness   245
12. A Note on Normality and Anxiety   255
13. Anxiety (*continued*)   275
14. Disease of the Nervous System   281
15. Walking   291
16. Mental Defect   299
17. Convulsions, Fits   303
18. Micturition Disturbances   315
19. Masturbation   323
20. Speech Disorders   329

PART 4 **Further Writings, 1932–1939**

1. Abstract: Psychoanalysis and Medicine, by F. Alexander, 1933 — 339
2. Abstract: Repression and Rationalisation, by H. Lundholm, 1934 — 341
3. Papular Urticaria and the Dynamics of Skin Sensation, 1934 — 343
4. Discussion: The Difficult Child by G. A. Auden, 1934 — 353
5. Abstract: A Contribution to the Problem of Psycho-physical Relations with Special Reference to Dermatology, by M. Barinbaum, 1935 — 357
6. The Manic Defence, 1935 — 359
7. The Teacher, the Parent and the Doctor, 1936 — 375
8. Letter to Robina Addis, April 1936 — 389
9. Contribution to a Discussion on Enuresis, 1936 — 391
10. Mental Hygiene of the Pre-School Child, 1936 — 397
11. Appetite and Emotional Disorder, 1936 — 413
12. Review: *Wayward Youth* by August Aichhorn, 1936 — 433
13. Review: *On the Bringing Up of Children* by Five Psycho-analysts, 1936 — 437
14. Review: *Child Psychiatry* by Leo Kanner, 1937 — 439
15. Letter to Roger Money-Kyrle, 13 May 1937 — 441
16. Notes on a Little Boy, 1938 — 443
17. Shyness and Nervous Disorders in Children, 1938 — 445
18. Skin Changes in Relation to Emotional Disorder, 1938 — 449
19. Letter to Mrs Neville Chamberlain, 10 November 1938 — 463
20. Letter to John Bowlby, 6 December 1938 — 465

Chronology — 467
References — 473
Contributors — 479
Credits — 481
Index — 487

Complete Contents of the Collected Works of D. W. Winnicott

VOLUME 2: 1939–1945

Editors' Note	xlvii
Introduction to Volume 2 CHRISTOPHER REEVES	3

PART 1 1939

1. Letter to the *British Medical Journal*, Circumcision, 14 January	25
2. Letter to the *British Medical Journal*, Pruritus and Psychology, 22 April	29
3. The Delinquent and Habitual Offender	31
4. The Deprived Mother	35
5. Early Disillusion	43
6. Letter to the *British Medical Journal*, Evacuation of Small Children, 16 December	47
7. The Psychology of Juvenile Rheumatism	49
8. Aggression, ca. 1939	65
9. Delinquency: Continued, ca. 1930s	73

PART 2 1940

1. Letter to Kate Friedlander, 8 January	79
2. Children and Their Mothers	81
3. Discussion of War Aims	87
4. Children in the War	95

PART 3 1941

1. Report on Q Camps	103
2. Letter to the *British Medical Journal*, Communal Feeding in Schools, 6 September	107
3. On Influencing and Being Influenced	109
4. Review: *The Moral Paradox of Peace and War* by Prof J. C. Flügel	115

5. Review: *The Cambridge Evacuation Survey* edited by Susan Isaacs   117

6. The Observation of Infants in a Set Situation   121

7. Meet to be Stolen From   141

PART 4 1942

1. Resolution K: On Scientific Aims in Psychoanalysis   145

2. Child Department Consultations   149

3. Letter to the *British Medical Journal*, Loneliness in Infancy, 17 October   165

4. Why Children Play   167

5. Review: *The Nursing Couple* by Merell P. Middlemore   171

PART 5 1943

1. A Doctor Looks at the Psychiatric Social Worker   177

2. Delinquency Research   195

3. Memorandum on 'The Relationship Between Clinical Paediatrics and Child Psychology'   201

4. Letter to the *Lancet*, Prefrontal Leucotomy, 10 April   207

5. Letter to the *Lancet*, Prefrontal Leucotomy, 15 May   209

6. Treatment of Mental Disease by Induction of Fits   211

7. Letter to the *British Medical Journal*, Responsibility and Freedom, 21 August   217

8. Getting to Know Your Baby   221

9. The Wearing of Masks in the Nursing of Premature and Older Infants   227

10. Letter to the *British Medical Journal*, Shock Treatment of Mental Disorder, 25 December   229

PART 6 1944

1. Letter to Roger North   233

2. Why Do Babies Cry?   237

3. Psychological Aspects of Birching	247
4. Letter to the *British Medical Journal*, Shock Therapy, 12 February	251
5. A Tendency in Therapeutics	255
6. Introduction to a Symposium on the Psycho-Analytic Contribution to the Theory of Shock Therapy	261
7. Kinds of Psychological Effect of Shock Therapy	265
8. What About Father?	271
9. Their Standards and Yours	277
10. What Do We Mean by a Normal Child?	281
11. Support for Normal Parents	287
12. Letter to Dr Marjorie Franklin, 19 October	291
13. Infant Feeding	293
14. The Problem of Homeless Children, with Clare Britton	299
15. Ocular Psychoneuroses of Childhood	313

PART 7 1945

1. The Only Child	323
2. The Evacuated Child	329
3. The Return of the Evacuated Child	335
4. Thinking and the Unconscious	341
5. Twins	343
6. Memorandum on Corporal Punishment	349
7. Home Again	353
8. Primitive Emotional Development	357
9. Evidence Given to the Home Office Committee on Children's Homes	369
10. Letter to the *British Medical Journal*, Physical Therapy in Mental Disorder, 22 December	379

11. Towards an Objective Study of Human Nature	381
12. Breast Feeding	389
Chronology	397
References	403
Contributors	407
Credits	409
Index	413

VOLUME 3: 1946–1951

Editors' Note	xlvii
Introduction to Volume 3	3
VINCENZO BONAMINIO AND PAOLO FABOZZI	

PART 1 1946

1. Children's Hostels in War and Peace	23
2. Educational Diagnosis	29
3. Letter to the *British Medical Journal,* Psychology in the Child's Education, 29 June	35
4. Letter to Lord Beveridge, 15 October	37
5. Letter to *The Times,* 6 November	39
6. Letter to Ella Sharpe, 13 November	41
7. Some Psychological Aspects of Juvenile Delinquency	43
8. Psychological Aspects of Juvenile Delinquency (n.d., ca. late 1940s)	49

PART 2 1947

1. Hate in the Countertransference	59
2. Physical Therapy of Mental Disorder	69
3. Residential Management as Treatment for Difficult Children	77
4. Further Thoughts on Babies as Persons	95
5. The Child and Sex	101
6. Letter to the *British Medical Journal,* Battle Neurosis Treated with Leucotomy, 13 December	113

Complete Contents of the Collected Works of D. W. Winnicott   xiii

PART 3 1948

1. Reparation in Respect of Mother's Organized Defence Against Depression — 117
2. Paediatrics and Psychiatry — 123
3. Letter to the *British Medical Journal,* 'Pathies in a State Service, 14 February — 141
4. The Gwrw Tree — 143
5. Letter to Anna Freud, 6 July — 147
6. Review: *The Psychology of the Unwanted Child* by Agatha H. Bowley — 149
7. Review: *Parents' Questions* by The Child Study Association of America — 151
8. Disorders of Childhood — 153
9. Review: *The Psychoanalytic Study of the Child, Volume 2* edited by Anna Freud, Willie Hoffer, Edward Glover, *et al.* — 157
10. Review: *The Personality of the Pre-School Child* by Professor Werner Wolff — 159
11. Obituary: Susan Isaacs — 161
12. Primary Introduction to External Reality: The Early Stages — 165
13. Environmental Needs; the Early Stages; Total Dependence and Essential Independence — 171

PART 4 1949

1. Letter to Paul Federn, 3 January — 179
2. Letter to the *British Medical Journal,* Taking Children's Temperatures, 6 January — 181
3. Letter to Marjorie Stone, 14 February — 183
4. The Infancy of Juliet — 185
5. Letter to Roger Money-Kyrle, 22 March — 195
6. Letter to Roger Money-Kyrle, 31 March — 197
7. Letter to Roger Money-Kyrle, 2 May — 199

8. Birth Memories, Birth Trauma, and Anxiety	201
9. Letter to Joan Riviere, 19 May	221
10. Letter to Roger Money-Kyrle, 13 June	223
11. Notes on the Discussion Held on Dr Winnicott's Paper 'The Birth Trauma'	225
12. Letter to Roger Money-Kyrle, 22 June	229
13. Letter to Roger Money-Kyrle, 24 June	231
14. Letter to Joan Riviere, 24 June	233
15. Review: *Handbook of Child Guidance* by Ernest Harms	235
16. Letter to *The Times*, Punishment and Crime: A Psychologist's View, 10 August	237
17. Letter to R. S. Hazlehurst, 1 September	239
18. Letter to S. H. Hodge, 1 September	241
19. Letter to the *British Medical Journal*, Paddington Green's Children's Hospital, 24 September	243
20. Mind and Its Relation to the Psyche-Soma	245
21. Leucotomy	259
22. Review: *Art Versus Illness* by Adrian Hill	265
23. A Man Looks at Motherhood	269
24. The Baby as a Going Concern	273
25. Where the Food Goes	277
26. The End of the Digestive Process	281
27. The Baby as a Person	285
28. Close-up of Mother Feeding Baby	289
29. The World in Small Doses	293
30. The Innate Morality of the Baby	299
31. Weaning	303
32. Young Children and Other People	307
33. Stealing and Telling Lies	313

34. The Impulse to Steal	319
35. Sex Education in Schools	323
36. Enuresis: Notes for a lecture to the Tavistock Children's Department (n.d., ca. 1949)	327

PART 5 1950

1. Letter to Clare Britton [Excerpt], early 1950	331
2. Aggression in Relation to Emotional Development	333
3. Letter to *The Times*, Neglected Children, 31 January	349
4. Letter to Otho W. S. Fitzgerald, 3 March	351
5. Childhood Psychosis	353
6. Letter to P. D. Scott, 11 May	357
7. Letter to *The Times*, Maladjusted Children: Damaging Effect of Delay, May 13	361
8. Review: *Infancy of Speech and Speech of Infancy* by Leopold Stein	363
9. Letter to Roger Money-Kyrle, 10 July	365
10. The Deprived Child and How He Can Be Compensated for Loss of Family Life	367
11. Letter to Roger Money-Kyrle, 8 August	381
12. Letter to Hannah 'Queen' Henry, 31 October	383
13. Letter to Roger Money-Kyrle, 16 November	385
14. Knowing and Learning	387
15. Instincts and Normal Difficulties	393
16. Growth and Development in Immaturity	397
17. Some Thoughts on the Meaning of the Word Democracy	407
18. 'Yes, But How Do We Know It's True?'	423

PART 6 1951

1. Review: *The Child and the Magistrate* by J. A. F. Watson	431
2. Letter to W. R. Bion, 22 January	433

3. Letter to James Strachey, 1 May — 435
4. The Foundation of Mental Health — 437
5. Visiting Children in Hospital — 441
6. Transitional Objects and Transitional Phenomena — 447
7. Review: *The Inner World of Man: with Psychological Drawings and Paintings* by Frances G. Wickes — 463
8. Letter to the *Lancet*, Leucotomy in Psychosomatic Disorders, 18 August — 465
9. Letter to the *British Medical Journal*, Ethics of Prefrontal Leucotomy, 25 August — 467
10. Review: *Jealousy in Children* by Edmund Ziman, M.D. — 469
11. Letter to *The Times*, Nursery Schools: A Definition of Functions, 8 September — 471
12. Review: *The Psychoanalytic Study of the Child, Volumes 3–4 and Volume 5* edited by Anna Freud, Willie Hoffer, and Edward Glover — 473
13. Letter to Edward Glover, 23 October — 475
14. Notes on the General Implications of Leucotomy — 477
15. Review: *On Not Being Able to Paint* by Marion Milner — 483
16. Review: *Problems of Infancy and Childhood* — 487
17. Review: *Papers on Psycho-Analysis* by Ernest Jones — 489
18. Review: *Infant Feeding and Feeding Difficulties* by Philip Rainsforth Evans and Ronald Mackeith — 491

Chronology — 495
References — 501
Contributors — 507
Credits — 509
Index — 515

VOLUME 4: 1952–1955

Editors' Note	xlvii
Introduction to Volume 4 DOMINIQUE SCARFONE	3

PART 1 1952

1. The Ordinary Devoted Mother and Her Baby: The First Week	21
2. The Ordinary Devoted Mother and Her Baby: Baby Bites	25
3. Letter to Hanna Segal, 21 February	29
4. Letter to The *Lancet*, Frontal Lobes of the Human Brain, 8 March	33
5. Psychoses and Child Care	35
6. Letter to Augusta Bonnard, 3 April	45
7. Letter to Willi Hoffer, 4 April	47
8. Letter to S. S. Davidson, 5 May	49
9. Letter to H. Ezriel, 20 June	51
10. Letter to Ernest Jones, 22 July	53
11. Anxiety Associated with Insecurity	55
12. Letter to Melanie Klein, 17 November	59
13. Letter to Roger Money-Kyrle, 27 November	63

PART 2 1953

1. Letter to Hanna Segal, 22 January	71
2. Letter to Herbert Rosenfeld, 22 January	73
3. Letter to Herbert Rosenfeld, 17 February	77
4. Symptom Tolerance in Paediatrics: A Case History	79
5. Letter to W. Clifford M. Scott, 19 March	97
6. Review in *British Medical Journal*: *Twins: A Study of Three Pairs of Identical Twins* by Dorothy Burlingham	101
7. Review in *New Era*: *A Study of Three Pairs of Identical Twins* by Dorothy Burlingham	103

8. The Unconscious — 107

9. Letter to Esther Bick, 11 June — 109

10. Review: *Maternal Care and Mental Health* by John Bowlby — 111

11. Review: *Psycho-Analysis and Child Psychiatry* by Edward Glover — 115

12. Review: *Problems of Infancy and Childhood* edited by Milton Senn — 117

13. Letter to Sylvia Payne, 7 October — 119

14. Letter to David Rapaport, 9 October — 121

15. Letter to Hannah Ries, 27 November — 123

16. Review: *Childhood and Society* by Erik H. Erikson — 125

17. Review: *Direct Analysis: Selected Papers* by John N. Rosen — 127

18. Review: *Psychoanalytic Studies of the Personality* by W. R. D. Fairbairn, with Masud Khan — 129

19. Two Adopted Children — 139

20. Mother, Teacher, and the Child's Needs — 151

21. Transitional Objects and Transitional Phenomena — 159

PART 3 1954

1. Letter to W. Clifford M. Scott, 27 January — 177

2. Letter to Charles Rycroft, 5 February — 179

3. Letter to *The Spectator*, A Psychiatrist's Choice, 12 February — 181

4. Letter to W. Clifford M. Scott, 26 February — 183

5. The Depressive Position in Normal Emotional Development — 185

6. Metapsychological and Clinical Aspects of Regression Within the Psycho-Analytical Set-Up — 201

7. Letter to Anna Freud, 18 March — 219

8. Letter to Betty Joseph, 13 April — 221

9. Letter to W. Clifford M. Scott, 13 April — 223

10. Letter to Sir David K. Henderson, 10 May — 227

11. Letter to John Bowlby, 11 May — 231

12. Review: *Child Psychotherapy* by S. R. Slavson — 233

Complete Contents of the Collected Works of D. W. Winnicott

13. Letter to Klara Frank, 20 May	235
14. Letter to Sir David K. Henderson, 20 May	237
15. Letter to Anna Freud and Melanie Klein, 3 June	241
16. Letter to Michael Fordham, 11 June	245
17. Review: *Aggression and Its Interpretation* by Lydia Jackson	247
18. Needs of the Under-Fives	249
19. Letter to Harry Guntrip, 20 July	257
20. Letter to *The Times*, Sponsored Television, 21 July	259
21. Letter to Harry Guntrip, 13 August	261
22. Review: *Clinical Management of Behavior Disorders in Children* by Harry Bakwin and Ruth Morris Bakwin	265
23. Letter to Thomas Stapleton, 20 September	267
24. Letter to Roger Money-Kyrle, 23 September	269
25. Letter to D. Chaplin, 18 October	271
26. Character Types: The Foolhardy and the Cautious: On *Funfairs, Thrills and Regressions* by Michael Balint	273
27. Letter to *The Times*, 'Pin-up' Pictures at Approved School, 1 November,	279
28. Play in the Analytic Situation	281
29. Withdrawal and Regression	283
30. Pitfalls in Adoption	291
31. Preface to *The First Treasured Possession* by Olive Stevenson	297

PART 4 **1955**

1. Holding and Interpretation: Fragment of an Analysis	303
Chronology	475
References	481
Contributors	485
Credits	487
Index	491

VOLUME 5: 1955–1959

Editors' Note	xlvii
Introduction to Volume 5	3
JENNIFER JOHNS AND MARCUS JOHNS	

PART 1 1955

1.	Letter to Roger Money-Kyrle, 10 February	19
2.	On Adoption	21
3.	Letter to Thomas Stapleton, 3 March	25
4.	Memorandum from Paddington Green Children's Hospital Psychology Department on Homosexuality and the Law	27
5.	Letter to Emilio Rodrigue, 17 March	31
6.	Letter to Roger Money-Kyrle, 17 March	33
7.	Private Practice	35
8.	Letter to Charles Rycroft, 21 April	43
9.	Group Influences and the Maladjusted Child: The School Aspect	45
10.	For Stepparents	55
11.	Clinical Varieties of Transference	61
12.	Adopted Children in Adolescence	67
13.	Letter to the *British Medical Journal*, Comforters, 13 August	77
14.	Letter to Michael Fordham, 26 September	79
15.	Letter to Hanna Segal, 6 October	81
16.	Letter to Wilfred R. Bion, 7 October	83
17.	Letter to Anna Freud, 18 November	87
18.	A Case Managed at Home	89
19.	Foreword to *Any Wife, Any Husband* by Dr Joan Graham	99
20.	First Experiments in Independence	101
21.	A Note on Regression and Reassurance	107
22.	Letter to Charles M. Schulz, 1955	109

23. The Toddler, the Second Adoption, Telling Children
    About Adoption, undated, ca. mid-1950s.   111

PART 2 1956

1. What Do We Know About Babies as Cloth Suckers?   115
2. Letter to the *British Medical Journal*, Prefrontal Leucotomy,
   28 January   119
3. Letter to Joan Riviere, 3 February   121
4. Fragments Concerning Varieties of Clinical Confusion   125
5. On 'A Study of Envy and Gratitude' by Melanie Klein   129
6. Letter to Enid Balint, 22 March   133
7. Psycho-Analysis and the Sense of Guilt   135
8. The Antisocial Tendency   149
9. Letter to Gabriel Casuso, 4 July   159
10. Letter to Oliver H. Lowry, 5 July   161
11. Paediatrics and Childhood Neurosis   165
12. Letter to Charles Rycroft, 7 October   171
13. Letter to Charles Rycroft, 17 October   173
14. Letter to J. Peter M. Tizard, 23 October   175
15. Letter to Barbara Lantos, 8 November   179
16. Primary Maternal Preoccupation   183
17. Notes on Adolescence, ca. 1956   189

PART 3 1957

1. Letter to Anna M. Kulka, 15 January   197
2. Letter to Charles Rycroft, 17 January   199
3. Letter to Thomas Main, 24 January   201
4. Address Introducing Margaret Mead, VIIIth Ernest
   Jones Lecture   203
5. Letter to Margaret Mead, 31 January   205

6. Letter to Thomas Main, 25 February	207
7. Letter to Melanie Klein, 7 March	209
8. Remarks on a Discussion of Balint's Paper on Technique	211
9. Letter to Michael Balint, 27 March	213
10. Letter to Michael Balint, 4 April	215
11. Letter to Tsuicheu Cheu, 4 April	217
12. Letter to *The Times*, I Qant Stand It, 11 April	219
13. Letter to Martin James, 17 April	221
14. Review: *Six Children* by Estelle J. Foote	223
15. The Contribution of Psycho-Analysis to Midwifery	225
16. Letter to Mary Applebey, 27 May	233
17. Foreword to *The Case as the Patient Sees It: Psychoanalysis*	235
18. Letter to Joan Riviere, 21 June	237
19. Letter to Prunella Briance, 15 July	239
20. The Capacity to Be Alone	241
21. On the Contribution of Direct Child Observation to Psycho-Analysis	249
22. Letter to Augusta Bonnard, 1 October	255
23. Hallucination and Dehallucination	257
24. Letter to Michael Balint, 3 October	261
25. Letter to Francesca Bion, 3 October	263
26. Integrative and Disruptive Factors in Family Life	265
27. Advising Parents	277
28. Letter to Augusta Bonnard, 7 November	285
29. Excitement in the Aetiology of Coronary Thrombosis	287
30. The Mother's Contribution to Society	293
31. Health Education Through Broadcasting	297
32. Preface to *Collected Papers: Through Paediatrics to Psychoanalysis*	301

PART 4 1958

1. Letter to Grantly Dick-Read, 15 January — 305
2. Letter to Marianne Baumann, 20 January — 307
3. Funeral Address for Ernest Jones — 309
4. Psychogenesis of a Beating Fantasy — 313
5. Review: *The Psychoanalytic Study of the Child, Volume 11* edited by Ruth S. Eissler, Anna Freud, Heinz Hartmann, and Ernst Kris — 317
6. The First Year of Life: Modern Views on the Emotional Development — 319
7. The Psychology of Separation — 333
8. Letter to Anna Freud, 14 May — 337
9. Where Angels Fear to Tread, or A Comment on Generic Teaching — 339
10. Letter to Marianne Baumann, 5 June — 345
11. Letter to Anna Freud, 8 June — 347
12. Letter to Joan Riviere, 13 June — 349
13. Child Analysis in the Latency Period — 351
14. Letter to R. D. Laing, 18 July — 361
15. Review: *The Psychoanalytic Study of the Child, Volume 12* edited by Ruth S. Eissler, Anna Freud, Heinz Hartmann, and Ernst Kris — 363
16. Letter to Herbert Rosenfeld, 16 October — 365
17. The Family Affected by Depressive Illness in One or Both Parents — 367
18. On 'Separation Anxiety' by John Bowlby — 379
19. Letter to Anna Freud, 7 November — 383
20. Letter to Victor Smirnoff, 19 November — 385
21. Obituary: Ernest Jones — 389
22. Obituary: Dr Ambrose Cyril Wilson — 399
23. Review: *The Doctor, His Patients, and the Illness* by M. Balint — 401

| 24. Transitional Objects and Transitional Phenomena | 405 |
| 25. Theoretical Statement of the Field of Child Psychiatry | 421 |

PART 5 1959

1. Review: *Envy and Gratitude* by Melanie Klein	433
2. Letter to Reginald Lightwood, 10 February	437
3. Letter to Miss Maw, 16 February	439
4. Memorandum on Gisburne House	441
5. Classification: Is There a Psycho-Analytic Contribution to Psychiatric Classification?	445
6. Letter to *The Times*, Nursery Schools Essential, 25 March	461
7. Letter to Donald Meltzer, 21 May	463
8. Letter to Kenneth Soddy, 9 June	465
9. Letter to Paul Halmos, 12 June	467
10. Nothing at the Centre	469
11. Letter to Dorothy E. M. Gardner, 13 July	473
12. Letter to Arthur J. Metcalfe, 14 July	475
13. Letter to Herman Gijsbert van der Waals, 23 July	477
14. Letter to A. Tommy M. Wilson, 23 September	479
15. Casework with Mentally Ill Children	481
16. Letter to Elliot Jaques, 13 October	493
17. Discussion of 'Grief and Mourning in Infancy' by John Bowlby	495
18. Letter to Paula Heimann, 5 November	501
19. Letter to Thomas Szasz, 19 November	503
20. Counter-Transference	505
21. The Effect of Psychotic Parents on the Emotional Development of the Child	516
22. The Fate of the Transitional Object	523
23. Review (film): *Going to Hospital with Mother* by James Robertson	529

24. Foreword to *Childbirth with Confidence* by Prunella Briance	533
25. Obituary: Oscar Friedmann	535
26. Clinical Material on the Theme of a Male Patient's Exploitation of His Female Self	539
27. A Clinical Approach to Family Problems: The Family	543

Chronology	547
References	553
Contributors	561
Credits	563
Index	567

VOLUME 6: 1960–1963

Editors' Note	xlvii
Introduction to Volume 6 ANGELA JOYCE	3

PART 1 1960

1. Saying 'No'	31
2. Letter to Michael Balint, 5 February	43
3. Letter to Jacques Lacan, 11 February	45
4. Jealousy	47
5. Letter to Merton J. Kahne, 19 February	63
6. The Effect of Psychosis on Family Life	65
7. What Irks?	73
8. The Relationship of a Mother to Her Baby at the Beginning	87
9. On Security	93
10. Aggression, Guilt and Reparation	97
11. Letter to Alexander Luria, 7 July	105
12. Letter to Ilse Hellman, 21 July	107
13. Letter to John Harvard-Watts, 28 July	109
14. Letter to Mr and Mrs Young, 28 July	111

15. Obituary: Melanie Klein — 113
16. Letter to Serge Lebovici, 8 November — 115
17. The Family and Emotional Maturity — 117
18. Letter to Wilfred Bion, 17 November — 125
19. Comments on Joseph Sandler's 'On the Concept of the Superego' — 127
20. String: A Technique of Communication — 135
21. The Theory of the Parent-Infant Relationship — 141
22. Ego Distortion in Terms of True and False Self — 159

PART 2 1961

1. Letter to Lydia James, 20 January — 175
2. Letter to Sir Aubrey Lewis, 26 January — 177
3. Memorandum on Organizational Aspects of Child Care at Paddington Green Children's Hospital — 179
4. Adolescence: Struggling Through the Doldrums — 187
5. Varieties of Psychotherapy — 197
6. Feeling Guilty — 205
7. Letter to Dr Joan FitzHerbert, 25 April — 211
8. Review: *The Concept of Love in Childcare* by T. S. Simey — 213
9. Psychoanalysis and Science: Friends or Relations? — 217
10. Review: *Clinical Child Psychiatry* by Kenneth Soddy — 223
11. Notes on the Time Factor in Treatment — 225
12. Comments on 'Problems of Research in Psycho-Analysis' by Joseph Sandler — 229
13. Letter to Masud Khan, 26 June — 233
14. Letter to Pearl King, 18 July — 235
15. Matti, *aet* 12½ Years: A Therapeutic Consultation — 237
16. Sakari: A Therapeutic Consultation — 241
17. Psycho-Neurosis in Childhood — 253

18. Letter to Harry Guntrip, 15 September ... 261
19. The Paediatric Department of Psychology ... 263
20. Letter to Sir Aubrey Lewis, 13 October ... 267
21. Envy: A Male Patient Near the End of His Analysis ... 269
22. Comments on the Report of the Committee on Punishment in Prisons and Borstals ... 273
23. Letter to Wilfred Bion, 16 November ... 279

PART 3 1962

1. Review: *The Psychoanalytic Study of the Child, Volume 15* edited by Ruth S. Eissler, Anna Freud, Heinz Hartmann, and Marianne Kris ... 283
2. The Aims of Psycho-Analytical Treatment ... 285
3. Letter to Benjamin Spock, 9 April ... 289
4. The Development of a Child's Sense of Right and Wrong ... 295
5. Training for Child Psychiatry ... 299
6. The Five-Year-Old ... 309
7. The Beginnings of a Formulation of an Appreciation and Criticism of Klein's Envy Statement ... 315
8. A Personal View of the Kleinian Contribution ... 325
9. Dependence in Infant-Care, in Child-Care and in the Psycho-Analytic Setting ... 333
10. Providing for the Child in Health and Crisis ... 343
11. The Development of the Capacity for Concern ... 351
12. The Psycho-Analyst and Child Psychiatry: A Matter of Economics ... 357
13. The Theory of the Parent-Infant Relationship: Further Remarks ... 359
14. The Theory of the Parent-Infant Relationship: Contributions to Discussion ... 363
15. Review: *Letters of Sigmund Freud, 1873–1939* edited by Ernest Jones ... 367

16. Review: *Psychologie du Premier Âge* by Marcel Bergeron   371

17. Review: *Un Cas de Psychose Infantile* by S. Lebovici and J. McDougall   373

18. Morals and Education   377

19. Ego Integration in Child Development   389

PART 4 1963

1. Review: *The Psychoanalytic Study of the Child, Volume 16* edited by Ruth S. Eissler, Anna Freud, Heinz Hartmann, and Marianne Kris   399

2. Letter to Ronald MacKeith, 31 January   401

3. A Note on a Case Involving Envy   403

4. Considerations in the Study of Homosexuality   407

5. The Mentally Ill in Your Caseload   409

6. Letter to Timothy Raison, 9 April   421

7. Struggling Through the Doldrums   423

8. Communicating and Not Communicating Leading to a Study of Certain Opposites   433

9. The Psychotherapy of Character Disorders   447

10. The Value of Depression   461

11. From Dependence Towards Independence in the Development of the Individual   469

12. Psychiatric Disorder in Terms of Infantile Maturational Processes   479

13. Hospital Care Supplementing Intensive Psychotherapy in Adolescence   491

14. The Tree   499

15. D. W. W.'s Dream Related to Reviewing Jung   501

16. Review: *The Non-Human Environment in Normal Development and in Schizophrenia* by Harold F. Searles   505

17. Review: *Childhood Schizophrenia* by William Goldfarb   509

18. Perversions and Pregenital Fantasy   511

19. Two Notes on the Use of Silence	513
20. Further Clinical Material on the Theme of a Male Patient's Exploitation of His Female Self	519
21. Fear of Breakdown	523
Chronology	533
References	539
Contributors	545
Credits	547
Index	551

VOLUME 7: 1964–1966

Editors' Note	xlvii
Introduction to Volume 7	3
ANNA FERRUTA	

PART 1 1964

1. The Concept of the False Self	27
2. Review: *Heal the Hurt Child* by Hertha Riese	33
3. Letter to *New Society*, Love or Skill?, 23 March	37
4. The Neonate and His Mother	41
5. Deductions Drawn from a Psychotherapeutic Interview with an Adolescent	51
6. Psycho-Somatic Illness in Its Positive and Negative Aspects	67
7. Youth Will Not Sleep	79
8. Letter to Renata Gaddini, 26 June	83
9. The Importance of the Setting in Meeting Regression in Psycho-Analysis	85
10. Letter to *The Observer*, All of Mother, 25 October	91
11. Letter to John O. Wisdom, 26 October	95
12. Foreword to *The Widow's Child* by Margaret Torrie	99
13. Letter to *The Observer*, All of Mother, 8 November	101
14. This Feminism	103

15. Letter to Mrs B. J. Knopf, 26 November	113
16. Review: *Memories, Dreams, Reflections* by C. G. Jung	115
17. Introduction to the *Child, the Family, and the Outside World*	125
18. Roots of Aggression	129

PART 2 1965

1. New Light on Children's Thinking	139
2. Letter to Michael Fordham, 2 February	145
3. Letter to Humberto Nagera, 15 February	147
4. The Price of Disregarding Psychoanalytic Research	149
5. Do Progressive Schools Give Too Much Freedom to the Child?	157
6. Notes Made in the Train	163
7. The Concept of Trauma in Relation to the Development of the Individual Within the Family	169
8. Letter to Michael Fordham, 24 June	189
9. Letter to Michael Fordham, 15 July	191
10. Comment on Obsessional Neurosis and 'Frankie'	193
11. Further Comments on Obsessional Neurosis and Frankie	197
12. The Child, the Family and the Offender	203
13. Clinical Material: Theme of 'Two', also theme of 'Black'	207
14. Review: *Childhood and Society* by Erik H. Erikson	213
15. Letter to Charles Anthony Storr, 30 September	215
16. Review: *Normality and Pathology in Childhood* by Anna Freud	217
17. Letter to Martin James, 7 October	227
18. The Psychology of Madness	229
19. Case Notes for a Psychoanalytic Seminar: Withdrawal, Regression, Male Identification	239
20. A 70th Birthday Present	243

Complete Contents of the Collected Works of D. W. Winnicott   xxxi

21. Dissociation Revealed in a Therapeutic Consultation — 245
22. The Value of the Therapeutic Consultation — 273
23. A Child Psychiatry Case Illustrating Delayed Reaction to Loss — 279
24. Introduction to *The Maturational Processes and the Facilitating Environment* — 305
25. Preface to *The Family and Individual Development* — 309
26. Review: *Shared Fate* by H. David Kirk — 311

PART 3 1966

1. Letter to *The Times*, George III, 17 January — 315
2. The Split-off Male and Female Elements to Be Found in Men and Women — 317
3. The Ordinary Devoted Mother — 331
4. Letter to *The Times*, Psychiatric Care, 3 March — 339
5. Letter to Hans Thorner, 17 March — 341
6. Letter to Herbert Rosenfeld, 17 March — 343
7. Social Aspects of Autism — 345
8. Autism — 349
9. Letter to *The Times*, Why Courts Must Act Swiftly, 26 March — 365
10. Review: *Dibs: In Search of Self* by Virginia M. Axline — 367
11. Letter to *The Times*, 'Blood-Tie' Child, 4 April — 369
12. Letter to a Confidant, 15 April — 371
13. Letter to Lili E. Peller, 15 April — 373
14. Review: *The Psychoanalytic Study of the Child*, Volume 20 edited by Ruth S. Eissler, Anna Freud, Heinz Hartmann, and Marianne Kris — 375
15. Letter to Sylvia Payne, 26 May — 377
16. On Cardiac Neurosis in Children — 379
17. The Child in the Family Group — 387
18. Review: *Infantile Autism* by Bernard Rimland — 397

19. Letter to Renata Gaddini, 13 September — 399

20. Review: *Adolescents and Morality* by E. M. Eppel and M. Eppel — 401

21. Letter to William Gillespie, 29 September — 403

22. Review: *Absent: School Refusal as an Expression of Disturbed Family Relationships* by Max B. Clyne — 405

23. On the Occasion of the Publication of the *Standard Edition* of Freud — 407

24. Letter to Donald Meltzer, 25 October — 411

25. Review: *Your Child Is a Person* by S. Chess, A. Thomas, and H. G. Birch — 415

26. Review: *Asthma: Attitude and Milieu* by Aaron Lask — 417

27. Preface to Renata Gaddini's Italian Translation of *The Family and Individual Development* — 419

28. Letter to Renata Gaddini, 21 November — 423

29. The Unconscious — 425

30. Review: *Adoption Policy and Practice* by Iris Goodacre — 427

31. The Location of Cultural Experience — 429

32. The Absence of a Sense of Guilt — 437

33. Letter to a Patient, 13 December — 447

34. The Beginning of the Individual — 449

35. Letter to D. N. Parfitt, 22 December — 455

36. Discussion of 'The Clinical Handling of the Analyst's Response' by Ian Alger — 457

37. An Allotted Spanner in the Works — 459

Chronology — 461
References — 467
Contributors — 473
Credits — 475
Index — 479

Complete Contents of the Collected Works of D. W. Winnicott   xxxiii

VOLUME 8: 1967–1968

Editors' Note	xlvii
Introduction to Volume 8 ANN HORNE	3

PART 1 1967

1. Letter to Mrs P. Aitken, 13 January	33
2. D. W. W. on D. W. W.	35
3. The Association for Child Psychology and Psychiatry Observed as a Group Phenomenon	49
4. The Concept of a Healthy Individual	65
5. Letter to Renata Gaddini, 9 March	79
6. Environmental Health in Infancy	81
7. Review: *The Successful Step-Parent* by Helen Thomson	89
8. Delinquency as a Sign of Hope	91
9. The Non-Pharmacological Treatment of Psychosis in Childhood	99
10. Review: *A Home from Home* by Sheila Stewart	105
11. A Tribute on the Occasion of Willi Hoffer's Seventieth Birthday	107
12. Foreword to *The Hands of the Living God* by Marion Milner	115
13. Winnicott's Wisdom: The Meaning of Mother Love	117
14. Obituary: James Strachey	123
15. Review: *Absent: School Refusal as an Expression of Disturbed Family Relationships* by Max B. Clyne	129
16. Winnicott's Wisdom: How a Baby Begins to Feel Sorry and to Make Amends	131
17. Winnicott's Wisdom: Why Do Babies Cry?	137
18. Letter to a Colleague, 4 September	143
19. Letter to Renata Gaddini, 4 September	145
20. Letter to Margaret Torrie, 4 September	147

21. Letter to Margaret Torrie, 5 September	149
22. Winnicott's Wisdom: Hobgoblins and Good Habits	151
23. Letter to Wilfred R. Bion, 5 October	157
24. Letter to Gillian Nelson, 6 October	159
25. The Aetiology of Infantile Schizophrenia in Terms of Adaptive Failure	161
26. Letter to Charles Clay Dahlberg, 24 October	167
27. Playing: Creative Activity and the Search for the Self	169
28. Review: *How to Survive Parenthood* by Eda J. LeShan	181
29. The Concept of Clinical Regression Compared with that of Defence Organization	183
30. Trips into Partisanship	191
31. Letter to Arthur Miller, 13 November	195
32. Letter to Renata Gaddini, 21 November	197
33. Letter to Marjorie Spence, 23 November	199
34. Letter to Marjorie Spence, 27 November	201
35. Review: A Collection of Children's Books by Multiple Authors	203
36. Letter to R. S. W. Dowling, 8 December	205
37. Addendum to 'The Location of Cultural Experience'	207
38. Mirror-Role of Mother and Family in Child Development	211

PART 2 1968

1. The Place Where We Live	221
2. Communication Between Infant and Mother, and Mother and Infant, Compared and Contrasted	227
3. Physical and Emotional Disturbances in an Adolescent Girl	239
4. Chards Pil …	245
5. The Use of the Word 'Use'	249
6. Interpretation in Psycho-Analysis	253

7.	Letter to Donald Gough, 6 March	259
8.	Foreword to *Disturbed Children* by Robert J. N. Tod	261
9.	Playing and Culture	263
10.	*Sum*, I Am	267
11.	Review: *Vulnerable Children: Three Studies of Children in Conflict* by Lindy Burton	275
12.	The Effect of Loss on the Young	277
13.	Review: *The Psychoanalytic Study of the Child, Volume 22* edited by Ruth S. Eissler, Anna Freud, Heinz Hartmann, and Marianne Kris	279
14.	A Link Between Paediatrics and Child Psychology: Clinical Observations	283
15.	Playing: A Theoretical Statement	299
16.	Children Learning	313
17.	Letter to L. Joseph Stone, 18 June	319
18.	Review: *Human Aggression* by Anthony Storr	321
19.	Sleep Refusal in Children	323
20.	Letter to Mrs T., 6 September	327
21.	Roots of Aggression	329
22.	Foreword to *Susan Isaacs* by D. E. M. Gardener	333
23.	Letter to Adam Limentani, 27 September	335
24.	Letter to Renata Gaddini, 21 October	337
25.	Review: *Children in Distress* by Alec Clegg and Barbara Megson	339
26.	Breast-feeding as Communication	341
27.	First Interview with Child May Start Resumption of Maturation	349
28.	The Use of an Object and Relating Through Identifications	355
29.	Clinical Illustration of 'The Use of an Object'	365
30.	Further Clinical Illustration of 'The Use of an Object'	369
31.	Letter to Joyce Coles, 22? November	379
32.	Letter to Joyce Coles, 25? November	381

33. Letter to Karl and Sheila Britton, 25 November … 383

34. Letter to Joyce Coles, 26? November … 385

35. Letter to Joyce Coles, 29 November … 387

36. Letter to Joyce Coles, 1? December … 389

37. Letter to Joyce Coles, 4 December … 391

38. Comments on My Paper 'The Use of an Object' … 393

39. Letter to Karl Britton, 7? December … 397

40. Letter to Joyce Coles, 8 December … 399

41. Letter to Renata Gaddini, 9? December … 401

42. Letter to Joyce Coles, 10? December … 403

43. Letter to Joyce Coles, 14 December … 405

44. Letter to Karl and Sheila Britton, 14 December … 407

45. Foreword to *Therapy in Child Care* by Barbara Dockar-Drysdale … 409

46. Review: *The Psychology of Childhood and Adolescence* by C. I. Sandström … 411

47. The Squiggle Game … 413

48. Thinking and Symbol-Formation … 441

Chronology … 445
References … 451
Contributors … 457
Credits … 459
Index … 463

VOLUME 9: 1969–1971

Editors' Note … xlvii
Introduction to Volume 9 … 3
  ARNE JEMSTEDT

PART 1 1969

1. Letter to Michael Rosenbluth, 3 January … 23

2. Letter to F. Robert Rodman, 10 January … 25

3. Letter to an American Correspondent, 14 January	29
4. The Use of an Object in the Context of *Moses and Monotheism*	33
5. Letter to Renata Gaddini, 19 January	39
6. Letter to Anna Freud, 20 January	41
7. Letter to Michael P. Collinson, 10 March	43
8. Contribution to a Symposium on Envy and Jealousy	47
9. Some Principles of Child Analysis	51
10. Letter to Michael B. Conran, 8 May	53
11. Letter to Agnes Wilkinson, 9 June	57
12. Letter to William W. Sargant, 24 June	59
13. Letter to *Child Care News*, Behaviour Therapy, June	63
14. Physiotherapy and Human Relations	67
15. Development of the Theme of the Mother's Unconscious as Discovered in Psycho-Analytic Practice	75
16. Freedom	79
17. The Threat to Freedom	83
18. Moon Landing	89
19. Letter to Helm Stierlin, 31 July	91
20. Review: *Indications for Child Analysis and Other Papers* by Anna Freud	93
21. Additional Note on Psycho-Somatic Disorder	95
22. Letter to Robert Tod, 6 November	99
23. The Pill	101
24. Letter to Renata Gaddini and Her Family, 15 November	111
25. Berlin Walls	115
26. The Building Up of Trust	121
27. Preface to *Dialogue with Sammy* by S. Lebovici and J. McDougall	129
28. The Mother-Infant Experience of Mutuality	131

29. Mother's Madness Appearing in the Clinical Material as an Ego-Alien Factor — 141

30. Answers to Comments on 'The Split-Off Male and Female Elements' — 149

31. Psychologists as a Group — 155

32. Commentary on *Play Therapy* by Virginia Axline — 159

PART 2 1970

1. Letter to Peter Giovacchini, 5 March — 167
2. Letter to Michael Fordham, 10 March — 169
3. Child Psychiatry, Social Work and Alternative Care — 171
4. A Personal Statement on Child Psychiatry — 175
5. Contribution to the Final Number of *Case Conference* — 179
6. The Place of the Monarchy — 181
7. Letter to Renata Gaddini, 31 August — 189
8. Cure — 191
9. Residential Care as Therapy — 199
10. Individuation — 207
11. Living Creatively — 213
12. Basis for Self in Body — 225
13. Two Further Clinical Examples — 235
14. Day Dreaming — 247
15. Dependence in Child Care — 249

PART 3 1971

1. Letter to John Davis, 1 January — 255
2. Letter to Jeannine Kalmanovitch, 7 January — 257
3. Letter to Jeannine Kalmanovitch, 19 January — 259
4. Introduction to *Playing and Reality* — 261
5. Transitional Objects and Transitional Phenomena — 265

6. Dreaming, Fantasying and Living: A Case-History Describing a Primary Dissociation — 289

7. Creativity and Its Origins — 299

8. Interrelating Apart from Instinctual Drive and in Terms of Cross-Identifications — 319

9. Contemporary Concepts of Adolescent Development and Their Implications for Higher Education — 337

10. Tailpiece to *Playing and Reality* — 349

11. Not Less Than Everything (Extracts), ca. 1968–71 — 351

12. Notes for the Vienna Congress — 355

PART 4 Undated Work and Winnicott's 'Ideas' File

1. Ideas and Definitions — 359

2. The Day-Dreamer — 361

3. Notes for a Discussion on Technique in Analysis of Psychotics — 365

4. Knowing and Not Knowing: A Clinical Example — 367

5. A Point in Technique — 369

6. Note on Infant Observation — 371

7. Found Objects and Waifs — 373

8. Notes on Play — 375

9. Cleopatra Anamnesis Imphiccough — 381

10. The Niffle — 383

11. A Note on the Mother-Foetus Relationship — 389

12. Outline for a Study in the Sociology of Knowledge — 391

13. Ditty on Enoch Powell — 395

Chronology — 397
References — 403
Contributors — 409
Credits — 411
Index — 415

VOLUME 10: *Therapeutic Consultations in Child Psychiatry*

Editors' Note	xlvii
Introduction to Volume 10	3
MARCO ARMELLINI	
Acknowledgements	23

Therapeutic Consultations in Child Psychiatry

PART 1

Introduction	27
1. 'Iiro' *aet* 9 Years 9 Months	37
2. 'Robin' *aet* 5 Years	57
3. 'Eliza' *aet* 7½ Years	83
4. 'Bob' *aet* 6 Years	113
5. 'Robert' *aet* 9 Years	141
6. 'Rosemary' *aet* 10 Years	157
7. 'Alfred' *aet* 10 Years	165

PART 2

Introduction	189
8. 'Charles' *aet* 9 Years	191
9. 'Ashton' *aet* 12 Years	215
10. 'Albert' *aet* 7 Years 9 Months	235
11. 'Hesta' *aet* 16 Years	255
12. 'Milton' *aet* 8 Years	277

PART 3

Introduction	305
13. 'Ada' *aet* 8 Years	309
14. 'Cecil' *aet* 21 Months at First Consultation	337
15. 'Mark' *aet* 12 Years	371
16. 'Peter' *aet* 13 Years	405

17. 'Ruth' *aet* 8 Years ... 421
18. 'Mrs X' *aet* 30 Years ... 443
19. 'Lily' *aet* 5 Years ... 453
20. 'Jason' *aet* 8 Years 9 Months ... 455
21. 'George' *aet* 13 Years ... 497

    Appendices ... 517
    Chronology ... 537
    References ... 543
    Contributors ... 545
    Credits ... 547
    Index ... 549

VOLUME 11: *Human Nature* and *The Piggle*

Editors' Note ... xlvii
Introduction to Volume 11 ... 3
    STEVEN GROARKE

PART 1 *Human Nature*

Preface ... 25
Editorial note ... 27
Acknowledgements ... 29
Introduction ... 31

PART I The Human Child Examined: Soma, Psyche, Mind

Introduction ... 35

1. The Psyche-Soma and the Mind ... 39
    Somatic Health ... 39
    Psyche Health ... 40
    Intellect and Health ... 40

2. Ill-Health ... 43
    Somatic Ill-Health ... 43
    Psyche Ill-Health ... 44

3. Inter-Relationship of Body Disease and Psychological Disorder ... 47
    The Effect of the Body and Its Health on the Psyche ... 47
    Heredity ... 47
    Congenital Disorder ... 48
    Deficiencies of Intake ... 49

Elimination Defects	50
Accidents	50
A Category for the Not-Yet-Known	50
Allergy	51
The Effect of the Psyche on the Body and Its Functioning	51

4. The Psycho-Somatic Field — 53

PART II The Emotional Development of the Human Being

Introduction — 59

1. Interpersonal Relationships — 63
First Part of the Statement	63
The Family	65
Instinct	65
Love Relationships	72

2. The Concept of Health Using Instinct Theory — 75
Imaginative Elaboration of Function	75
The Psyche	76
The Soul	76
Excited and Quiet States	77
The Oedipus Complex	78
Restatement	79
Infantile Sexuality	80
Reality and Fantasy	81
The Unconscious	82
Summary	83
Chart Showing Psychology of Small Boy in Terms of Instinct Theory	84
Defences Against Anxiety—Castration Threat	84
Breakdown of Defences	85

PART III Establishment of Unit Status

Introduction: Emotional Development Characteristic of Infancy — 89

1. The Depressive Position — 91
Concern, Guilt and Inner Personal Psychic Reality	91
The Depressive Position: Recapitulation	97
Repression Reconsidered	99
The Management of Bad Forces and Objects	99
Inner Richness and Complexity	101

2. Development of the Theme of the Inner World — 103
Introduction	103
Paranoid Way of Life	103
Depression and the 'Depressive Position'	104
The Manic Defence	105

3. Various Types of Psycho-Therapy Material — 107

4. Hypochondriacal Anxiety — 113

PART IV From Instinct Theory to Ego Theory

Introduction: Primitive Emotional Development — 117

1. Establishment of Relationship with External Reality — 119
   Excited and Quiet Relationships — 119
   The Value of Illusion and Transitional States — 123
   Failure in Initial Contact — 125
   Primary Creativity — 126
   The Mother's Importance — 128
   The Baby at Birth — 129
   The Philosophy of 'Real' — 130

2. Integration — 133

3. Dwelling of Psyche in Body — 139
   Body Experience — 139
   Paranoia and Naiveté — 141

4. The Earliest States — 143
   Diagram of the Environment-Individual Set-Up — 143
   Action of Gravity — 147

5. A Primary State of Being: Pre-Primitive Stages — 149

6. Chaos — 153

7. The Intellectual Function — 157

8. Withdrawal and Regression — 159

9. The Birth Experience — 161

10. Environment — 169

11. Psycho-Somatic Disorder Reconsidered — 175
    Asthma — 175
    Gastric Ulcer — 177

Appendix — 179
   Synopsis I — 179
   Synopsis II — 182

PART 2 *The Piggle: An Account of the Psychoanalytic Treatment of a Little Girl*
EDITED BY ISHAK RAMZY

Preface by Clare Winnicott and R. D. Shepherd	187
Editor's Foreword by Ishak Ramzy	189
Introduction by D. W. Winnicott	193
1. The Patient	197
2. First Consultation	199
3. Second Consultation	207
4. Third Consultation	217
5. Fourth Consultation	227
6. Fifth Consultation	235
7. Sixth Consultation	241
8. Seventh Consultation	249
9. Eighth Consultation	255
10. Ninth Consultation	263
11. Tenth Consultation	271
12. Eleventh Consultation	279
13. Twelfth Consultation	287
14. Thirteenth Consultation	297
15. Fourteenth Consultation	305
16. Fifteenth Consultation	309
17. Sixteenth Consultation	315
Afterword: By the Parents of the Piggle	317
Chronology	319
References	325
Contributors	327
Index	329

Complete Contents of the Collected Works of D. W. Winnicott

VOLUME 12: Appendices and Bibliographies

Note on the Compilation, Structure, and Contents
of the *Collected Works*   liii
    ROBERT ADÈS

Introduction to Volume 12: Appendices and Bibliographies   3
    ROBERT ADÈS

PART 1 Winnicott's Publications

1. Chronological Bibliography of Works by D. W. Winnicott   25
2. Alphabetical Bibliography of Works by D. W. Winnicott   81
3. Complete Back Catalogue of the Published Books
of D. W. Winnicott   123
4. Winnicott's Plans for Books   151
5. Reference Lists from Books in Winnicott's Back Catalogue: 159
   a. *Collected Papers: Through Paediatrics to Psychoanalysis* (1958)   159
   b. *Holding and Interpretation: Fragment of an Analysis* (1986)   162
   c. *The Maturational Processes and the Facilitating Environment* (1965)   163
   d. *Playing and Reality* (1971)   166

PART 2 Winnicott's Correspondence

1. Chronological Bibliography of Letters by D. W. Winnicott   173
2. Alphabetical Bibliography of Letters by D. W. Winnicott   185
3. Short Biographies of Winnicott's Correspondents   193

PART 3 Winnicott's Lectures, Broadcasts, and Audio Recordings

1. Winnicott's Lectures   213
2. Winnicott's Broadcasts   233
3. Index of Available Audio Recordings   239
   Introduction to Winnicott's Broadcasts   239
       ANNE KARPF
   The Ordinary Devoted Mother and Her Baby   239
   The Ordinary Devoted Mother and Her Children   239
   Further Audio Material   240

4. Original Broadcast Scripts — 241
   a. *The New Baby:* Looking Forward to Baby's Arrival (1945) — 241
   b. *The New Baby:* Getting to Know Your Baby (1945) — 245
   c. Problems of Management: Training Babies (1949) — 249
   d. The Ordinary Devoted Mother and Her Baby: My Fan Mail (1952) — 253

PART 4 Guide to New Material in the *Collected Works*

1. Works Published for the First Time — 259

2. Letters Published for the First Time — 263

3. Works First Published in a Winnicott Edition — 267

4. Remarks on Some Chapter Revised for the *Collected Works* — 273

PART 5 Selected Drawings and Signatures

1. Selected Drawings — 279

2. Selected Signatures — 289

   D. W. W.: A Reflection — 295
   CLARE WINNICOTT

   Reference List of the *Collected Works* — 311
   Chronology — 343
   Contributors — 349
   Credits — 351
   Complete Index of the *Collected Works* — 353

EDITORS' NOTE

The *Collected Works* comprises eleven volumes of previously published and new texts and a selection of letters, presented in chronological order following either the date of delivery, writing, or first publication, and an accompanying volume of end material. Some undateable items have been grouped together as the final part of Volume 9. For more information on the structure and organisation of the *Collected Works*, see the Note in Volume 12.

This entire collection is also available online, together with many of Winnicott's original audio recordings and an introduction to his collection of broadcasts to parents by journalist and author Anne Karpf, at www.oxfordclinicalpsych.com/winnicott/.

In compiling these collected works, the editors made all reasonable efforts to preserve Winnicott's original writings and publications with minimal editorial intervention. For this reason, some points of style, such as citation format, figure numbering, and spelling vary from piece to piece. For the convenience of the reader, figure numbers have been added in instances where the original figures were unnumbered. All editorial notes are marked with lowercase roman numerals and, in the print edition, appear as footnotes. Winnicott's own notes are marked with Arabic numerals and appear as endnotes. Editorial interpolations in the original text and notes appear in square brackets. Cross-references to works appearing elsewhere in the *Collected Works* have been added to aid the reader. These references are indicated by an abbreviation that includes volume, part, and chapter numbers (e.g., "CW 2:7:8" for Volume 2, Part 7, Chapter 8). Although the *Collected Works* is as complete as possible a collection of Winnicott's work, it does not include works which remain inaccessible or which are protected by confidentiality restrictions.

The Collected Works of D. W. Winnicott

Volume 3, 1946–1951

CONTENTS

Introduction to Volume 3   3
VINCENZO BONAMINIO AND PAOLO FABOZZI

PART 1 1946

1. Children's Hostels in War and Peace   23
2. Educational Diagnosis   29
3. Letter to the *British Medical Journal*, Psychology in the Child's Education, 29 June   35
4. Letter to Lord Beveridge, 15 October   37
5. Letter to *The Times*, 6 November   39
6. Letter to Ella Sharpe, 13 November   41
7. Some Psychological Aspects of Juvenile Delinquency   43
8. Psychological Aspects of Juvenile Delinquency (n.d., ca. late 1940s)   49

PART 2 1947

1. Hate in the Countertransference   59
2. Physical Therapy of Mental Disorder   69
3. Residential Management as Treatment for Difficult Children   77
4. Further Thoughts on Babies as Persons   95
5. The Child and Sex   101
6. Letter to the *British Medical Journal*, Battle Neurosis Treated with Leucotomy, 13 December   113

PART 3 1948

1. Reparation in Respect of Mother's Organized Defence Against Depression   117

2. Paediatrics and Psychiatry	123
3. Letter to the *British Medical Journal*, 'Pathies in a State Service, 14 February	141
4. The Gwrw Tree	143
5. Letter to Anna Freud, 6 July	147
6. Review: *The Psychology of the Unwanted Child* by Agatha H. Bowley	149
7. Review: *Parents' Questions* by the staff of The Child Study Association of America	151
8. Disorders of Childhood	153
9. Review: *The Psychoanalytic Study of the Child, Volume 2*, edited by Anna Freud, Willie Hoffer, Edward Glover, *et al.*	157
10. Review: *The Personality of the Preschool Child* by Professor Werner Wolff	159
11. Obituary: Susan Isaacs	161
12. Primary Introduction to External Reality: The Early Stages	165
13. Environmental Needs; the Early Stages; Total Dependence and Essential Independence	171

PART 4 1949

1. Letter to Paul Federn, 3 January	179
2. Letter to the *British Medical Journal*, Taking Children's Temperatures, 6 January	181
3. Letter to Marjorie Stone, 14 February	183
4. The Infancy of Juliet	185
5. Letter to Roger Money-Kyrle, 22 March	195
6. Letter to Roger Money-Kyrle, 31 March	197
7. Letter to Roger Money-Kyrle, 2 May	199
8. Birth Memories, Birth Trauma, and Anxiety	201
9. Letter to Joan Riviere, 19 May	221
10. Letter to Roger Money-Kyrle, 13 June	223

11. Notes on the Discussion Held on Dr Winnicott's Paper 'The Birth Trauma' — 225

12. Letter to Roger Money-Kyrle, 22 June — 229

13. Letter to Roger Money-Kyrle, 24 June — 231

14. Letter to Joan Riviere, 24 June — 233

15. Review: *Handbook of Child Guidance* edited by Ernest Harms — 235

16. Letter to *The Times*, Punishment and Crime: A Psychologist's View, 10 August — 237

17. Letter to R. S. Hazlehurst, 1 September — 239

18. Letter to S. H. Hodge, 1 September — 241

19. Letter to the *British Medical Journal*, Paddington Green Children's Hospital, 24 September — 243

20. Mind and Its Relation to the Psyche-Soma — 245

21. Leucotomy — 259

22. Review: *Art Versus Illness* by Adrian Hill — 265

23. A Man Looks at Motherhood — 269

24. The Baby as a Going Concern — 273

25. Where the Food Goes — 277

26. The End of the Digestive Process — 281

27. The Baby as a Person — 285

28. Close-up of Mother Feeding Baby — 289

29. The World in Small Doses — 293

30. The Innate Morality of the Baby — 299

31. Weaning — 303

32. Young Children and Other People — 307

33. Stealing and Telling Lies — 313

34. The Impulse to Steal — 319

35. Sex Education in Schools — 323

36. Enuresis: Notes for a Lecture to the Tavistock Children's Department (n.d., ca. 1949)   327

PART 5 **1950**

1. Letter to Clare Britton [excerpt], early 1950   331
2. Aggression in Relation to Emotional Development   333
3. Letter to *The Times*, Neglected Children, 31 January   349
4. Letter to Otho W. S. Fitzgerald, 3 March   351
5. Childhood Psychosis   353
6. Letter to P. D. Scott, 11 May   357
7. Letter to *The Times*, Maladjusted Children: Damaging Effect of Delay, May 13   361
8. Review: *The Infancy of Speech and the Speech of Infancy* by Leopold Stein   363
9. Letter to Roger Money-Kyrle, 10 July   365
10. The Deprived Child and How He Can Be Compensated for Loss of Family Life   367
11. Letter to Roger Money-Kyrle, 8 August   381
12. Letter to Hannah 'Queen' Henry, 30 October   383
13. Letter to Roger Money-Kyrle, 16 November   385
14. Knowing and Learning   387
15. Instincts and Normal Difficulties   393
16. Growth and Development in Immaturity   397
17. Some Thoughts on the Meaning of the Word Democracy   407
18. 'Yes, But How Do We Know It's True?'   423

PART 6 **1951**

1. Review: *The Child and the Magistrate* by J. A. F. Watson   431
2. Letter to W. R. Bion, 22 January   433
3. Letter to James Strachey, 1 May   435

4. The Foundation of Mental Health	437
5. Visiting Children in Hospital	441
6. Transitional Objects and Transitional Phenomena	447
7. Review: *The Inner World of Man: With Psychological Drawings and Paintings* by Frances G. Wickes	463
8. Letter to *The Lancet*, Leucotomy in Psychosomatic Disorders, 18 August	465
9. Letter to the *British Medical Journal*, Ethics of Prefrontal Leucotomy, 25 August	467
10. Review: *Jealousy in Children* by Edmund Ziman, M.D.	469
11. Letter to *The Times*, Nursery Schools: A Definition of Functions, 8 September	471
12. Review: *The Psychoanalytic Study of the Child, Volumes 3–4 and Volume 5* edited by Anna Freud, Wille Hoffer, and Edward Glover	473
13. Letter to Edward Glover, 23 October	475
14. Notes on the General Implications of Leucotomy	477
15. Review: *On Not Being Able To Paint* by Marion Milner	483
16. Review: *Problems of Infancy and Childhood*	487
17. Review: *Papers on Psycho-Analysis* by Ernest Jones	489
18. Review: *Infant Feeding and Feeding Difficulties* by Philip Evans and Ronald MacKeith	491
Chronology	495
References	501
Contributors	507
Credits	509
Index	515

Volume 3

1946–1951

Introduction to Volume 3
SOWING CREATIVE SEEDS FOR FUTURE CLINICAL DEVELOPMENT

Vincenzo Bonaminio and Paolo Fabozzi

Hate in the Countertransference

Hate. This is the first time that a *feeling* bursts into psychoanalytic discourse with such disruptive effect on the metapsychological terrain, at a time when both theoretical and clinical thinking were predominantly taken up with the drives.[i]

This feeling emerges directly in the very title of the paper, as though Winnicott wanted from the outset to make a vehement statement of personal intent. Also ground-breaking is that this *negative* feeling is related immediately to the analyst, and this constitutes a radical challenge to the prevailing model in which transference was seen as the central configuration of psychoanalytic work, with countertransference[ii] standing in the way of the analyst's engaging with the flow of the patient's free associations.

In this paper, Winnicott anticipates later developments in the concept of countertransference, taking it as a given, as an acquisition from his own clinical work. He describes this as ordinary countertransference: 'The identifications and tendencies belonging to an analyst's personal experience and personal development which provide the positive setting for his analytic work and make his work different in quality from that of any other analyst' [CW 3:2:1].

---

[i] Winnicott's idiosyncratic and freely disrespectful way of writing in comparison with the established' *écriture* of the time has been pointed out elsewhere (Bonaminio, 2005).

[ii] Countertransference was yet to acquire the dignity and the official recognition that it was accorded following Paula Heimann's seminal 1950 paper 'On Counter-transference'.

Winnicott is implying a displacement of the centre of gravity of psychoanalysis from the patient onto the analyst. When he gets to the heart of his argument, the reader is further unsettled by the statement that, in the case of some psychotic patients, analytic work cannot be judged as completed unless the analyst has put his countertransference feelings at the disposal of the patient. His very extensive clinical work, especially with psychotic, schizoid, borderline, and other severely ill patients, is presumably the source of these revolutionary ideas.

He issues an emotional challenge to the analyst:

> This coincidence of love and hate to which I am referring is something distinct from the aggressive component complicating the primitive love impulse, and implies that in the history of the patient there was an environmental failure at the time of the first object-finding instinctual impulses.
>
> If the analyst is going to have crude feelings imputed to him he is best forewarned and so forearmed, for he must tolerate being placed in that position. Above all *he must not deny hate that really exists in himself. Hate that is justified in the present setting has to be sorted out and kept in storage and available for eventual interpretation.* [CW 3:2:1, emphasis added]

The radical suggestion that the analyst must offer something of himself to the patient was unprecedented. We cannot know Winnicott's personal motive for choosing hate with which to begin this reversal of psychoanalytic perspective, but we might speculate that it had partly to do with the transformation of the neutrality previously attributed to the analyst's position.

More significantly, perhaps, it demands a search for authenticity in the feelings of both analyst and patient, an issue that echoes through other works in this volume. It fleshes out a theme in Winnicott's seminal work of 1945, 'Primitive Emotional Development' [CW 2:7:8], which Ogden (2001) describes as a kind of master plan from which flow all those currents of research that Winnicott would carry forward, in different directions yet with a surprising germinative unity, over the next twenty-five years. In 'Ego Distortion in Terms of True and False Self' [6:1:22], he again emphasised the importance of putting something of one's self at the disposal of the patient. He continued to develop this idea, which reached its fullest elaboration in his late paper 'The Use of an Object' [CW 8:2:28].

A New Semantics of Aggression

'Hate in the Countertransference' was written the year after Klein's 'Notes on Some Schizoid Mechanisms' (1946). Her paper contains two strands. On the one hand, it is a synthesis and a systemization of the preceding decade's research. She describes a mind that functions and develops from a primitive paranoid-schizoid position towards a more organizing depressive position.

On the other hand, it is an intuition of the theory of projective identification, perhaps her most revolutionary concept of this period. Here, Klein grasps the fact that the psychic activity of the individual is displaced onto the other, who, for the first time, is conceptualised as an object containing an inside.

This crucial transition in Kleinian theory gives primacy to the emphatically conflictual dialectic between the libidinal drives and the aggressive impulses of the child in relation to the mother's breast. Specifically, she conceptualises the aggressive impulses of the child in terms of object relations. In a direct challenge to the Freudian concept of the death drive, Klein strips this of its conjectural implications as a biological and philosophical matrix and deflects it onto the child's inborn psychological framework. In order to express this inborn destructive impulse, the infant attacks the mother's breast, the bad breast, so as to be free of it and to maintain the relationship with the opposite pole of the split, the ideal breast.

By contrast, Winnicott does not conceptualise a primary aggression, either as an expression of the death drive or (in the more descriptive terms of academic psychology) as a reaction to frustration. He visualises the roots of aggression as being an expression of that 'primitive . . . motility potential' [CW 3:5:2] which has its origins in the first movements of the foetus within the womb. Although Winnicott does not explicitly mention the significance ascribed by the mother to these signs of life, this plays an essential role: it is the mother who will see in the infant's earliest integration either erotic potential or signs of aggressiveness.[iii]

Winnicott's view of aggression is described both experientially and clinically when he introduces his concept of the fundamental developmental difference between the stages of concern and pre-concern. The aggressiveness of pre-concern is inherent in ruthless love. It embodies not an attack on the object but a potential for motility in the processes of maturation. It is only when the child is firmly anchored in the stage of concern that aggressiveness is directed against the object.

For Winnicott, there exists, therefore, an ontogenesis, a kind of natural history of aggressiveness. In states of profound narcissistic withdrawal, although aggression may appear primitive, it is never primary; it is always the result of something that the object or the environment has done to the subject. It is not that Winnicott is positing a naïve, Rousseau-esque conception of the primordial goodness of the individual ruined by society. It is that love and hate take shape within the continuous interplay between what is offered by the environment and the varyingly reactive responses of the individual.

[iii] It would be a mistake to imagine that Winnicott is thinking of the mother on her own in relation to the baby. Despite being the principal agent of the baby's care, she is seen as existing within a structure provided by the holding functions of the father.

Viewing the Child: A Radical New Perspective

At the beginning of his 1945 paper 'Primitive Emotional Development' [CW 2:7:8], Winnicott makes a bold methodological statement: since he was interested in the child and the infant, he has decided to study psychosis psychoanalytically. His vision of the earliest stage of emotional development is based on his conviction that the analysis of psychotic, depressed, and hypochondriacal patients does not require a modification of Freudian technique—provided that 'the transference situation inherent in such work' is taken into account.

The methodological premise of basing the study of primary development on the analyses of psychotic patients yields its greatest results in the identification and analysis of the three principal processes in emotional development: integration (starting from a condition of primary unintegration), personalization (the localization of the self in the body), and the assessment of spatial and temporal dimensions (the construction of the relationship with reality).

This conceptual organization of primary development is highly innovative, as is the proposal that integration is a slow and gradual process of construction, occurring as instinctual experiences are combined with the 'technique' of maternal care. Furthermore, there is a fundamental break with earlier theorisations in Winnicott's conception and description of the relationship with external reality as a *capacity* that necessitates a slow and gradual process of construction, as well as the indispensable contribution of the maternal figure. This is the first appearance of various central winnicottian *Leitmotifs*: the establishment of an authentic relationship with external reality, the distinction and productive exchange between reality and fantasy, and the construction of the sense of being real.

In the 1945 paper, Winnicott has yet to elaborate fully the contribution of the mother's psychic functioning to the baby's development. However, the following passage allows us to understand the broader theoretical and clinical view being outlined as part of this thinking:

> In terms of baby and mother's breast . . . the baby has instinctual urges and predatory ideas. The mother has a breast and the power to produce milk, and the idea that she would like to be attacked by a hungry baby. These two phenomena do not come into relation with each other till the mother and child *live an experience together*. The mother being mature and physically able has to be the one with tolerance and understanding, so that it is she who produces a situation that may with luck result in the first tie the infant makes with an external object, an object that is external to the self from the infant's point of view. [CW 2:7:8]

With the image of a mother and baby who '*live an experience together*', Winnicott is preparing to construct a very specific situation: in presenting the baby with the breast, the mother must allow the baby to feel that he has created the experience himself.[iv] The potential for this psychic function (that is also fundamental to the relationship with external reality) lies in the possibility that an *overlap* may be created between something that stems from the mother and something that originates from the baby's nascent psyche.

Here, we witness the gestation of other fundamental Winnicottian concepts: transitional objects and phenomena, the subjective object, the intermediate area, potential space. With the idea that the mother 'would like to be attacked by a hungry baby', he introduces into the psychoanalytic field in embryonic form the point of view that considers the mother's *psychic functioning* as crucial. In broadening his focus then to include the experience of the baby who encounters the mother's experience, Winnicott calls to our attention the patient's experience (in the transference) which meets and generates effects upon the experience that the analyst has with the patient.

What unites the three situations described in 'Hate in the Countertransference' [CW 3:2:1] is that the object (the mother or analyst) must face and work through reactions to 'pressures' from the subject (the baby or patient). The technical implication—that the analyst must 'bear strain'—opens up another unexplored field: the object's response to the subject's unconscious movements due to a tension that arises from primitive defensive processes. Winnicott explicitly establishes this crucial connection when he states that the analyst 'is in the position of the mother of an infant unborn or newly born'. Every detail of technique then becomes vitally important and assumes a therapeutic value for those patients 'whose very early experiences have been so deficient or distorted that the analyst has to be the first in the patient's life to supply certain environmental essentials'.

The Emergence of a Different View of the Relation Between Subject and Object

From the situations just described, two issues arise that profoundly change the way of approaching psychoanalysis. Firstly, Winnicott highlights the patient's unconscious work on the analyst's unconscious and thus on his mental functioning. Secondly, he introduces a methodological modification: he suggests

---

[iv] 'I think of the process as if two lines came from opposite directions, liable to come near each other. If they overlap there is a moment of *illusion*—a bit of experience which the infant can take as *either* his hallucination *or* a thing belonging to external reality' [CW 2:7:8].

that we need to consider the functioning of the analyst's mind as a tool of psychoanalytic investigation.

There seems to be a bridge here between the 1945 essay and the one written in 1947 [CW 3:2:1]. The source of Winnicott's investigation of earliest infancy is his experience of transference situations encountered with psychotic patients. His attention to the *psychic and unconscious relationship* between mother and newborn permits him to grasp aspects of the transference-countertransference relationship, of the mental functioning of seriously ill patients, and of the origin of psychosis.

In 'Hate in the Countertransference', we can see the co-existence of three levels: theoretical, clinical, and technical. At the level of theory, he offers many reasons to hypothesize the precedence of the mother's hate over that of the newborn, thereby dislodging from the model of the earliest stages of mental functioning the idea of an innate death instinct. From a clinical point of view, he implies that, in order for the psychotic patient to acquire the capacity to distinguish hate from love, he must first enter into contact with an object capable of feeling hate towards him. Technically, he is positing the coexistence of three forms of countertransference: one as a blind spot; another that constitutes the specific identity of that individual analyst; and a third, objective form that exists in reaction to the personality of that particular patient.

In this essay, it becomes evident that Winnicott's vision of psychic functioning is founded on the radical and innovative principle that the unconscious functioning of the object, as well as its transformations caused by the unconscious of the subject, must be investigated and retransformed in order that the subject may embark on a psychic transformation. The idea that he is engaged simply in magnifying the importance of the environment is clearly superficial and misleading. This is no mere introduction of the analyst's arbitrary subjectivity into the clinical situation. It involves the construction of a space that, until then, did not exist. In highlighting the phenomena created by the reciprocal action of the patient's unconscious on the unconscious of the analyst, he is maintaining that it is possible to observe such phenomena, that it is necessary to analyze them, and that it is legitimate to utilize them in understanding psychic functioning and the transformation accomplished through psychoanalysis.

This might be seen as a simple clinical deepening of a Freudian intuition. What makes it a radical turning point, however, is its proposition that the birth and development of the mind depends not only on the work of intra-psychic construction, but also on unconscious *interpsychic* processes and that this is true also within the analytic relationship. This process involves not just a communication from unconscious to unconscious, but (in play) the capacity for mutual unconscious modification. The unconscious of one *puts forth a demand for psychic work on the unconscious of the other*; the matter is not merely one of tolerating and containing the emotional effect of the other, but of also *elaborating* what reaches the subject's unconscious from the unconscious of the object (Fabozzi, 2012). This is the intuition that Winnicott reveals in this work: the existence of a network of unconscious movements between subject and object that mark both analytic process and the development of the child's psyche. This network of unconscious movements activates the psychic activity of both analyst and mother, permitting the development of the patient's missing psychic functions and those of the neonate still *in statu nascendi*. The fruits of this theoretical-clinical position of Winnicott's will reach full maturity in his final works [CW 8:2:28; CW 9:1:15; CW 9:1:29].

Correlation Between Winnicott's Conception of Aggression and His Discovery and 'Invention' of Transitional Objects and Space

In 'Primitive Emotional Development' [CW 2:7:8] and 'Aggression in Relation to Emotional Development' [CW: 3:5:2], Winnicott introduces a fundamental link between aggression and the initiation of a relationship with external reality, a theme that continues to represent one of his principal threads of research as he explores the functions and meanings of the transitional object.

This concept has, of course, a monumental scope. In the first place, the object coalesces from a Platonic ideal of representation to become a concrete object. The term 'object' refers here to something that can be manipulated and, as such, assists in the child's progressive attribution of meanings as they take shape out of the nascent interior world. This is the starting point for his essential paradoxical vision:

> The following complex statement has to be made. The infant can employ a transitional object when the internal object is alive and real and good enough (not too persecutory). But this internal object depends for its qualities on the existence and aliveness and behaviour of the external object (breast, mother figure, general environmental care). [CW 4:2:21]

It is in this context that we can understand the revolutionary significance of the statement that the transitional object is 'the first not-me possession', originally as part of the child's emotional development, but also for the patient in analysis. In these three terms, joined together in a figurative phrase, are condensed further intersecting levels of experience. 'The first': the child creates a space where none existed before and which an outside observer has no capacity to grasp. 'Not-me': the differentiation between 'me' and 'not-me' represents the integration of the ego via a kind of opposition to the fundamental unity with the mother—an awareness of that which it is not. 'Possession': the pseudopod that in an inseparable entanglement of aggression and libido lays down the basis for the birth of the relationship with the object.

In an important letter to Money-Kyrle (27 November 1952 [CW 4:1:13]) Winnicott says that he prefers the term 'transitional' to 'intermediate'. It evokes an intrinsic dynamism, implying that both object and space are in continual movement and development. Hence, one of the principal functions of the transitional object: to act as a support for the to-ing and fro-ing between the edges of the internal and external worlds and between union and separation. Analogously, transitional space is not a fixed place but is continually recombining and restructuring itself in relation to the oscillations of the object.

Repositioning Primary Narcissism in the Context of the Early Infant–Mother Relationship

The newborn enters into a relation with the breast that was there, waiting to be discovered, and draws from it the sensation of having created it. Winnicott coins a new term—subjective object—to convey this from the baby's point of view. The baby experiences the breast in terms of an absence of separateness, deriving from it an *experience* of omnipotence.

It will be clear that Winnicott's model is not a repositing of the existence of primary narcissism because the presence and contribution of the object are crucial. The mother has a natural yet complex status as the supplier of the baby's need for both nourishment and illusion, and the capacity for illusion is created by her active adaptation to her baby. At first, she will not make conscious or unconscious demands on him; she will respect his needs, emotional states, rhythms, and processes of maturation so that he may discover the environment on the basis of his own spontaneous movements.

For this, the baby needs a mother of average predictability, neither unstable, incoherent, nor subject to exaggerated mood swings. In late pregnancy and during the early weeks of the baby's life, she must be able to tolerate states of regression and complex identifications—with herself as a baby, with her own mother, and with her own child. The baby gradually establishes a relation to external reality through her gradual de-adaptation from his needs (which brings a degree of frustration) and through the baby's own discovery of a transitional object that will acquire specific functions and meanings, placing him in a particular area of reality and experience.

The transitional object constitutes the beginning of the process that will enable him to recognise the external nature of objects. It functions as a bridge: between child and mother, at those points when the mother is absent; between the subjective object and the objective object; between what is internal and what is external. It is the first external object, and it also represents the beginning of symbolism: it stands for the mother and, at the same time, for the Self of the child.

What is crucial is its material quality. The child can experience it through the senses. Its forms and deformations, its smells and new subtleties, are what first define its 'not-me' nature. But for the transitional object to exist, the environment must guarantee its psychic existence. In a sense, the gaze of the observer defines the nature of the transitional object. The mother must refrain from confronting the child with the dilemma of whether its reality is internal or external and allow him not to answer a question that is not to be asked about the source of the transitional object (whether it was created or found).

This will enable the transitional object to remain situated in a paradoxical space, a notional psychic place hitherto unexplored by psychoanalysis. This is the intermediate area of experience, the area of illusion, of potential space (Fabozzi, 2006) that engenders a chain of developmental potentialities. Thanks to the constitution of a separateness, the child can fill up this distance by introducing an experience that symbolically allows him or her to establish a new union with the mother. Separation is thus transformed into a bond, continuity into contiguousness, distance into closeness. When the psychic and emotional prerequisites have been achieved, this leads on to developmental frustration, which can give rise to a creative gesture, a game, a movement towards the structuring of a symbol. This will 'fill' and give form to the space, which is always on the point of losing and regaining its character as potential.

Winnicott's Unique Semantic of Potential

Giannakoulas and Hernandez (2001) suggest that the 'limits' of potential space are constituted by four 'dialectical dynamisms': the mother's movements of identification with herself and with the newborn within the primary maternal preoccupation; the paradoxical nature of the transitional object; the mother's function as a mirror, which introduces elements of similarity and difference; and the use of the object, a crucial experience in which the child destroys the object just when it is on the point of becoming real and then experiences the object's survival. There is a circularity that binds subject, object, and potential space and allows the dialectical movement between separation and union that is realised through playing and creativity.

It is perhaps too simplistic to say that the psychoanalytic process takes place within the same sort of transitional space. The space generated within the analytic relationship is not fixed but continually recreated by the reciprocal contribution of analyst and patient. Its topology is neither predictable nor able to be prescribed in any normative, abstract way. Here, the persona of the analyst comes into play. If he is capable of grasping what the patient offers, embryonically and potentially, he will facilitate and contribute to the creation of this space; an unforeseen and unforeseeable place within the analytic field.

The same conception applies to the dreamlike function of the analyst—Bion's *reverie*, an oneiric state of wakefulness (1962, p. 35), Winnicott's *unending dream* [CW 11:1], Bollas's *dreaming position of the analyst* (1997, p. 12), or Khan's *dreaming ego* (1974, p. 36). This is not a *posture* deliberately chosen by the analyst. It is created unexpectedly, something that the analyst must be capable of grasping and the patient of receiving in order to give life and form to the 'play' between the two partners in the analytic relationship. This spontaneous space, continuously revealed, is the location for the communicative exchanges, both between Self and object and between the patient and himself.

It is also crucial to Winnicott's 'capacity to be alone in the presence of the other' [CW 5:3:20], a concept that couples union and separateness, dependency and autonomy, both in the development of the child and in the analytic situation. This idea revolutionises a wide range of theories, including the whole range of separation anxieties, panic attacks, and phobias. Clinical experience shows that one of the factors underlying these forms of psychopathology, which lie within a vast spectrum, is the absence of this significant developmental step. During a panic attack, for example, the patient feels alone in facing the catastrophic threat of death; he has failed to establish the capacity to be alone in the presence of the other. Similarly, the claustro-agoraphobic patient feels lost in infinite space, like an astronaut who inadvertently severs the umbilical link to the spaceship and is left floating in the void for eternity.

For both Winnicott and Klein, these psychopathological dispositions are defences against the earliest anxieties. Unlike Klein, Winnicott defines this 'falling for ever' [CW 6:3:19] in terms of primitive agonies experienced by the infant when the environment does not fulfil its function of good-enough holding. However, it would be a misrepresentation of Winnicott's thinking to see the role of the environment as simply succeeding or failing to foster growth. In his theoretical-clinical thinking he explores a much deeper and more complex range of psychopathology that is attributable to specific forms of excess, intrusion, unpredictability, infiltration, or colonisation. When the environment, and in particular the mother's unconscious, subjects the child to these experiences, he will defend himself with well-organised, sophisticated defences that Winnicott defines at various levels.

Authenticity and Falseness: A Unifying View

Although the papers in this volume each have their own specificity, they are unified by this issue, which is both central and peculiar to Winncott's work. 'Reparation in Respect of Mother's Organized Defence Against Depression' constitutes a landmark in this line of thinking and crystallises the nucleus of his contribution and its innovative scope. Ground-breaking in its clinical observations and remarkable for various important features, its density may account for why it has remained relatively neglected, even in the Winnicott-inspired literature.

> Early in my career a little boy came to hospital by himself and said to me 'Please, Doctor, mother complains of a pain in my stomach', and this drew my attention usefully to the part mother can play'. [CW 3:3:1]

With this simple anecdote, Winnicott shows the reader a new conception of the child's somatic illness as a part of a structuring relation with the mother. A few lines further on, we find the revolutionary statement:

> Probably I get a specially clear view of this problem in a children's outpatient department because such a department is really a *clinic for management of hypochondria in mothers* . . . . There is no sharp dividing line between the frank hypochondria of a depressed woman and a mother's genuine concern for a child. [CW 3:3:1]

From a theoretical perspective this radical assertion represents a decisive and explicit shift. Winnicott is saying that the centre of gravity of psychology and psychopathology may reside not within the confines of the individual, but within the other who treats the child as an extension of itself. Paraphrasing Freud's famous statement 'the Ego is not master in its own house', we might say that for Winnicott the child's self is not master in its own house in as much as it is occupied and colonised by the self of the mother. So the structuring relation with the mother as environment affects both the normal development of the child and its psychopathological aspect. The role of the clinician is to judge the shift from normality to pathology.

In line with Anna Freud, Winnicott observes how an alteration in the relation of the child to his environment is organised into infantile neurosis as the result of an interiorization of the object. Anna Freud states that in judging the degree of normality or pathology in the child it is crucial to discover whether the child's 'disturbance' can be shifted through an intervention in the environment or whether it has already been absorbed into the ego, becoming a constitutive if ego-dystonic part of it.

Anna Freud, Klein, and Winnicott may use different theoretical models and idioms, but, as consummate clinicians, they are all guided by clinical practice, and they pursue what are in many respects convergent lines of thinking. However, whereas Klein's vision of pathology tends towards the extreme end of the spectrum (the infant is, so to speak, a little psychotic), Winnicott reformulates this issue in a radically different way in his essay 'Paediatrics and Psychiatry' [CW 3:3:2]. Almost impudently with respect to Klein (whom he does not explicitly mention), he asserts:

> At this point I have learned to expect a misunderstanding unless deliberate care is taken to avoid it. It has often been said to me: the idea that mad

people are like babies, or small children, simply isn't true. Can I make it clear that I do not suggest that the insane are behaving like infants any more than that neurotics are just like older children. Ordinary healthy children are not neurotic (though they can be) and ordinary babies are not mad.

In fact this line of thinking originates well before 1948. It is implied, for instance, in 'The Manic Defence' [CW 1:4:6]. Here, Winnicott describes the manic defence as the denial (Freud's *Verleugnung*) of internal reality and of the sensations related to depression and suspended animation. This implies a basic dissociation within the personality. He developed this idea 10 years later, in 1945, through the concept of 'integration and non-integration', and, in 'Ego Distortion in Terms of True and False Self' [CW 6:1:22], he arrived at a final definition of 'a dissociation in internal reality'. This idea of a basic dissociation in personality is not the same as repression or splitting, both of which imply an ego to do the work. It forecloses the child's further development if the integration facilitated by the environment cannot be made or is blocked. Only 'After integration the child starts to have a self' [CW 5:1:9].

In 'Reparation in Respect of Mother's Organized Defence Against Depression' [CW 3:3:1], Winnicott refers to the 'false reparation' that we meet in clinical practice. It is false because it occurs in relation not to the patient's guilt, but to the external other. This theory, very radical in the context of the Kleinian ideas of the time, gives rise to his clinical discoveries concerning dissociation in connection with the false self [CW 6:1:22]. However, the central core of the configuration has a more comprehensive relevance. It is capable of explaining, along a continuum, both primitive psychopathological phenomena in the early structuring of the self and the later schizoid phenomena with which Winnicott's concept of dissociation was initially associated.

At the beginning of the 1948 paper Winnicott writes:

> This false reparation appears through the *patient's identification with the mother* and the dominating factor is not the patient's own guilt but the mother's organized defence against depression and unconscious guilt.
>
> ... the depression of the child can be the mother's depression in reflection. The child uses the mother's depression as an escape from his or her own; this provides a false restitution and reparation in relation to the mother, and this hampers the development of a personal restitution[v] capacity...

---

[v] The terms 'restitution', 'reparation', and 'guilt' reflect the influence of the Kleinian concepts of the period with which Winnicott established a dialogue while at the same time attempting the search for an idiom of his own that would explain these clinical phenomena in a different way. The terms 'reparation' and 'guilt' are part of the concept of the depressive position, but the terms 'restitution' and particularly *personal* restitution' allude to the process of the development of the true self in contrast to that of false reparation and hence false analysis.

> ... It will be seen that these children in extreme cases have *a task which can never be accomplished*. Their task is first *to deal with mother's mood*. If they succeed in the immediate task, they do no more than succeed in creating an atmosphere in which they can *start on their own lives*. [CW 3:3:1, emphasis added]

Here, Winnicott is starting to describe the psychic work done on behalf of the *other* within the self, through identification. The degree of this work varies, but at its most extreme it may extend to occupation of the self by the other.[vi]

Close to the end of his scientific career, Winnicott concludes the journey begun with 'Hate in the Countertransference'. In 1967, he discusses the aetiological factors proposed by his theory of emotional development, which include the 'mother's capacity to adapt to the infant's needs through her healthy ability to identify with the baby' [CW 8:1:25]. He notes:

> It seems necessary to add to this the concept of the mother's *unconscious* (repressed) hate of the child. Parents naturally love and hate their babies, in varying degrees. This does not do damage. At all ages, and in earliest infancy especially, the effect of the repressed death wish towards the baby is harmful, and it is beyond the baby's capacity to deal with this. At a later stage than this one that concerns us here, one can see a child all the time making efforts *in order to arrive at the starting post*—that is, to counteract the parents' unconscious wish (covered by reaction formation) that the child should be dead.

The child's effort to arrive at the starting post by managing the occupation of the potential self by the parents' unconscious hampers the development of personal capacities. This is similar to the task of the depressed child in dealing with the mother's moods in order to create an atmosphere in which he can begin a life of his own, as first described in 'Reparation in Respect of Mother's Organized Defence Against Depression' [CW 3:3:1].

The Maturational Process of Integration

At the beginning, the individual is like a bubble. If the pressure from outside actively adapts to the pressure within, then the bubble is the significant thing; that is to say, the infant self. If, however, the environmental pressure is greater or less than the pressure within the bubble, then it is not the bubble that is

---

[vi] The 'presence' in the self of this depressed object is discussed by André Green in his paper 'The Dead Mother' (1980). '[The] "dead mother" ... is a mother who remains alive, but who is, so to speak, psychically "dead" in the eyes of the young child in her care' (p. 142).

important but the environment. The bubble adapts to the outside pressure [CW 3:4:8].

These words are taken from the analysis of a patient to whom Winnicott conveys his gratitude for having given such figurative expression to what was previously an embryonic concept of psychic life. They emphasise the role of the environmental pressure that disturbs, interferes with or interrupts the maturational physiological processes of emotional development. The centrality of the concept of reaction runs through all of his work and is strongly related to concepts of 'going on being', psychic continuity and the consequences of its interruption.

The essay 'Birth Memories, Birth Trauma and Anxiety' is Winnicott's formulation of the theoretical origin of psychic life. In it, he applies the concept of 'reaction' to the very earliest stages:

> There's certainly before birth the beginning of an emotional development, and it is likely that there is before birth a capacity for false and unhealthy forward movement in emotional development; in health environmental disturbances of a certain degree are valuable stimuli, but beyond a certain degree these disturbances are unhelpful in that they bring about a *reaction*. At this very early stage of development there is not sufficient ego strength for there to be a reaction without loss of identity. [CW 3:4:8]

The intuition of the phenomenon of reaction existing pre-birth is an exquisitely Winnicottian observation. In this essay, he also clarifies the recurring heuristic significance, for him, of the adjective 'theoretical'. The concept of the 'theoretical first feed', for example, is a normative fiction. It is used to establish the potential frame of reference within which the business of the individual's emotional development would unfold in a state of health were there not intervening factors or environmental impingements. Depending on their intensity, such impediments may be reabsorbed into the bubble or they may compel psychic work of a reactive kind.

How does Winnicott approach the origin of psychic life? Of course, his enormous experience as a paediatrician helps him with the task of tracing the germinative seeds of psychic experience from the foetal stage onwards, but it is the analytic situation that forms the laboratory par excellence in which his hypotheses can assume substance through emotional participation with the patient. Here, he is exploring the limits of an intermediate area between physiological and psychic traumatic reactions in the light of psychic life. One can only be astonished and fascinated by the fact that many of the contemporary thematics of prenatal and neonatal psychology had already been tackled by Winnicott. What can seem like a naïve lack of inhibition in this area in fact reflects the certainty of someone with a store of observational and psychoanalytic clinical material at his disposal. It is this experience that produces his concepts of the development of the

Self, the fear of breakdown, holding, handling, object-presenting, and the False Self.

In 'Birth Trauma, Birth Memories and Anxiety' he writes:

> Thus, in the natural process *the birth experience is an exaggerated sample of something already known to the infant.* For the time being, during birth, the infant is a reactor and the important thing is the environment; and then after birth there is a return to a state of affairs in which the important thing is the infant, whatever that means. In health the infant is prepared before birth for some environmental impingement, and already has had the experience of a natural return from reacting to a state of not having to react, which is the only state in which the self can begin to be. [CW 3:4:8]

The role of experience is a vector of growth. The progressive exchange between the environment and the foetus, then later the baby, enables the coalescing of the psychic functions of the human being. This line of thinking culminates (in this volume) with the extraordinary paper 'Mind and Its Relation to the Psyche-Soma' [CW 3:4:20]. For Winnicott, mind is always an organised defence; it is the structural precipitate of the baby's reactions to the environment, and it sanctions the fundamental dissociation of the personality. Once the mind has been constituted, the psyche-soma loses its wholeness; the dissociation between intellect and emotions has become behavioural, and the whole range of schizoid and dissociative pathology originates from this fundamental splitting of the personality.

This essay develops the insights presented initially in 'Primitive Emotional Development' and establishes the foundation for the successive elaborations of the false self and 'Basis for Self in Body' [CW 9:2:12]. In this paper, he uses the expressions 'false entity' and 'easy identification with the environmental aspect of all relationships', which precisely evoke the processes underlying the development of the false self, and the expression 'true self' makes its first appearance.

The ideas and insights of this period, 1947 to 1951, provide the foundation for the creative developments of the decades to come.

Conclusion

This third volume, which brings together many of Winnicott's fundamental papers, is a treasure trove of ideas, intuitions, clinical observations, and underlying threads. These link sketches of theory which gradually take shape and become part of a more complex corpus, continually open to changes and revisions. What strikes the reader—or at least what struck us as authors of this Introduction—is the inner coherence of Winnicott's thinking, his courage in carrying forward his insights and the intellectual honesty that characterises the whole of his work.

The essays included here constitute the source for the future germination of many themes, and they characterize that quiet genius, sometimes chaotic, that distinguishes Winnicott's unique way of working in psychoanalysis. Due to limitations of space, we have been unable to discuss some of the writings that would have taken us in different directions, but, in the end, these always relate, in one way or another, to the issues that we have highlighted.

As Winnicott himself said at the end of his clinical career, his legacy has yet to be fully understood. In 'The Use of an Object' he writes:

> I cannot assume that the way in which my ideas have been developed has been followed by others, but I should like to point out there has been a sequence, and the order that there may be in the sequence belongs to the evolution of my work. [CW 8:2:28]

Our purpose has been not to guide or drive our readers—Winnicott would have wrinkled his nose at this idea—but to leave them free to find their own way, guided by their own personal feelings and inclinations. In other words, we hope to offer an object that they can create and recreate at will.

References

Bion, W. R. (1962). *Learning from experience.* London: Heinemann.
Bollas, C. (1997). *Cracking up: The work of unconscious experience.* London: Routledge.
Bonaminio, V. (2005). L'uso delle parole e la scrittura in Winnicott. *Rivista di Psicoanalisi, 50*, 259–274.
Fabozzi, P. (2006). Spazio potenziale tra vincolo e creatività. In *Il vincolo*, Centro Italiano di Psicologia Analitica (Ed.) (pp. 213–226). Milan: Rafaello Cortina.
Fabozzi, P. (2012). A silent yet radical future revolution: Winnicott's innovative perspective. *Psychoanalytic Quarterly, 81*, 601–626.
Giannakoulas, A., & Hernandez, M. (2001). On the construction of potential space. In M. Bertolini, A. Giannakoulas, & M. Hernandez (Eds.), *Squiggles and spaces. Volume 1: Revisiting the work of D. W. Winnicott.* London/Philadelphia: Whurr.
Green, A. (1980). The dead mother. In *Life narcissism, death narcissism.* London: Free Association Books, trans. Andrew Weller, 2001.
Heimann, P. (1950). On counter-transference. *International Journal of Psycho-Analysis, 31*, 81–84.
Khan, M. M. R. (1974). *The privacy of the self.* London: Hogarth.
Klein, M. (1946). Notes on some schizoid mechanisms. *International Journal of Psycho-Analysis, 27*, 99–110.
Ogden T. (2001). Reading Winnicott. *Psychoanalytic Quarterly, 70*, 299–323.
Winnicott, D. W. (1945). Primitive emotional development.
Winnicott, D. W. (1948). Paediatrics and psychiatry.
Winnicott, D. W. (1949). Hate in the countertransference [1947].
Winnicott, D. W. (1953). Transitional objects and transitional phenomena.

Winnicott, D. W. (1954). Mind and its relation to the psyche-soma [1949].
Winnicott, D. W. (1958). The manic defence [1935].
Winnicott, D. W. (1958a). Aggression in relation to emotional development [1950].
Winnicott, D. W. (1958b). Birth memories, birth trauma and anxiety [1949].
Winnicott, D. W. (1958c). The capacity to be alone.
Winnicott, D. W. (1958d). Reparation in respect of mother's organized defence against depression [1948].
Winnicott, D. W. (1965). Ego distortion in terms of true and false self [1960].
Winnicott, D. W. (1965). Ego integration in child development.
Winnicott, D. W. (1965). Group influences and the maladjusted child: The school aspect [1955].
Winnicott, D. W. (1968). The aetiology of infantile schizophrenia in terms of adaptive failures [1967].
Winnicott, D. W. (1969). The use of an object and relating through identifications [1968].
Winnicott, D. W. (1971). Basis for self in body [1970].
Winnicott, D. W. (1972). Mother's madness appearing in the clinical material as an ego-alien factor [1969].
Winnicott, D. W. (1988). *Human nature*. C. Bollas, M. Davis, & R. Shepherd (Eds.).
Winnicott, D. W. (1989). Development of the theme of the mother's unconscious as discovered in psycho-analytic practice [1969].

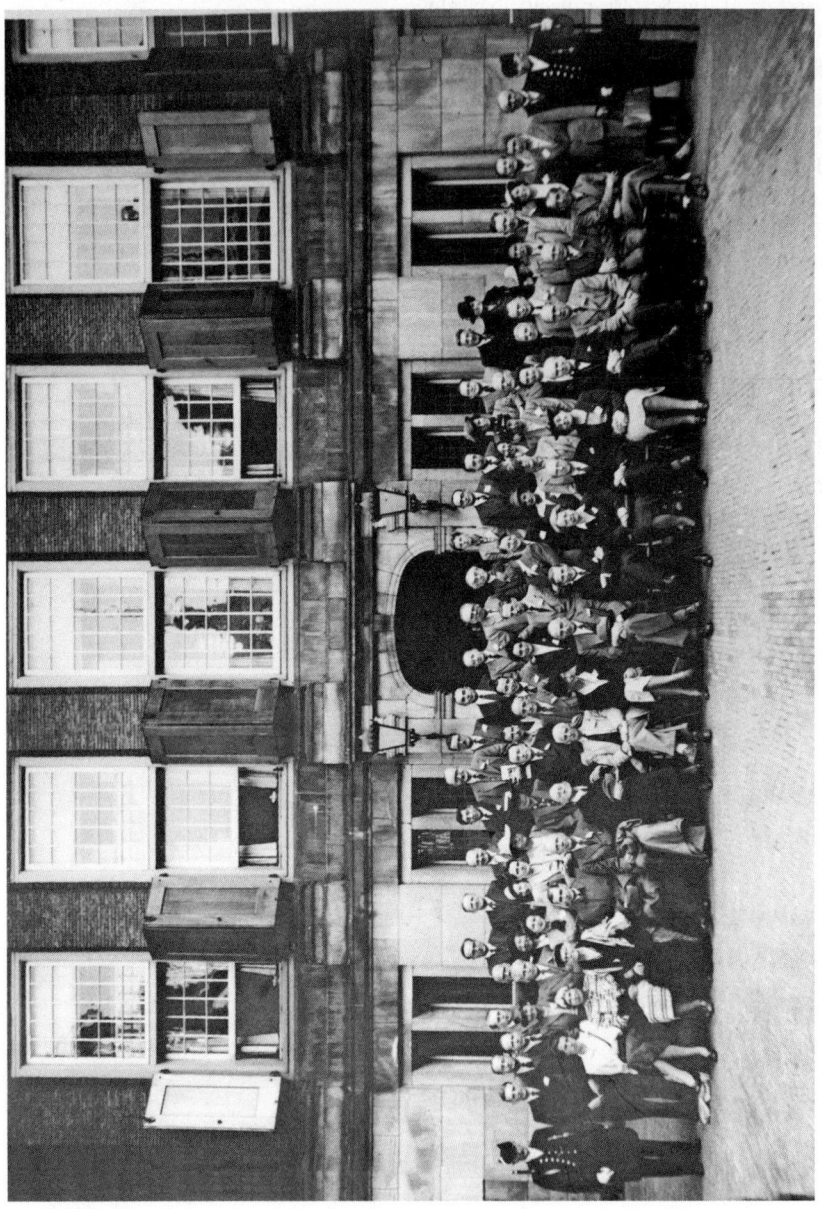

FIGURE 1 In August 1951, Winnicott attended the Seventeenth Congress of the International Psychoanalytical Association, Amsterdam. In this photograph of attendees, Winnicott appears on the far left of the back row, second from the end.

From the Donald Woods Winnicott Archive, in the care of the Wellcome Library, London, courtesy of the Winnicott Trust.

PART 1

1946

1

Children's Hostels in War and Peace

Revised and first published in *British Journal of Medical Psychology*, 1948, 21(3), 175–180. Also published in *The child and the outside world: Studies in developing relationships* (pp. 117–121). London: Tavistock, 1957; and C. Winnicott, R. Shepherd, & M. Davis (Eds.), *Deprivation and delinquency* (pp. 73–77). London: Tavistock, 1984.

A contribution to the symposium 'Lessons for Child Psychiatry', given at a meeting of the Medical Section of the British Psychological Society on 27 February 1946.

Evacuation produced its own problems and wartime its own solutions to problems. Can we make use, in peace, of the results of what was so painfully experienced in time of acute stress and awareness of common danger?

Probably very little that was new in psychological theory came out of the evacuation experience, but there is little doubt that because of it things became known to very large numbers of people who would otherwise have remained ignorant. Especially did the general public become aware of the fact of antisocial behaviour, from bed-wetting to train-wrecking.

It has been truly said that the fact of antisocial behaviour is in itself a stabilising factor in society, it is (in one way of speaking) a return of the repressed, a reminder of individual spontaneity or impulsiveness, and of society's denial of the unconscious to which instinct is relegated.

For my part, I was fortunate in being employed by a county council (from 1939 to 1946) in connection with a group of five hostels for children who were difficult to billet. In the course of this work,[1] which involved a visit each week to the county, I had detailed knowledge of 285 children, most of whom were observed over a period of years. Our job was to cope with the immediate problem and we succeeded or failed in so far as we did or did not relieve those in charge of the local evacuation arrangements of difficulties which threatened the success of their work. Now the war is over, there is still some value to be got out of the experience we went through, especially out of this fact of the public's new awareness of antisocial tendencies as psychological phenomena.

Of course, we must avoid seeming to suggest that hostels (or boarding-schools for maladjusted children, as they are officially called now) are a panacea for emotional disturbance of children. We tend to think of hostel management simply because the alternative is merely to do nothing at all through the shortage of psychotherapists. But this tendency has to be checked. With this proviso it can be said that there are children who urgently need to be cared for in some kind of home. In my clinic at the Paddington Green Children's Hospital (a medical out-patient department) there is a proportion of cases absolutely needing hostel management.

There are two broad categories of such children in peacetime: children whose homes do not exist or whose parents cannot form a stable background in which a child can develop, and children with an existing home which, nevertheless, contains a mentally ill parent. Such children appear in our peacetime clinics, and we find they need just what the children who were difficult to billet needed. Their home environment has failed them. Let us say that what these children need is *environmental stability, personal* management, and *continuity* of management. We assume an ordinary standard of physical care.

To ensure personal management the staffing of a hostel must be adequate, and the wardens must be able to stand the emotional strain that belongs to the proper care of any child, but especially to the care of children whose own homes have failed to bear such strain. Because of this the wardens need constant support from psychiatrist and psychiatric social worker.[2] The children (unselfconsciously) look to the hostel, or failing that to society in a wider sense, to provide the framework for their lives that their own homes have failed to give them. Inadequate staffing not only makes personal management impossible, but also it leads to ill-health and breakdowns in the staff, and therefore interferes with continuity of personal relationship, which is essential in this work.

A psychiatrist who is in charge of a clinic from which cases are referred to hostels should be responsible for a hostel himself, so that he may keep in touch with the special problems involved in such work. The same is true of magistrates at juvenile courts, who would do well to sit on hostel committees.

Psychotherapy

In dealing with antisocial children in clinics it is useless just to recommend psychotherapy. The first essential is to get each child properly placed, and proper placing in itself works as a therapy in a fair proportion of cases, given time. Psychotherapy can be added. It is essential to get the therapy arranged tactfully. If a psychotherapist is available, and if the hostel wardens actually want to help with regard to a child, then individual psychotherapy can be added. But there is a complication which cannot be ignored; in the good care of a child of this type the child has to become almost a part of the warden, and if someone else is giving treatment the child is apt to lose something vital in his relation to the warden (or some member of the staff), and the psychotherapist cannot easily make up for this in spite of the fact that he can give deeper understanding. Wardens, if they are good at this special type of job, must tend to dislike psychotherapy of the children in their care. In the same way good parents hate their children to be undergoing analysis, even when they seek it and co-operate fully.

The psychiatric social worker and myself, in this scheme, kept in intimate contact with the wardens both in regard to their personal problems, and to the children and the problems of their management as they arose. This contrasts with ordinary clinic work in which the psychiatrist can do best in a direct personal relation to each child patient, and to the parents.

Provision of Hostels

We must not be surprised to find ministries issuing edicts in favour of hostels, and also to meet children in need of hostels, and yet to find nothing happening, even to find hostels everywhere closing down. The contact between the supply and the need is only to be provided by men and women who are able and willing to live an experience with the children, willing to let a group steal a few years of their lives. Those of us who are clinically involved with these children must all the time play a part in bringing together the three things—official policy, wardens, and children—and must not expect anything good really to happen apart from our own personal voluntary deliberate efforts. Even in State Medicine the ideas and the clinical contacts belong to the clinician, without whom the best scheme is void.

Placing

The obvious method to be adopted by a large body (such as the London County Council, or a ministry) is to work the distribution of cases from a central bureau which keeps in touch with the various groups of hostels. If I have a child in my clinic needing a hostel (and it is always urgent), I am to send a report including Intelligence Quotient and school report to the central bureau, from which each case is to be distributed according to routine. But I do not play the game, nor do the parents, except when the child is so awful that the only need is to be rid of him immediately. In this mass-production arrangement something personal is lacking. The fact is that if a child comes under my care I cannot just put his or her name on a list somewhere. Doctors and parents must be allowed to maintain interest in the placing of their children; they must actually find out that what is provided is good.

There must be some personal link between clinic and hostel; someone must know someone. If no one knows any one then suspicion develops, because *in the imagination* there are bad parents, bad doctors, bad wardens, bad hostels, even bad ministries. And by bad I mean malicious. If a doctor or a hostel warden is not known as good, he is easily felt to be malevolent.

It will be apparent that our convalescent homes are unsuitable for these children, usually physically healthy, who need long-term management by specially chosen wardens supported by the psychiatric social worker and psychiatrist. Moreover, hospital-trained nurses seem to be rendered unsuitable for this work by their professional training; and many paediatricians turn a blind eye to psychology.

Prevention of Delinquency

This work is prophylactic work for the Home Office, whose main job it is to implement the law. For some reason or other I have met opposition to this idea from doctors who work for the Home Office. But hostels for evacuees all over the country succeeded in preventing many children from reaching the courts, thereby saving immense sums of money as well as producing citizens instead of habitual offenders; and from our point of view as doctors, the important thing is that the children have been under the Ministry of Health, that is, they have been recognised as ill. One can only hope that the Ministry of Education, which is now taking over [written in 1945] will do as well during peacetime as the Ministry of Health did during the war, in this prophylactic work for the Home Office.

Main Thesis

It happened that by my two appointments I was in touch with the London need for hostels at the same time as I was involved in the provision of hostels in an evacuation area. As physician to a London children's hospital, I was struck by the way in which this wartime provision solved the peacetime problem of management of the early antisocial case.

In sixteen instances I was able to draft London out-patient children to the hostels which I was visiting as psychiatrist. It came about by the chance that I held the two appointments, and it seemed to me to be a good arrangement, one that could be adapted to peace conditions. Because of my position I could be the link between the child, the parents or relatives, and the hostel wardens, and also between the child's past, present, and future.

The value of this work is not to be assessed only by the degree of relief of the psychiatric illness of each child. The value lies also in the provision of a place where the physician could care for these children who, without such provision, must degenerate at hospital or at home, causing great distress to adults, and badly affecting other children.

It is a sad reflection that many of the wartime hostels have closed down, and now there is no serious attempt to provide the hostel accommodation urgently needed for the early antisocial case. As for mad children, for them there is practically no provision. Officially, they do not exist.

Notes

1. A description of this work from different angles can be read in: (a) Britton & Winnicott, 'The Problem of Homeless Children' [CW 2:6:14]; (b) Britton & Winnicott, 'Residential Management as Treatment for Difficult Children: The Evolution of a Wartime Hostels Scheme' (*Human Relations*, 1947). These two papers have been dovetailed together to form 'Residential Management as Treatment for Difficult Children'. [CW 3:2:3]
2. It would seem to be the psychiatrist's job to be to some extent responsible for the staffing because the mental and physical state of the staff is the main thing in the therapy. A hostel whose staff is appointed and managed by one authority and whose children are under the care of another is unlikely to be successful.

2

Educational Diagnosis

Originally published in the *National Froebel Foundation Bulletin*, 1946, 41, 3. Also published in *The child and the outside world: Studies in developing relationships* (pp. 29–34). London: Tavistock, 1957; and *The child, the family, and the outside world* (pp. 205–210). Harmondsworth, UK: Penguin, 1964.

What is there that a doctor can usefully say to a teacher? Obviously he cannot teach him how to teach, and no one wants a teacher to take up a therapeutic attitude towards pupils. Pupils are not patients. At least, they are not patients in relation to the teacher while they are being taught.

When a doctor surveys the field of education, he soon finds himself asking a question: the whole of a doctor's work is based on diagnosis; what in teaching corresponds to this in medical practice?

Diagnosis is so important to a doctor that there was once a tendency in medical schools to ignore the subject of therapy, or to relegate it to a corner where it can easily be forgotten. At the height of this phase of medical education, which was reached perhaps three or four decades ago, people spoke with enthusiasm about a new phase in medical education in which therapy would be the main thing taught. We are now presented with remarkable methods of therapy: penicillin, safe surgery, immunization against diphtheria, and so on, and the public is deluded into thinking that the practice of medicine is thereby improved, little knowing that these very improvements threaten the foundation of good medicine, which is accurate diagnosis. If an individual is ill and feverish, and is given an anti-biotic, and gets well, he thinks he is well served, but sociologically the case is a tragedy, because the doctor is relieved of the necessity of making a diagnosis by the fact of the patient's response to the drug, blindly administered. Diagnosis on a scientific basis is the most precious part of our medical heritage, and distinguishes the medical profession from the faith healers, and the osteopaths, and all the other people we consult when we want a quick cure.

The question is, what do we see when we look at the teaching profession that corresponds with this business of diagnosis? It is quite possible that I am wrong, but I feel bound to say that I can see but little in teaching that is truly equivalent to the deliberate diagnosis of doctors. In my dealings with the teaching profession I am frequently disturbed in mind by the way in which the general mass of children are educated without first being diagnosed. Obvious exceptions spring to the mind, but I think the general statement is true. At any rate, it may be useful for a doctor to show what in his opinion could be gained from something equivalent to diagnosis, if it were seriously undertaken in the teaching world.

First of all, what is already being done in this direction? There is one way in which diagnosis comes in in every school; if a child is objectionable the tendency is for that child to be got rid of, either expelled, or removed by indirect pressure. This may be good for the school, but bad for the child, and most teachers would agree that the best thing is for such children to be eliminated at the beginning, when the Committee or the Headmaster or Headmistress 'finds it unfortunately impossible to take another child at the moment'. However, it is extremely difficult for a Head to be certain that in refusing to admit doubtful cases he at the same time is not keeping out specially interesting children. If there were a scientific method available for selection of pupils, it would doubtless be used.

Scientific method is at hand for measuring available intelligence, the Intelligence Quotient (I.Q.). The various tests are well known and are employed on an increasing scale, though sometimes they are used as if they meant more than they can ever do. An I.Q. can be valuable at both ends of the scale. It is helpful to know by these carefully prepared tests that a child who is not doing well is able to reach an average attainment, thus showing that it is his emotional difficulties that are holding him up, if not actually a fault in the method of teaching; and it is also helpful to know that a child is so far below the average intellectually that he almost certainly has a poor brain which cannot benefit from education designed for children with good brains. In the case of mental defectives the diagnosis is usually fairly obvious before the test is made. There is general recognition that the provision of special schools for the backward, and of occupation centres for the very backward, is an essential part of any education scheme.

So far so good. Diagnosis is being made in so far as scientific method is available. However, most teachers feel that it is natural for their classes to contain both clever and less clever children, and they naturally adapt themselves to the varying needs of their pupils in so far as the classes are not too big for them to be able to do individual work. What troubles teachers is not so much the varying *intellectual* capacity of their children, as their varying *emotional* needs. Even with regard to teaching, some children thrive on having things rammed down their throats, whereas others only learn at their own pace, and in their own way, almost in secret. With regard to discipline, groups vary greatly, and no hard and fast rule works. If kindness works in one school, it fails in another: freedom, kindness, and tolerance can produce casualties, just as an atmosphere of strictness can. And then there is the question of the emotional needs of various sorts of children—the amount of reliance on the personality of the teacher, and the mature and primitive feelings that develop in the children towards the person of the teacher. All these things vary, and although the ordinary good teacher manages to sort them out, there is often a feeling that a few children have to be denied what they obviously need for the sake of the many others, who would be disturbed if the school were to be adapted to the special needs of one or two. These are very big problems that are occupying the minds of teachers day in, day out, and a doctor's suggestion is that more could be done than is being done at present along the lines of diagnosis. Perhaps the trouble is that classification is not yet properly worked out. The following suggestions might help.

In any group of children there are those whose homes are satisfactory and those whose homes are unsatisfactory. The former naturally use their homes for their emotional development. In their case the most important testing out and acting out is done at home, the parents of such children being able and willing to take responsibility. The children come to school for something to be added to their lives; they want to learn lessons. Even if learning is irksome, they want so many hours a day of hard work which will enable them to get through examinations, which can lead to their eventually working in a job like their parents. They expect organization of games, because this cannot be done at home, but playing in the ordinary sense of the word is something which belongs to home, and the fringe of home life. By contrast, the other children come to school for another purpose. They come with the idea that school might possibly provide what their home has failed to provide. They do not come to school to learn, but to find a home from home. This means that they seek a stable emotional situation in which they can exercise their own emotional lability, a group of which they can gradually become a part, a group that can be tested out as to its ability to withstand aggression and to tolerate aggressive ideas. How strange that these two kinds of children find themselves in the same classroom! It should surely be possible to have different types of schools, not by chance, but by planning, adapted to these extreme diagnostic groupings.

Teachers find themselves by temperament more suitable for one or other type of management. The first group of children cries out for teaching proper, with the emphasis on scholastic instruction, and it is with children living in their own satisfactory homes (or with good homes to go back to in the case of boarding-school children) that the most satisfactory teaching is done. On the other hand, with the other group of children without satisfactory homes, the need is for organized school life with suitable staffing arrangements, regular meals, supervision of clothing, management of children's moods and of their extremes of compliance and non-cooperation. The emphasis here is on *management*. In this type of work teachers should be chosen for stability of character, or because of their own satisfactory private lives, rather than because of their ability to put across arithmetic. This cannot be done except in small groups; if there are too many children in the care of one teacher, how can each child be known personally, how can provision be made for day to day changes, and how can a teacher sort out such things as maniacal outbursts, unconsciously determined, from the more conscious testing of authority? In extreme cases the step has to be taken of providing these children with an alternative to home life in the shape of a hostel, this alone giving the school a chance to do some actual teaching. In small hostels there is immense gain from the fact that, because of the smallness of the group, each child can be totally managed over a long period of time in a personal way by a small constant staff. The relation of the staff to what remains of each child's home life is in itself a tricky and time-absorbing business, which further proves the need for the avoidance of large groups in the management of these children.

A sorting out along these lines occurs naturally in private school selection, because there are all types of schools, and all types of masters and mistresses, and gradually through agencies and hearsay parents more or less sort out themselves, and the children find themselves in suitable schools. However, where day schools have to be provided by the State, the matter is quite different. The State has to act in a relatively blind way. Children have to be provided with schooling near the neighbourhood in which they live, and it is difficult to see how there can ever be enough schools in each neighbourhood for these extremes to be catered for. The State can grasp the difference between a mental defective and an intelligent child, and can take note of anti-social behaviour, but the application of anything so subtle as a sorting out of the children who have good homes from those who have not is extremely difficult. If the State attempts to sort out good from bad homes some gross errors will be made, and these errors will necessarily interfere with the especially good parents who are unconventional and who do not plan for appearances.

In spite of these difficulties, it seems to be worth while to draw attention to this sort of fact. Extremes sometimes usefully illustrate ideas. It is easy to say that a child who is anti-social and whose home has failed for one reason or another needs special management, and this can help us to see that so-called 'normal' children can already be divided into those whose homes are coping, and for whom education is a welcome addition, and those who expect from their school the essential qualities lacking in their own home.

The subject is even more complex because of the fact that some of the children who could be classified with those who lack a good home actually have a good home of which they are not able to make use, because of their own personal difficulties. Many families of several children have one who is unmanageable at home. It is a justifiable simplification, however, to make a division between those children whose homes can cope with them and those whose homes cannot cope with them, for the sake of illustrating a point. It would be necessary in a further development of this theme to make a further distinction between those children whose homes have failed them after making a good start, and those children who have had no satisfactory consistent personal introduction to the world at all, not even in early infancy. Along with these latter children will be those whose parents could have given these necessary things had not something interrupted the process, such as an operation, a long stay in hospital, a mother having suddenly to leave the child because of illness, and so on.

In a few words I have tried to show that teaching could very well base itself, as good medical practice does, on diagnosis. I have chosen only one kind of classification in order to make my meaning clear. This does not mean that there are not other and perhaps more important ways of sorting children. Sorting according to age and according to sex has certainly been much discussed among teachers. Further sorting could usefully be done according to psychiatric types. How strange to teach withdrawn and preoccupied children along with the extroverted and those whose goods are in the shop window! How strange to give the same teaching to a child in a depressive phase as is given to that child when the phase has given way to a more care-free mood! How strange to have one technique for the harnessing of true excitement and for the management of the ephemeral and unstable contra-depressive swing, or elated mood!

Of course, teachers do intuitively adapt themselves and their methods of teaching to the various and varying conditions that they meet with. In a sense this idea of classification and diagnosis is already even stale. Yet the suggestion is made here that teaching should be officially based on diagnosis, just as good medical practice is, and that intuitive understanding on the part of the specially talented teachers is not good enough for the profession as a whole. This is particularly important in view of the spread of State planning, which tends always to interfere with the talents of individuals, and to produce quantitative increase of accepted theory and practice.

3

Letter to the *British Medical Journal*
PSYCHOLOGY IN THE CHILD'S EDUCATION

> Originally published in *British Medical Journal*, 'Psychology in the child's education'. 29 June 1946, 1(4460), 998.

SIR: The letter from Dr E. Stungo (June 15, p. 930) stimulates me to make comment. We can easily agree that children are the citizens of the future and deserve the best we can give them, but why is it that when we start planning we so easily start on the wrong foot?

The main suggestion in the letter is to the effect that children should be taught as the Nazi children were taught, only taught citizenship. How easy to say, and how difficult to put into practice! Dr Stungo leaves out the real source of good citizenship, which is in the life of the child in his own home, including the first relationship, that between infant and mother. On the basis of a good first relationship, more complex relationships can be developed gradually at home, and if all goes well the wider world is approached through the family's external relationships. If these things fail, citizenship (or something else) has to be taught, and a job it is.

If doctors are to interest themselves in this business of producing citizens they can start immediately by refraining from all avoidable interference with infants and small children. Neither should any physical treatment be undertaken that can *possibly be avoided*, nor should infants and small children be taken from home except in case of dire necessity. Small children in hospitals should be visited so frequently that they never cease to be sad, which means that they do not lose the thread of home life; and they should be sent home as quickly as possible. Moreover, there should be a stop to the general practice of taking over responsibility from parents who would like to retain responsibility: it is possible to give help without in any way making parents feel they are not fit to act on their own judgment.

Doctors and psychiatrists should remember that parents and teachers cannot wait for psychology to get to know everything. Parents and teachers have to deal with whole problems, and this is specially true of mothers with their infants. We understand some very important things about emotional development, but there is very much we do not yet know, or but dimly see. Let us not imagine we can tell a mother how to be a mother or a teacher how to teach. We can help each to understand this and that, and we can make their mothering and teaching jobs more conscious and more interesting; but all the time parents and teachers will have to carry on intuitively and without being able to account for all that they do.

Dr Stungo says 'children learn something of love, charity, sacrifice, humility, modesty, good and evil from religious instruction ... they should be taught to appreciate the nature of hate, envy, greed, spite, guilt, and temper ...'. In my opinion children know more about all these things than we do, and we could spend our time letting them teach us with a good deal of profit.—I am, etc.,

London, W.1.   D. W. WINNICOTT.

4

Letter to Lord Beveridge

Originally published in Rodman, F. R. (Ed.), *The spontaneous gesture. Selected letters of D. W. Winnicott* (Letter 5, p. 8). Cambridge, MA: Harvard University Press, 1987.

William Beveridge (1879–1963), economist and social reformer, was the author of a report on the state of the health services in the United Kingdom that led to the introduction of the National Health Service.

15 October 1946

Dear Lord Beveridge,

Can you help me out of a difficulty. I am very impressed with the views you hold on our treatment of Germany and for this reason wish to support you strongly. However, as a thinking kind of practising doctor (paediatrician-psychiatrist) I feel that the nationalisation of doctors is destructive of the best in our profession, and one of the chief things that has brought about this is the clause in your famous Report. So from my point of view you are the main cause of a bad thing.

I think your suggestion that the medical profession should be nationalised was made in good faith, and that you were truly ignorant of the harm your suggestion must do. It was true ignorance that allowed you to make medical practice subservient to politics instead of to science, but ignorance cannot absolve you of my hatred.

How can I reconcile my admiration of your new work on behalf of our democratic value, and my hatred of you because of your irresponsible suggestions in respect of doctors?

If you can find time to answer this letter please do not assume that I talk lightly and without true knowledge of medical practice. As a psycho-analyst I have been able to deepen and widen my own considerable experience by intimate knowledge of the feelings of others.

The public cannot of course be expected to understand these things, and very few understand what they stand to lose by the turning of doctors into civil servants; but in your position you cannot be absolved, and I must at any rate be honest with myself and express to you yourself the hate that rises naturally in me, alongside my other feelings for you and your work.

Yours truly,
D. W. Winnicott, F.R.C.P.

5

Letter to *The Times*

Originally published in Rodman, F. R. (Ed.), *The spontaneous gesture. Selected letters of D. W. Winnicott* (Letter 6, p. 9). Cambridge, MA: Harvard University Press, 1987.

This letter was not published by *The Times*.

6 November 1946

Sir: The National Health Service Bill has been reported in its various stages but for some reason it has scarcely been discussed in your columns; nevertheless it is bound to be far-reaching in its effects. Perhaps, now that it is practically law a letter might be allowed suggesting that a total state medical service can have severe ill-effects.

For instance, one result is that medical practice is now to be subservient not to science but to politics. Whatever gains come from the new scheme these must essentially be out-weighed by the loss of what has been won by the great scientist doctors of our history, and maintained by generations of practitioners in face of continuous public demand for faith-healing and magic.

Already a Minister of Health (without scientific training) has been the one to decide not to include osteopathy and faith-healing in the state medical service. From the doctor's point of view this is exactly as bad as if he had decided the other way. That such decisions should rest with whomever the parliamentary majority happens to give charge of housing, health and a few other odd items, is a depressing thought.

It seems to me to have been the duty and privilege of a paper with the standing of the Times to have put this issue clearly before the public: a body of people, untrained in scientific method but elected because of the complexion of their political views, had finally destroyed a good thing out of ignorance.

I am etc.
D. W. Winnicott

6

Letter to Ella Sharpe

Originally published in Rodman, F. R. (Ed.), *The spontaneous gesture. Selected letters of D. W. Winnicott* (Letter 7, p. 10). Cambridge, MA: Harvard University Press, 1987.

Ella Freeman Sharpe (1857–1947) was a British psychoanalyst and a member of the Middle Group.

13 November 1946

Dear Miss Sharpe,

I am very grateful to you indeed for writing about Wednesday's meeting. The subject had to be almost insulted by the fact that I had to speak only for half an hour,[i] when really the original plan in my mind was for six or more discussions.

As a matter of fact, I am not certain that I agree with you about psycho-analysis as an art. Out of your very wide experience there is something that you want to say, and which you express in this way. But from my point of view I enjoy true psycho-analytic work more than the other kinds, and the reason is to some extent bound up with the fact that in psycho-analysis the art is less and the technique based on scientific considerations more. Therefore, when I hear you speak about psycho-analysis as an art I find myself in difficulties; not wishing to completely disagree with you, but fearing lest this comment which you make should be given too much importance. There is obviously plenty of room for discussion here, but I thought I would let you know what I feel, because I usually find [when] I talk on non-analytic aspects of psychiatric work, that [people think] I am making an indirect comment on true analysis which I am not making.

---

[i] Winnicott had spoken to open a discussion on 'Consultation Technique' at the BPAS on 6 November.

7

Some Psychological Aspects of Juvenile Delinquency

Originally published in *New Era in Home and School*, 1946, 27(10), 295. Also published in *Delinquency Research*, 1946, 24(5); and *The child and the outside world: Studies in developing relationships* (pp. 181–187). London: Tavistock, 1957; and, in revised form, in *The child, the family, and the outside world* (pp. 227–231, as 'Aspects of juvenile delinquency'). Harmondsworth, UK: Penguin, 1964; and in C. Winnicott, R. Shepherd, & M. Davis (Eds.), *Deprivation and delinquency* (pp. 113–119). London: Tavistock, 1984.

An address given by invitation to magistrates.

I find I want to give a simple and yet not untrue description of one aspect of delinquency, a description that links delinquency with deprivation of home life. This could prove helpful to those who wish to understand the roots of the delinquent's problem.

First I invite consideration of the word unconscious. This talk is addressed to magistrates, who are, by training, accustomed to weighing up evidence, to thinking things out as well as feeling things. Now Freud contributed something really useful here. He showed that if we substitute thinking-out for feeling we cannot leave out the unconscious without making gross errors; in fact not without making fools of ourselves. The unconscious may be a nuisance for those who like everything tidy and simple, but it definitely cannot be left out of account by planners and thinkers.

Man the feeler, man the intuitive, far from leaving the unconscious out of account, has always been swayed by his unconscious. But man the thinker has not yet realised that he can both think and also at the same time include the unconscious in his thinking. Thinking people, having tried logic and having found it shallow, have started on a reaction towards unreason, which is a dangerous tendency indeed. The strange thing is to what a degree front-rank thinkers, even scientists, have failed to make use of this particular scientific advance. Do we not see economists leaving out of account unconscious greed, politicians ignoring repressed hate, doctors unable to recognise the depression and hypochondria that underlie such illnesses as rheumatism and that impair the industrial machine? We even have magistrates who fail to see that thieves are unconsciously looking for something more important than bicycles and fountain pens.

Every magistrate is fully aware of the fact that thieves have unconscious motives. First, however, I want to state and emphasise quite a different application of the same principle. I want to ask for consideration of the unconscious in its relation to the job of being a magistrate, this job being the implementing of the law.

It is because I am so anxious to see psychological methods used in the investigation of court cases, and in the management of antisocial children, that I want to make an attack on one of the biggest threats to an advance in that direction; this threat comes from the adoption of a sentimental attitude towards crime. If advances seem to come but are based on sentimentality, they are valueless; reaction must surely set in, and the advances had better never have been made. In sentimentality there is repressed or unconscious hate, and this repression is unhealthy. Sooner or later the hate turns up.

Crime produces public revenge feelings. Public revenge would add up to a dangerous thing were it not for the law and those who implement it. First and foremost in court work, the magistrate gives expression to public revenge feelings, and only by so doing can the foundation be laid for a humane treatment of the offender.

I find that there can be very strong resentment over this idea. Many people, if asked, may claim that they do not want to punish criminals, that they would rather see them treated. But my suggestion, one based on very definite premises, is that no offence can be committed without an addition being made to the general pool of unconscious public revenge feelings. It is one function of the law to protect the criminal against this same unconscious, and therefore blind, revenge. Society feels frustrated, but it allows the offender to be dealt with in the courts, after the passage of time and the cooling of passion; some satisfaction follows when justice is done. There is a real danger lest those who want to see offenders treated as ill people (as they are indeed) will be thwarted just as they are seeming to succeed, through not taking into account the unconscious revenge potential. There would be danger in the adoption of a purely therapeutic aim on the magisterial bench.

This having been said, I can go on to what interests me so very much more, the understanding of crime as a psychological illness.[i] It is a huge and complex

---

[i] The version of this article reproduced in *The Child, the Family, and the Outside World* (1964), began here.

subject, but I will try to say something simple about antisocial children, and the relation of delinquency to deprivation of home life.

You know that in investigation of the several pupils in an approved school diagnosis may range from normal (or healthy) to schizophrenic. However, something binds together all delinquents. What is it?

In an ordinary family, a man and woman, husband and wife, take joint responsibility for their children. Babies are born, mother (supported by father) brings each child along, studying the personality of each, coping with each one's personal problem as it affects society in its smallest unit, the family and the home.

What is the normal child like? Does he just eat and grow and smile sweetly? No, that is not what he is like. A normal child, if he has confidence in father and mother, pulls out all the stops. In the course of time he tries out his power to disrupt, to destroy, to frighten, to wear down, to waste, to wangle, and to appropriate. Everything that takes people to the courts (or to the asylums, for that matter) has its normal equivalent in infancy and early childhood, in the relation of the child to his own home. If the home can stand up to all the child can do to disrupt it, he settles down to play; but business first, the tests must be made, and especially so if there is some doubt as to the stability of the parental set-up and the home (by which I mean so much more than house). At first the child needs to be conscious of a framework if he is to feel free, and if he is to be able to play, to draw his own pictures, to be an irresponsible child.

Why should this be? The fact is that the early stages of emotional development are full of potential conflict and disruption. The relation to external reality is not yet firmly rooted; the personality is not yet well integrated; primitive love has a destructive aim, and the small child has not yet learned to tolerate and cope with instincts. He can come to manage these things, and more, if his surroundings are stable and personal. At the start he absolutely needs to live in a circle of love and strength (with consequent tolerance) if he is not to be too fearful of his own thoughts and of his imaginings to make progress in his emotional development.

Now what happens if the home fails a child before he has got the idea of a framework as part of his own nature? The popular idea is that, finding himself 'free' he proceeds to enjoy himself. This is far from the truth. Finding the framework of his life broken, he no longer feels free. He becomes anxious, and if he has hope he proceeds to look for a framework elsewhere than at home. The child whose home fails to give a feeling of security looks outside his home for the four walls; he still has hope, and he looks to grandparents, uncles and aunts, friends of the family, school. He seeks an external stability without which he may go mad. Provided at the proper time, this stability might have grown into the child like the bones in his body, so that gradually in the course of the first months and years of his life he would have passed on to independence from dependence and a need to be managed. Often a child gets from relations and school what he missed in his own actual home.

The antisocial child is merely looking a little farther afield, looking to society instead of to his own family or school to provide the stability he needs if he is to pass through the early and quite essential stages of his emotional growth.

I put it this way. When a child steals sugar he is looking for the good mother, his own, from whom he has a right to take what sweetness is there. In fact this sweetness is his, for he invented her and her sweetness out of his own capacity to love, out of his own primary creativity, whatever that is. He is also looking for his father, one might say, who will protect mother from his attacks on her, attacks made in the exercise of primitive love. When a child steals outside his own home he is still looking for his mother, but he is seeking with more sense of frustration, and increasingly needing to find at the same time the paternal authority that can and will put a limit to the actual effect of his impulsive behaviour, and to the acting out of the ideas that come to him when he is in a state of excitement. In full-blown delinquency it is difficult for us as observers, because what meets us is the child's acute need for the strict father, who will protect mother when she is found. The strict father that the child evokes may also be loving, but he must first be strict and strong. Only when the strict and strong father figure is in evidence can the child regain his primitive love impulses, his sense of guilt, and his wish to mend. Unless he gets into trouble, the delinquent can only become progressively more and more inhibited in love, and consequently more and more depressed and depersonalised, and eventually unable to feel the reality of things at all, except the reality of violence.

Delinquency indicates that some hope remains. You will see that it is not *necessarily* an illness of the child when he behaves antisocially, and antisocial behaviour is at times no more than an S.O.S. for control by strong, loving, confident people. Most delinquents are to some extent ill, however, and the word illness becomes appropriate through the fact that in many cases the sense of security did not come into the child's life early enough to be incorporated into his beliefs. While under strong management, an antisocial child may seem to be all right; but give him freedom and he soon feels the threat of madness. So he offends against society (without knowing what he is doing) in order to reestablish control from outside.

The normal child, helped in the initial stages by his own home, grows a capacity to control himself. He develops what is sometimes called an 'internal environment', with a tendency to find good surroundings. The antisocial, ill child, not having had the chance to grow a good 'internal environment', absolutely needs control from without if he is to be happy at all, and if he is to be able to play or work. In between these two extremes of normal and antisocial ill children are children who can still achieve a belief in stability if a continuous experience of control by loving persons can be given them over a period of years. A child of 6 or 7 stands a much better chance of getting help in this way than one of 10 or 11.

In the war many of us had experience of just this belated provision of a stable environment for children deprived of home life, in the hostels for evacuated children, especially for those who were difficult to billet. These have been under the Ministry of Health. In the war years, children with antisocial tendencies were treated as ill. I am glad to say these hostels are not all closing down now, and they have been transferred to the care of the Ministry of Education. These hostels do prophylactic work for the Home Office. They can treat delinquency as an illness the more easily because most of the children have not yet come before the Juvenile Courts. Here, surely, is the place for the treatment of delinquency as an illness of the individual, and here, surely, is the place for research, and opportunity to gain experience. We all know the fine work done in some approved schools, but the fact that most of the children in them have been convicted in a court makes for difficulty.

In these hostels, sometimes called boarding-homes for maladjusted children, there is an opportunity for those who see antisocial behaviour as the S.O.S. of an ill child to play their part, and so to learn. Each hostel or group of hostels under the Ministry of Health in wartime had a committee of management, and in the group with which I was connected the lay committee really interested itself in, and took responsibility for, the details of the hostel work. Surely many magistrates could be elected to such committees, and so get into close contact with the actual management of children who have not yet come before the Juvenile Courts. It is not enough to visit approved schools or hostels, or to hear people talking. The only interesting way is to take some responsibility, even if indirectly, by intelligently supporting those who manage boys and girls who tend towards antisocial behaviour.

In such hostels for the so-called maladjusted one is free to work with a therapeutic aim, and this makes a lot of difference. Failures will eventually come to the courts, but successes become citizens.

Of course, the work done in these small and properly staffed hostels is done by the wardens. These wardens have to start as the right kind, but they need education and opportunities for discussing their work as they go along, and also they need someone in between them and that impersonal thing called a ministry. In the scheme I knew, this was the job of the psychiatric social worker and the psychiatrist. These in turn needed a committee which could grow with the scheme, and profit from experience. It is on this sort of committee that a magistrate could profitably serve.

Now to return to the theme of children deprived of home life. Apart from being neglected (in which case they reach the Juvenile Courts as delinquents) they can be dealt with in two ways. They can be given personal psychotherapy, or they can be provided with a strong stable environment with personal care and love, and gradually increasing doses of freedom. As a matter of fact, without this latter the former (personal psychotherapy) is not likely to succeed. And with the provision of a suitable home-substitute, psychotherapy may become unnecessary, which is fortunate because it is practically never available. It will be years before properly-trained psychoanalysts are available even in moderate numbers for giving the personal treatments that are so urgently needed in many cases.

Personal psychotherapy is directed towards enabling the child to complete his or her emotional development. This means many things, including establishing a good capacity for feeling the reality of real things, both external and internal, and establishing the integration of the individual personality. Full emotional development means this and more. After these primitive things, there follow the first feelings of concern and guilt, and the early impulses to make reparation. And in the family itself there are the first triangular situations, and all the complex interpersonal relationships that belong to life at home.

Further, if this all goes well, and if the child becomes able to manage himself and his relationship to grown-ups and to other children, he still has to begin dealing with complications, such as a mother who is depressed, a father with maniacal episodes, a brother with a cruel streak, a sister with fits. The more we think of these things the more we understand why infants and little children absolutely need the background of their own family, and if possible a stability of physical surroundings as well; and from such considerations we see that children deprived of home life must either be provided with something personal and stable when they are yet young enough to make use of it to some extent, or else they must force us later to provide stability in the shape of an approved school, or, in the last resort, four walls in the shape of a prison cell.[ii]

[ii] [Added 1964]: In this way I come back to the idea of 'holding', and of meeting dependence. Rather than to be compelled to hold an ill child or adult who is antisocial, how much better to 'hold' an infant well at the beginning.

8

Psychological Aspects of Juvenile Delinquency

An undated talk probably given to probation officers.

Ladies & Gentleman,

Dr Mannheim has asked me to speak to you for three parts of an hour,[i] and I am grateful to him, but I cannot escape the difficulty which belongs to any giver of a single lecture. The fact is that I do not know you, and by the time I do know you my chance will be gone.

Although I have taken the trouble to write out what I shall say to you I do invite you to interrupt me because there is not the least reason why I should stick to my lines, and I would rather drop one bomb within the target area than to range widely over foggy territory entailing landing difficulties.

Another difficulty is that my terms of reference are wide. The Psychological Aspects of Juvenile Delinquency could constitute a complete university course. No doubt you have heard & thought a great deal of many such aspects. I must choose some definite thing for today's discussion, and I hope you will not think that I am neglecting all the other kinds of things that might be said.

One other thing to clear the ground: there are certain things about the origins of antisocial behaviour which I know I do not understand, and which, as far as I know, no one understands. Some, who intuitively and empathically understand in feeling, sympathise, enter into the delinquent child's feelings, might write a play or a poem about a criminal, thus revealing insight. But such insight is of but little use to us. When we study the *poem* we might as well study a *child*, in fact we can learn more from the child, or from a study of

---

[i] Dr Hermann Mannheim was Lecturer in Criminology at the London School of Economics (LSE) from 1935 to 1946, and Reader in Criminology at the University of London from 1946 until his retirement in 1955. He was extensively involved in the training of probation officers at LSE, at Rainer House, and at the Institute for the Study and Treatment of Delinquency.

the author who has this insight. What we want is an intellectual, or is it intellectualistic understanding, which we can pass on to each other in word form, and which adds to the store of scientific knowledge.

I have chosen to pass in review the possible treatments of an antisocial child (or grown up) and to illustrate one by some case material.

The various treatments of such a child indicates various reactions in ourselves to antisocial behaviour. We may be inclined to a

$$\begin{Bmatrix} \text{moral} \\ \text{legal} \\ \text{psychological} \end{Bmatrix} \text{approach}$$

and whichever we favour we must always remember the existence of the other two.

Moral
A boy steals your bicycle:

A) You are hurt by this by direct loss and inconvenience
B) you are disturbed by this by the evidence it gives of the child's lack of effective conscience.

Legal
You apply to the law for redress

A) because you are angry
B) because you want to do more than get redress over an item, you hope the law will do for the child instead of a conscience, and so prevent further troubles
C) because you want to protect the child against your hate and revenge. This implies identification with him.

Psychological
Through identification with the child you want

A) to experiment with manipulation of environment
B) to do away with the fears and the despair which underlie the antisocial symptoms
C) to understand the motivation of crime

The first thing to understand if you start in any aspect of the psychological approach is that as the bicycle stolen is not always yours, and as the psychological approach means your identification with the criminal, and as the psychological approach is neither moral nor legal, *you will be unpopular*. To some extent you will be condemned by the moralist and considered antisocial by the police. This is inevitable, and if you cannot see this or cannot allow for it I strongly advise you to stick to the moral or legal aspects of the subject.

(I have deliberately left out the sentimental approach, though much could be said about it. Enough to say that the greatest dangers to the social reformer come from the sentimental quarter.)

Of the moral and legal approach I need not say anything here. Three kinds of psychological approach have been mentioned and I propose to say something of each.

A) Manipulation of Environment

External factors. The first thing that strikes a practical worker in this field is the quantity of the bad external factors that are to be found in this particular class of psychological cause, both of the 'past, finished', and of the 'continuing' varieties, (though not so much of the 'recent shock'). This stimulates people to try to do something about it, by prevention or by making the home lives of the children more satisfactory. Such effects are usually foredoomed. There is nothing so easy as this in psychotherapy.

A) Whatever the reality of the bad external factor, in any one case the child is affected internally by it, the structure of his emotional makeup has been modified in an effort to cope with the external factor, and unless the structure is to some extent pulled down and rebuilt the child's character is relatively unaffected by environmental inputs.

B) Have you ever tried altering environments?

Boy of 11: truant, vagrant, thief, liar, is the illegitimate son of a perfectly good mother whose legitimate family she has brought up perfectly well. The boy cannot stand the idea of being illegitimate. What do you do about altering his illegitimacy?

Boy, 13: persistent eneuretic and gloomy, suffered the loss of his mother when he was 7. He was not very well served by his relations, and his father did not know how to keep the home together. What do you do? One cannot marry all the widows to give their children good homes and even then one cannot undo the effect of mother's death.

The father of a boy is a hardened criminal, has been to prison and has taught the boy to admire criminal technique. What do you do? You cannot annul this.

C) Sooner or later you stop wasting energy in trying to alter the people at home and you start on the more promising labour of providing a suitable home for the children—either for the unbilletables or for the already convicted, who gravitate to Remand Homes.

There is an enormous field for practical and useful work only if you do it.

1) You must be prepared to be unpopular and 2) you must be prepared to be worn out by the work, which is exactly not by chance but inherently. The best probation officers tend to die young from sheer exhaustion.

Say you are to manage a home for billet failures, these things are required of you. You will be in charge of and be held responsible for a group of (say) boys who potentially:

  pilfer
  make mess
  play truant
  use foul language
  get excited and {break things up / hit and hurt each other seriously / indulge in sexual orgies, homosexual and heterosexual}
  go begging round the neighbourhood, invent tales of ill treatment and neglect
  tend to set homes on fire
  prefer the roof to the other parts of the house
  are incapable of more than very limited constructive play or work, in fact if they can persevere they are to that extent not typical delinquents and to that extent capable of being helped by wise education.

A ringleader entering the scenes soon collects round him a small group of friends who organise a crime incident in whatever direction the ringleader leads. One crime excites the whole group, and in no time there is an outbreak of incidents till police action settles the matter—especially if the ringleader is removed.

The boys will be loveable and will love you, but they will definitely and certainly let you down at important moments. They will eventually learn—either to go to a Remand Home or else, if the very best has happened, to go to work. But in any case they will not come and thank you for what you have done, being unable to believe in you. If you are kind there is a trick in it. If you are fierce, that's what they expect. If you are brutal they fall in love with you. Their relationship to individuals is determined more by fear than by love. Yet characteristically, they believe there is something good somewhere and they constantly raise your hopes as well as their own by their optimism. After all, stealing implies a belief in something good, even though this can never be found without being spoilt thereby.

When you have settled down to your new job you will find you are treated as a criminal by the police. For them you either support them and their methods or else you are against them. If you protect your charges from the police you are part and parcel of this criminal behaviour. For instance, say one of your boys steals an electric torch. He will almost certainly let you know, for it happens that almost all the crime among your boys is recounted in the dormitory the same evening and these boys all split on each other constantly, well, you get the boy to own up and as he seems a little bit sorry you take him in the shop and you say: 'Mr Jones, this boy has stolen this torch, he is sorry, and he returns it unharmed. Will you please let it pass this time?' Even if Mr Jones says 'Righto!' this does not make your action legal. You are doing something illegal which you can describe in more accurate legal language than I can. But you will be wise to recognise that whenever you do not drag in the police you are a criminal. And even if you do save the boy much harm by your action, he or one of his friends will split on you, and you will never get thanked by anyone. You had better get a gramophone record saying thank you, thank you, thank you …, and in the evenings put it on for your own comfort.

You will try to lessen your troubles by getting your committee to share the burden. They too will be blamed for the boys' misdemeanours when they play bridge, go shopping and sit on more respectable committees, and they won't like it. They will just simply fail to come to grips with the real problems, and will play the passenger. How you will value the exceptions to this rule!

One of your hardest jobs will be to tolerate the lack of real constructive play or work. What will be the result of your efforts?

Divide your boys into these classes:

1. At one diagnostic end are those who are habitual offenders, whose compulsive antisocial trends make them into ringleaders, and who are perhaps unaltered by any treatment. The anxiety and depression and fear of madness and all the uncomfortable things underlying their antisocial behaviour has been lost in the primitive pull towards crime, and the enjoyment to be got from a technique that soon becomes specialised and complex and even beautiful, like the finger work of a violinist or the mental agility of the mathematics don. These boys come and go, and the sooner they go the better.
2. At the other end are boys who are unbilletable more because they cannot find ordinarily tolerant billets than because of character disturbance. These boys can be sorted out and sent to suitable billets or sent back home before wrong treatment has embittered them.
3. In between these two extremes is the main mass of the potentially delinquent, and you may expect to find in those children a steady development and strengthening of character. To some extent they can make use of the second chance you give them to discover a world that is somewhat although not altogether trustworthy.

B)

You may have quite another tendency, to approach the subject from the psychological angle. You may wish to alleviate the pain which you can detect in the delinquent, even beneath his at times maniacal excitability. This, however, requires of you a discipline—it requires that you should train to investigate the psychology of the children themselves. This means that you recognise the unconscious.

Investigation of the unconscious is called psycho-analysis, and so much work was done on such investigation by Sigmund Freud that no one can get anywhere today without first hearing all that Freud had to say on the subject and without working in the institute which does its best to carry on and develop Freud's ideas. I must stress this—Psychoanalysis is the name of the method by which the total personality can be investigated and understood. There is not psychoanalysis *and* various other methods. If Jung or someone else has something valuable that psychoanalysis has not got, then psychoanalysis is just deficient at present, and must eventually incorporate it. It is of no value to say there is psychoanalysis (Freud) and Individual Analysis (Adler) and Psychological Analysis (Jung).

If I have time I will say something about an investigation of a delinquent boy, with whom I had 7 contacts. This investigation is very satisfactory in so far as it resembles psycho-analysis and in so far as I can bring psycho-analytical theory to bear on what happened in those seven visits. It is also unsatisfactory in so far as it did not go on until the boy achieved maturity and emotional development.

I could wish to describe to you a psycho-analysis of a delinquent, but:

A) Such psycho-analyses are rare.
B) None has ever been done to completion as far as I know.
C) Even a year's psycho-analysis is terribly difficult to describe because of abundance of material, and to be complete an analysis must have gone on certainly more than a year.
D) As you are not trained in the technique of psycho-analysis, I should have to train you in such technique and instruct you in the theory in order to convey to you complete analytic material.

On the other hand, if you understand what psycho-analysis is, I actually can give you a glimpse of the psychology of one delinquent by describing a short and only partially successful treatment. My only fear is that by such a description you may be side-tracked from the belief in the unconscious which I want you to have because I shall show you unconscious material brought to light apparently easily. The point is that this material is tolerated by the patient in this sort of treatment only in the treatment hour, and because of the support of my being there, and a great deal of work has to be done before the most deeply unavailable feelings are generally tolerated.

For purposes of orientation I must preface the case material by these remarks:

1) The boy who steals has a belief in something good, and a hope of finding it, else he would be mad or depressed. He has experienced a good relationship sometime or other and has lost it, probably not through inhibition but because of some factor external to himself.
2) If he finds the good thing or person he will certainly hurt it; this is a sort of final test of a good thing or person, that it can be hurt. Anyone can believe in being loved when nice—but what I want is someone who will be nice to me when I'm nasty as well as when I'm nice.
3) In any steady relationship between me and another individual it will be possible, if I keep my own desires out of it, to trace the development of the other's feelings to the development of what I mean to him. In this way the patient discovers in his relation to me forgotten relationships, and in time will help discover types of relationship which he has never known about although they are his.

Anxieties which belong to such relationships become bearable when understood as they turn up in the analytic situation, though they could not alter while the patient was unaware of their meaning. I hope you observe the difference between this thing and reliving *in the analytic situation* of repressed human relationships and symptoms, for the one is psycho-analysis, and brings about a real maturing of the personality, while the others are productive of results only in so far as one type of relationship is taken for granted and used in the treatment.

PART 2

1947

Hate in the Countertransference

Originally published in *International Journal of Psychoanalysis*, 1949, 30, 69–74. Also published in *Collected papers: Through paediatrics to psycho-analysis* (pp. 194–203). London: Tavistock, 1958.

Based on a paper read to the British Psycho-Analytical Society, 5 February 1947.

In this paper I wish to examine one aspect of the whole subject of ambivalence, namely, hate in the countertransference. I believe that the task of the analyst (call him a research analyst) who undertakes the analysis of a psychotic is seriously weighted by this phenomenon, and that analysis of psychotics becomes impossible unless the analyst's own hate is extremely well sorted-out and conscious. This is tantamount to saying that an analyst needs to be himself analysed, but it also asserts that the analysis of a psychotic is irksome as compared with that of a neurotic, and inherently so.

Apart from psycho-analytic treatment, the management of a psychotic is bound to be irksome. From time to time I have made acutely critical remarks about the modern trends in psychiatry, with the too easy electric shocks and the too drastic leucotomies. (Physical Therapy of Mental Disorder [CW 3:2:2], Leucotomy [CW 3:4:21]). Because of these criticisms that I have expressed I would like to be foremost in recognition of the extreme difficulty inherent in the task of the psychiatrist, and of the mental nurse in particular. Insane patients must always be a heavy emotional burden on those who care for them. One can forgive those engaged in this work if they do awful things. This does not mean, however, that we have to accept whatever is done by psychiatrists and neuro-surgeons as sound according to principles of science.

Therefore although what follows is about psycho-analysis, it really has value to the psychiatrist, even to one whose work does not in any way take him into the analytic type of relationship to patients.

To help the general psychiatrist the psycho-analyst must not only study for him the primitive stages of the emotional development of the ill individual, but also must study the nature of the emotional burden which the psychiatrist bears in doing his work. What we as analysts call the countertransference needs to be understood by the psychiatrist too. However much he loves his patients he cannot avoid hating them and fearing them, and the better he knows this the less will hate and fear be the motives determining what he does to his patients.

One could classify countertransference phenomena thus:

1. Abnormality in countertransference feelings, and set relationships and identifications that are under repression in the analyst. The comment on this is that the analyst needs more analysis, and we believe this is less of an issue among psycho-analysts than among psychotherapists in general.
2. The identifications and tendencies belonging to an analyst's personal experiences and personal development which provide the positive setting for his analytic work and make his work different in quality from that of any other analyst.
3. From these two I distinguish the truly objective countertransference, or if this is difficult, the analyst's love and hate in reaction to the actual personality and behaviour of the patient, based on objective observation.

I suggest that if an analyst is to analyse psychotics or antisocials he must be able to be so thoroughly aware of the countertransference that he can sort out and study his *objective* reactions to the patient. These will include hate. Countertransference phenomena will at times be the important things in the analysis.

I wish to suggest that the patient can only appreciate in the analyst what he himself is capable of feeling. In the matter of motive: the *obsessional* will tend to be thinking of the analyst as doing his work in a futile obsessional way. A *hypo-manic* patient who is incapable of being depressed, except in a severe mood swing, and in whose emotional development the depressive position has not been securely won, who cannot feel guilt in a deep way, or a sense of concern or responsibility, is unable to see the analyst's work as an attempt on the part of the analyst to make reparation in respect of his own (the analyst's) guilt feelings. A *neurotic* patient tends to see the analyst as ambivalent towards the patient, and to expect the analyst to show a splitting of love and hate; this patient, when in luck, gets the love, because someone else is getting the analyst's hate. Would it not follow that if a *psychotic* is in a 'coincident love-hate' state of feeling he experiences a deep conviction that the analyst is also only capable of the same crude and dangerous state of coincident love-hate relationship? Should the analyst show love, he will surely at the same moment kill the patient.

This coincidence of love and hate is something that characteristically recurs in the analysis of psychotics, giving rise to problems of management which can easily take the analyst beyond his resources. This coincidence of love and hate to which I am referring is something distinct from the aggressive component complicating the primitive love impulse, and implies that in the history of the patient there was an environmental failure at the time of the first object-finding instinctual impulses.

If the analyst is going to have crude feelings imputed to him he is best forewarned and so forearmed, for he must tolerate being placed in that position. Above all he must not deny hate that really exists in himself. Hate *that is justified* in the present setting has to be sorted out and kept in storage and available for eventual interpretation.

If we are to become able to be the analysts of psychotic patients we must have reached down to very primitive things in ourselves, and this is but another example of the fact that the answer to many obscure problems of psycho-analytic practice lies in further analysis of the analyst. (Psycho-analytic research is perhaps always to some extent an attempt on the part of an analyst to carry the work of his own analysis further than the point to which his own analyst could get him.)

A main task of the analyst of any patient is to maintain objectivity in regard to all that the patient brings, and a special case of this is the analyst's need to be able to hate the patient objectively.

Are there not many situations in our ordinary analytic work in which the analyst's hate is justified? A patient of mine, a very bad obsessional, was almost loathsome to me for some years. I felt bad about this until the analysis turned a corner and the patient became lovable, and then I realized that his unlikeableness had been an active symptom, unconsciously determined. It was indeed a wonderful day for me (much later on) when I could actually tell the patient that I and his friends had felt repelled by him, but that he had been too ill for us to let him know. This was also an important day for him, a tremendous advance in his adjustment to reality.

In the ordinary analysis the analyst has no difficulty with the management of his own hate. This hate remains latent. The main thing, of course, is that through his own analysis he has become free from vast reservoirs of unconscious hate belonging to the past and to inner conflicts. There are other reasons why hate remains unexpressed and even unfelt as such:

> Analysis is my chosen job, the way I feel I will best deal with my own guilt, the way I can express myself in a constructive way.
> I get paid, or I am in training to gain a place in society by psychoanalytic work.
> I am discovering things.

I get immediate rewards through identification with the patient, who is making progress, and I can see still greater rewards some way ahead, after the end of the treatment.

Moreover, as an analyst I have ways of expressing hate. Hate is expressed by the existence of the end of the 'hour!'

I think this is true even when there is no difficulty whatever, and when the patient is pleased to go. In many analyses these things can be taken for granted, so that they are scarcely mentioned, and the analytic work is done through verbal interpretation of the patient's emerging unconscious transference. The analyst takes over the role of one or other of the helpful figures of the patient's childhood. He cashes in on the success of those who did the dirty work when the patient was an infant.

These things are part of the description of ordinary psycho-analytic work, which is mostly concerned with patients whose symptoms have a neurotic quality.

In the analysis of psychotics, however, quite a different type and degree of strain is taken by the analyst, and it is precisely this different strain that I am trying to describe.

Recently for a period of a few days I found I was doing bad work. I made mistakes in respect of each one of my patients. The difficulty was in myself and it was partly personal but chiefly associated with a climax that I had reached in my relation to one particular psychotic (research) patient. The difficulty cleared up when I had what is sometimes called a 'healing' dream. (Incidentally I would add that during my analysis and in the years since the end of my analysis I have had a long series of these healing dreams which, although in many cases unpleasant, have each one of them marked my arrival at a new stage in emotional development.)

On this particular occasion I was aware of the meaning of the dream as I woke or even before I woke. The dream had two phases. In the first I was in the 'gods' in a theatre and looking down on the people a long way below in the stalls. I felt severe anxiety as if I might lose a limb. This was associated with the feeling I have had at the top of the Eiffel Tower that if I put my hand over the edge it would fall off on to the ground below. This would be ordinary castration anxiety.

In the next phase of the dream I was aware that the people in the stalls were watching a play and I was now related through them to what was going on on the stage. A new kind of anxiety now developed. What I knew was that I had no right side of my body at all. This was not a castration dream. It was a sense of not having that part of the body.

As I woke I was aware of having understood at a very deep level what was my difficulty at that particular time. The first part of the dream represented the ordinary anxieties that might develop in respect of unconscious fantasies of my neurotic patients. I would be in danger of losing my hand or my fingers if these patients should become interested in them. With this kind of anxiety I was familiar, and it was comparatively tolerable.

The second part of the dream, however, referred to my relation to the psychotic patient. This patient was requiring of me that I should have no relation to her body at all, not even an imaginative one; there was no body that she recognized as hers and if she existed at all she could only feel herself to be a mind. Any reference to her body produced paranoid anxieties, because to claim that she had a body was to persecute her. What she needed of me was that I should have only a mind speaking to her mind. At the culmination of my difficulties on the evening before the dream I had become irritated and had said that what she was needing of me was little better than hair-splitting. This had had a disastrous effect and it took many weeks for the analysis to recover from my lapse. The essential thing, however, was that I should understand my own anxiety and this was represented in the dream by the absence of the right side of my body when I tried to get into relation to the play that the people in the stalls were watching. This right side of my body was the side related to this particular patient and was therefore affected by her need to deny absolutely even an imaginative relationship of our bodies. This denial was producing in me this psychotic type of anxiety, much less tolerable than ordinary castration anxiety. Whatever other interpretations might be made in respect of this dream the result of my having dreamed it and remembered it was that I was able to take up this analysis again and even to heal the harm done to it by my irritability which had its origin in a reactive anxiety of a quality that was appropriate to my contact with a patient with no body.

The analyst must be prepared to bear strain without expecting the patient to know anything about what he is doing, perhaps over a long period of time. To do this he must be easily aware of his own fear and hate. He is in the position of the mother of an infant unborn or newly born. Eventually, he ought to be able to tell his patient what he has been through on the patient's behalf, but an analysis may never get as far as this. There may be too little good experience in the patient's past to work on. What if there be no satisfactory relationship of early infancy for the analyst to exploit in the transference?

There is a vast difference between those patients who have had satisfactory early experiences which can be discovered in the transference, and those whose very early experiences have been so deficient or distorted that the analyst has to be the first in the patient's life to supply certain environmental essentials. In the treatment of a patient of the latter kind all sorts of things in analytic technique become vitally important, things that can be taken for granted in the treatment of patients of the former type.

I asked a colleague whether he does analysis in the dark, and he said: 'Why, no! Surely our job is to provide an ordinary environment: and the dark would be extraordinary'. He was surprised at my question. He was orientated towards analysis of neurotics. But this provision and maintenance of an ordinary environment can be in itself a vitally important thing in the analysis of a psychotic, in fact it can be, at times, even more important than the verbal interpretations which also have to be given. For the neurotic the couch and warmth and comfort can be *symbolical* of the mother's love; for the psychotic it would be more true to say that these things *are* the analyst's physical expression of love. The couch *is* the analyst's lap or womb, and the warmth *is* the live warmth of the analyst's body. And so on.

There is, I hope, a progression in my statement of my subject. The analyst's hate is ordinarily latent and is easily kept so. In analysis of psychotics the analyst is under greater strain to keep his hate latent, and he can only do this by being thoroughly aware of it. I want to add that in certain stages of certain analyses the analyst's hate is actually sought by the patient, and what is then needed is hate that is objective. If the patient seeks objective or justified hate he must be able to reach it, else he cannot feel he can reach objective love.

It is perhaps relevant here to cite the case of the child of the broken home, or the child without parents. Such a child spends his time unconsciously looking for his parents. It is notoriously inadequate to take such a child into one's home and to love him. What happens is that after a while a child so adopted gains hope, and then he starts to test out the environment he has found, and to seek proof of his guardians' ability to hate objectively. It seems that he can believe in being loved only after reaching being hated.

During the Second World War a boy of nine came to a hostel for evacuated children, sent from London not because of bombs but because of truancy. I hoped to give him some treatment during his stay in the hostel, but his symptom won and he ran away as he had always done from everywhere since the age of six when he first ran away from home. However, I had established contact with him in one interview in which I could see and interpret through a drawing of his that in running away he was unconsciously saving the inside of his home and preserving his mother from assault, as well as trying to get away from his own inner world, which was full of persecutors.

I was not very surprised when he turned up in the police station very near my home. This was one of the few police stations that did not know him intimately. My wife very generously took him in and kept him for three months, three months of hell. He was the most lovable and most maddening of children, often stark staring mad. But fortunately we knew what to expect. We dealt with the first phase by giving him complete freedom and a shilling whenever he went out. He had only to ring up and we fetched him from whatever police station had taken charge of him.

Soon the expected change-over occurred, the truancy symptom turned round, and the boy started dramatizing the assault on the inside. It was really a whole-time job for the two of us together, and when I was out the worst episodes took place.

Interpretation had to be made at any minute of day or night, and often the only solution in a crisis was to make the correct interpretation, as if the boy were in analysis. It was the correct interpretation that he valued above everything.

The important thing for the purpose of this paper is the way in which the evolution of the boy's personality engendered hate in me, and what I did about it.

Did I hit him? The answer is no, I never hit. But I should have had to have done so if I had not known all about my hate and if I had not let him know about it too. At crises I would take him by bodily strength, without anger or blame, and put him outside the front door, whatever the weather or the time of day or night. There was a special bell he could ring, and he knew that if he rang it he would be readmitted and no word said about the past. He used this bell as soon as he had recovered from his maniacal attack.

The important thing is that each time, just as I put him outside the door, I told him something; I said that what had happened had made me hate him. This was easy because it was so true.

I think these words were important from the point of view of his progress, but they were mainly important in enabling me to tolerate the situation without letting out, without losing my temper and without every now and again murdering him.

This boy's full story cannot be told here. He went to an Approved School. His deeply rooted relation to us has remained one of the few stable things in his life. This episode from ordinary life can be used to illustrate the general topic of hate justified in the present; this is to be distinguished from hate that is only justified in another setting but which is tapped by some action of a patient.

Out of all the complexity of the problem of hate and its roots I want to rescue one thing, because I believe it has an importance for the analyst of psychotic patients. I suggest that the mother hates the baby before the baby hates the mother, and before the baby can know his mother hates him.

Before developing this theme I want to refer to Freud. In *Instincts and their Vicissitudes* (1915), where he says so much that is original and illuminating about hate, Freud says: 'We might at a pinch say of an instinct that it "loves" the objects after which it strives for purposes of satisfaction, but to say that it "hates" an object strikes us as odd, so we become aware that the attitudes of love and hate cannot be said to characterize the relation of instincts to their objects, but are reserved for the relations of the ego as a whole to objects. . . '. This I feel is true and important. Does this not mean that the personality must be integrated before an infant can be said to hate? However early integration may be achieved—perhaps integration occurs earliest at the height of excitement or rage—there is a theoretical earlier stage in which whatever the infant does that hurts is not done in hate. I have used the term 'ruthless love' in describing this stage. Is this acceptable? As the infant becomes able to feel to be a whole person, so does the word hate develop meaning as a description of a certain group of his feelings.

The mother, however, hates her infant from the word go. I believe Freud thought it possible that a mother may in certain circumstances have only love for her boy baby; but we may doubt this. We know about a mother's love and we appreciate its reality and power. Let me give some of the reasons why a mother hates her baby, even a boy:

> The baby is not her own (mental) conception.
> The baby is not the one of childhood play, father's child, brother's child, etc.
> The baby is not magically produced.
> The baby is a danger to her body in pregnancy and at birth.
> The baby is an interference with her private life, a challenge to preoccupation.
> To a greater or lesser extent a mother feels that her own mother demands a baby, so that her baby is produced to placate her mother.
> The baby hurts her nipples even by suckling, which is at first a chewing activity.
> He is ruthless, treats her as scum, an unpaid servant, a slave.
> She has to love him, excretions and all, at any rate at the beginning, till he has doubts about himself.
> He tries to hurt her, periodically bites her, all in love.
> He shows disillusionment about her.
> His excited love is cupboard love, so that having got what he wants he throws her away like orange peel.
> The baby at first must dominate, he must be protected from coincidences, life must unfold at the baby's rate and all this needs his mother's continuous and detailed study. For instance, she must not be anxious when holding him, etc.
> At first he does not know at all what she does or what she sacrifices for him. Especially he cannot allow for her hate.
> He is suspicious, refuses her good food, and makes her doubt herself, but eats well with his aunt.
> After an awful morning with him she goes out, and he smiles at a stranger, who says: 'Isn't he sweet?'
> If she fails him at the start she knows he will pay her out for ever.
> He excites her but frustrates—she mustn't eat him or trade in sex with him.

I think that in the analysis of psychotics, and in the ultimate stages of the analysis, even of a normal person, the analyst must find himself in a position comparable to that of the mother of a new-born baby. When deeply regressed the patient cannot identify with the analyst or appreciate his point of view any more than the foetus or newly born infant can sympathize with the mother.

A mother has to be able to tolerate hating her baby without doing anything about it. She cannot express it to him. If, for fear of what she may do, she cannot hate appropriately when hurt by her child she must fall back on masochism, and I think it is this that gives rise to the false theory of a natural masochism in women. The most remarkable thing about a mother is her ability to be hurt so much by her baby and to hate so much without paying the child out, and her ability to wait for rewards that may or may not come at a later date. Perhaps she is helped by some of the nursery rhymes she sings, which her baby enjoys but fortunately does not understand?

> 'Rockabye Baby, on the tree top,
> When the wind blows the cradle will rock,
> When the bough breaks the cradle will fall,
> Down will come baby, cradle and all'.

I think of a mother (or father) playing with a small infant; the infant enjoying the play and not knowing that the parent is expressing hate in the words, perhaps in terms of birth symbolism. This is not a sentimental rhyme. Sentimentality is useless for parents, as it contains a denial of hate, and sentimentality in a mother is no good at all from the infant's point of view.

It seems to me doubtful whether a human child as he develops is capable of tolerating the full extent of his own hate in a sentimental environment. He needs hate to hate.

If this is true, a psychotic patient in analysis cannot be expected to tolerate his hate of the analyst unless the analyst can hate him.

If all this is accepted there remains for discussion the question of the interpretation of the analyst's hate to the patient. This is obviously a matter fraught with danger, and it needs the most careful timing. But I believe an analysis is incomplete if even towards the end it has not been possible for the analyst to tell the patient what he, the analyst, did unbeknown for the patient whilst he was ill, in the early stages. Until this interpretation is made the patient is kept to some extent in the position of infant—one who cannot understand what he owes to his mother.

An analyst has to display all the patience and tolerance and reliability of a mother devoted to her infant; has to recognize the patient's wishes as needs; has to put aside other interests in order to be available and to be punctual and objective; and has to seem to want to give what is really only given because of the patient's needs.

There may be a long initial period in which the analyst's point of view cannot be appreciated (even unconsciously) by the patient. Acknowledgement cannot be expected because, at the primitive root of the patient that is being looked for, there is no capacity for identification with the analyst; and certainly the patient cannot see that the analyst's hate is often engendered by the very things the patient does in his crude way of loving.

In the analysis (research analysis) or in ordinary management of the more psychotic type of patient, a great strain is put on the analyst (psychiatrist, mental nurse) and it is important to study the ways in which anxiety of psychotic quality and also hate are produced in those who work with severely ill psychiatric patients. Only in this way can there be any hope of the avoidance of therapy that is adapted to the needs of the therapist rather than to the needs of the patient.

2

Physical Therapy of Mental Disorder

Originally published in *British Medical Journal*, 1947, 1(4506), 688–689. Also published in C. Winnicott, R. Shepherd, & M. Davis (Eds.), *Psycho-analytic explorations* (pp. 534–541, part of 'Physical therapy of mental disorder: Convulsion therapy'). Cambridge, MA: Harvard University Press, 1989.

An abridgement of a paper read before the British Psychological Society Medical Section, 27 November 1946.

The full title of this talk was 'Some Reasons for a Personal Prejudice Against the So-called Physical Therapies of Mental Disorder'. By representing my ideas in this form I admit that I prejudge the situation. This may be an unscientific approach, but perhaps it is a suitable one in the case of such unscientific methods of treating the disordered mind. My objections are not to the brutality of the methods. Compared with psychiatric illness, even a broken back is not much, and a broken leg nothing. Moreover, with good care these accidents can be so reduced as to be negligible. I of course assume the good faith of those who practise the arts against which I am prejudiced. I know of no case whatever in which I would ascribe the giving of physical therapy to any but the ordinary motives of the practising physician.

Science in Medical Practice

A doctor is consulted because someone suffers. Patients, and especially relatives, demand therapy; but the doctor is trained in the scientific method, and his job is to apply science. By so doing he disappoints even if he gives relief to his patient. But he serves the community by being part of a bulwark against superstition. It is open to anyone to go to a quack for magical relief, but it is the doctor who is expected to represent science, or objectivity, and to be not afraid to do nothing if science cannot help. Diagnosis is based on scientific knowledge; the basis of therapy should be the same.

Scientific Psychology

A scientific approach to mental phenomena follows on acceptance of the theory that mental disorder is a disorder of emotional development, that the basis of mental health is laid down on what is inborn, from birth, by the course of development of the personality and development of the individual's emotional contacts with external reality. Through Freud's formulations and work, especially his method for objective investigation of unconscious phenomena, there has been a steady development of psychological insight.

The development of scientific psychology could briefly be described in three stages: the first bringing understanding of neurotic ambivalence, the second bringing understanding of depression and hypochondria, and the third bringing understanding of the more primitive mental states which reappear in the insanities.

First came the elucidation of the disturbed relationships between people and the disturbances in people of their instinctual functions as a result of their unconscious conflicts. The work was done from the sorting out of love and hate as it emerged in the transference situation. Following this, as it appears to me, the patient's conscious and unconscious fantasy about himself began to become analysed: his depression and conscious sense of guilt became his sense of something wrong inside himself, and the psychology of hypochondria became the psychology of the results of loving and hating. The incorporation and discharge of objects came into the analytic interpretation. Melanie Klein's work made all this possible, and mania as an alternative to depression was seen to be an extreme example of hypomania as a denial of depression.

The new work on depression naturally linked up with the examination of the integration of the personality itself, and phenomena of integration and reality appreciation, etc., began to be able to be dealt with in the transference developments and to be brought into relation to instincts. These developments have enabled psychology to encroach on the domain of the alienist, the doctor who manages the insanity case.

Convulsion Therapy

Along with this steady progress of psychological science there has been a development of the practice of convulsion therapy. My main objection to convulsion therapy is that it comes as *an escape from the acceptance of the psychology of the unconscious* and from the implications of the psychological developments of the past fifty years.

It is well known that there are several techniques, but from my point of view the electric technique is worse than the others because of the ease with which it can be done. Moreover, electricity has special significance for the unconscious, and paranoid and schizoid persons are well known to mix up the idea of electricity with ideas of magical influence. Such considerations do not necessarily make E.C.T. bad, but they certainly put us very much on guard when we interpret results, and when we meet the prejudice in favour of E.C.T. that is common among psychiatrists today. Whatever the technique, convulsion therapy is empirical. No one has the slightest idea how it works, when it does work. It is true that empiricism carries no final objection. However, scientists hate empiricism and regard it as a stimulus to research.

Our responsibility is great. What is done here in England tends to be done blindly in many parts of the world, especially where there is no access to libraries or training in psycho-analytic method or free scientific discussion. The sociological ill effect of a therapy has to be considered as well as the immediate effect on individuals.

Theory of Mental Health

The march of psychology, because of psycho-analysis, is towards the completion of the theory of mental disorder as a disturbance of emotional development. The basis of mental health is being laid down in infancy, in the developing relationship between infant and mother, and even in a more primitive way between the infant and his subjective mother, and more primitively still in the infant's self-establishment. The result of this theory is the fruitful one that the prevention of mental disorder is a new task of paediatrics. In contrast, the result of the empirical therapy of mentally ill people by physical methods is a relatively unfruitful one; it is that more and more neurologists must be found who are qualified to give people fits. These are two sociological results that can be compared one with the other.

Many besides myself have deplored the fact that convulsion therapy inevitably leads away from the psychological approach to a biochemical and a neurological one. Convulsion therapy attracts to mental hospitals people with first-rate qualifications for dealing with the complexities of insulin shock and of all the biochemical changes that need study in this kind of work. The physical therapies in general draw to psychiatry physically minded young doctors, and it is always unlikely that men and women who have reached a high degree of postgraduate training on the physical side will be willing or able to start again and to go into psychology at its beginning. Leucotomy in an extreme degree attracts the wrong kind of doctor to psychiatry. To my mind the modern acceptance of leucotomy is the direct result of the acceptance of empirical shock therapy.

If the sociological results of convulsion therapy are bad the sociological results of leucotomy are deplorable. I think leucotomy is the worst honest error in the history of medical practice. In mental hospitals the result of leucotomy is a new accession of power to the neurosurgeon, an unqualified practitioner from the point of view of the psychologist. Let us not be deceived by his very high degree of skill as a neurosurgeon, this having nothing to do with the case. If one deplores leucotomy and its collaterals one must deplore the convulsion therapies that paved the way for it. The feeling against leucotomy is too great to find expression—the general public and doctors alike are too appalled by this application of empirical method to do anything about it. And they are afraid that if they raise objections the psychiatrists will cease to relieve them of the awful burden of insane relatives and patients.

Let me apply the formula I devised earlier on. Now, instead of private suffering with demand for magical treatment being met by the doctor who applies science, it has become true to say that society's suffering (on account of its mentally ill members) leads to the use of the doctor (because of his being supposed to act according to scientific principles) to cover a panic application of magic. Leucotomy should be a quack remedy, available for those who ask for 'cures'.

From this subject of leucotomy with its irreversible brain changes I come back to convulsion therapy with a feeling of relief. At least here no damage is done (so we blandly assume). If it should turn out that the effects, good and bad, of E.C.T. are, after all, psychological effects, no one individual has been really hurt, and the convulsion subject can still employ psychotherapy if it should come his way. He can even recover spontaneously in the course of time, with good management, if he is so disposed.

Objections to Convulsion Therapy

To condense my views so far expressed I would say I would not give convulsion therapy, because (1) I would not have it done to myself; (2) it draws to psychiatry the wrong kind of doctors, skilled in the wrong way; (3) it undermines the public's justification for relying on doctors to keep their scientific heads in face of the demand for magic; (4) this form of therapy done here in England leads to mass treatments by the same methods of treatment all over the world; (5) physical methods of treatment represent a tendency away from scientific psychology. Here I would like to add a new point—which is that the chief indication for E.C.T. seems to be involutional melancholia and the lesser depressions.

Now, *depression is the illness of valuable people.* At the borderline depression is the breakdown of people who are overburdened with responsibility or loss. On this side of the line is the valuable person, often a good mother, who burdens herself with too much concern. On the other side is the same phenomenon, but less conscious, and this is depression. In depression at least the patient suffers for her own illness. E.C.T. is at present being applied to the valuable people, and if this is recognised it no doubt makes the psychiatrist very concerned indeed as to his own suitability for his task. Few of us are innocent of depression, and if we have escaped it we may have done so by a contra-depressive defence which is more abnormal than the frank depression phase of a patient.

Psychological Effects of Convulsion Therapy

Having thus summarised my prejudice I would like to give my guess as to the future developments in the psychology of convulsion therapy. I think that psycho-analysts and those trained in that sort of way should work at present on the assumption that all the results of E.C.T.—good, bad, and indifferent—are psychological results. The immense field of the psychological effects of the idea of E.C.T. has been seriously neglected. To discuss this it is not necessary to have given E.C.T. to a thousand patients, or indeed to have given any at all. What we need to do is to pool experiences of the feelings and ideas found during analysis of patients who have had convulsion therapy, and of patients who are in touch with fellow patients who have undergone convulsion therapy.

Need for Research

I give two lines of approach. The subject that urgently needs research and discussion is that of the patient's conscious and unconscious reactions to (*a*) the idea of E.C.T., etc.; (*b*) the experience of submission to convulsion therapy; and (*c*) the actual fit. Here are some suggestions.

>   (*a*) *Reaction to the idea of being given a fit.*—I suppose a *normal* person hates the idea. It must be for this reason that psychiatrists do not have fits given to themselves whenever they feel a bit depressed. *Anxious* people are likely to be able to become frightened at the *idea* of the fits, in the same way as they can become frightened at the idea of anything. In contrast they may be especially brave in relation to the actual experience. *Obsessional* patients' difficulties are greatly increased when the idea of convulsion therapy is put before them. The organised defence against spontaneity and

uncontrol is liable to be strengthened. Obsessional doubt is liable to find a setting in the problem whether to give or to withhold permission. Guilt will be felt whichever line is taken. In organised *paranoia* the fits are easily felt to be part of the hostile attack that is expected. In one patient, a girl who had a delusion that someone was trying to destroy her brain, this form of therapy was felt to be absolute confirmation of her delusion. In cases with thought-transference delusions and the fantasies that so readily get mixed up with theories of electrical phenomena and malicious influence, it can well be imagined that electrical shock therapy has a special significance.

(b) *Reaction to the experience of being given fits.*—In cases with a tendency to *conversion hysteria* a partial knowledge of brain-functioning is easily used in rationalisation of paralyses and paraesthesiae following convulsion therapy. *Depressive people* equate the convulsion with dying, and easily feel absolved by having experienced what it is like to meet death. They hanker after convulsion therapy. In some cases each successive convulsion becomes more dreaded, and the last one is equated with death, and recovery from it gives a new lease of life because of the emotional experience. *Suicidal* impulses can be met by the convulsion. By this seeming experience of death a suicidal patient can use convulsion therapy as an alternative to suicide. This is comparable to the relief that a suicidal patient can get through a genuine suicidal attempt—one from which the patient recovers through successful intervention.

(c) *Reaction to the fit itself.*—In what may be called *introversion neurosis* the patient has organised a secret inner world in which relationships are good, and this has been done at the expense of trust in the external world in which are placed the bad relationships. It is probable that in these cases the actual fit is felt as a threat to the artificially good inner world, and in consequence a rearrangement has to take place with less complete secret hoarding of good relationships within.

This approach is tentative and admittedly incomplete, but I give it to indicate the way the results of shock therapy may be examined as psychological phenomena. It is just here that research is most urgently needed. Curiously enough, it is also just here that there is an unwillingness on the part of practitioners of convulsion therapy to investigate. Much of the objection to convulsion therapy would disappear if the mechanism by which results are obtained were understood. The main trouble is that false theories are built around the assumption that the mechanism by which change is brought about is a physical one, and these theories have already paved the way for the wide employment of leucotomy—and who knows what may follow?

Society's Unconscious Reactions to Insanity

I also want to put forward the idea that these physical therapies express society's unconscious reaction to insanity. This is by far the most difficult thing I have to say. I have reason to believe that the good results that can come from these physical therapies depend on this—that by them expression is given in an acceptable (because hidden) form to the unconscious distress society experiences in face of mental illness. By unconscious I really mean unconscious, and I mean repressed and unavailable to consciousness. Massive guilt feelings and fear and consequent hate are roused in people who are concerned with mentally ill persons, and I think this unconscious hate also underlay the cruelty to mental patients that notoriously coloured the management of the insane up to recent times.

Tail-piece

As a last word I would like to say why I have no hope that these arguments will make any sudden difference to the now established practice of psychiatry. Mental disorder can be maddening to nurse. Abolition of shock therapy tomorrow would place on the doctors and nurses of mental hospitals an emotional burden which they could not suddenly take, and there will be those who claim that this alone justifies the method. I see this argument, and respect it. Nevertheless, there seems to be a need for someone to register a strong objection to easy and seductive methods which tend to lead away from the difficult path that must be walked by those who try to understand human nature and to eschew magic.

3

Residential Management as Treatment for Difficult Children
With Clare Britton

> Originally published in *The child and the outside world: Studies in developing relationships* (pp. 98–116). London: Tavistock, 1957. Also published in C. Winnicott, R. Shepherd, & M. Davis (Eds.), *Deprivation and delinquency* (pp. 54–72). London: Tavistock, 1984. This article is a combination of 'Residential Management as Treatment for Difficult Children: The Evolution of a Wartime Hostels Scheme' (with Clare Britton), *Human Relations*, 1947, 1(1), 87–97, with some parts of 'The Problem of Homeless Children' (with Clare Britton), *New Education Fellowship Monograph*, No. 1, 1944 [CW 2:6:14].

The Evolution of a Wartime Hostels Scheme

It fell to the lot of the authors to play a part in a wartime scheme that grew up in a certain county in Britain around the problems presented by children evacuated from London and other big cities. It is well known that a proportion of evacuated children failed to settle in their billets; and that whereas some of those went back home to the air-raids, many of them stayed on and were a nuisance unless given special conditions of management. As visiting psychiatrist and resident psychiatric social worker, we formed a small psychiatric team employed to make a scheme of this kind work in our county. Our job was to see that the available resources were actually brought to bear on the problems that arose: one of us (D. W. W.), as a paediatrician and child psychiatrist whose main work had been in London, was able to relate such problems as were specifically related to the war situation to the corresponding problems of peacetime experience.

The scheme that developed was necessarily complex, and it would be difficult to say that one cog in the wheel was more important than any other. We are, therefore, describing what happened, because we have been asked to do so and without claiming to be specially responsible for its good points; the views expressed are our own and are given without reference to the other participants in the scheme.

It could perhaps be said that in our job of seeing that the children concerned actually did get cared for and treated we also had to keep the total situation in view; because in every case there was a need for much more to be done than could, in fact, be done; and in each case, therefore, the assessment of the total situation had an important practical bearing. It is this relationship between the work done with each child and the total situation that we especially wish to describe.

It should be mentioned that there was no attempt to make this particular scheme a special case or a pilot model. No grant from a research organisation was sought or accepted. It is not claimed that the scheme with which we happened to be connected was specially good or successful, or that it was better in our county than in other counties. Probably, indeed, the arrangement that grew up in this particular county would have been unsuitable for any other county; and what occurred can be taken as an example of natural adaptation to circumstances.

In fact, a significant feature of such wartime schemes as a whole was the lack of rigid planning, which made it possible for each Ministry of Health Region (indeed, of each county in each region) to adapt to local needs; with the result that at the end of the war there were as many types of scheme as there were counties. This might be thought to be a failure of over-all planning, but in this matter we suggest that opportunity to adapt is of more value than prevision. If a rigid scheme is devised and put into operation, there is an uneconomic forcing of situations where local circumstances do not admit of adaptation; more important still, the people who are attracted to the task of applying a set scheme are very different from those who are attracted by the task of developing a scheme themselves. The attitude of the Ministry of Health, which was responsible for dealing with these matters, seems to us to have called for a creative originality, and therefore for a live interest on the part of all those who had to produce work, and work schemes, according to local needs.[1]

In all work that concerns the care of human beings it is the worker with originality and a live sense of responsibility that is needed. When, as in this task, the human beings are children, children who lack an environment specifically adapted to their individual needs, then the worker who loves to follow a rigid plan is unqualified for the task. Any large plan for the care of children deprived of adequate home life must, therefore, be of a type which allows for the fullest degree of local adaptation, and which attracts free-minded people to work it.

The Developing Problem

Children evacuated from the big cities were sent to ordinary people's homes. It soon became evident that a proportion of these boys and girls were difficult to billet, quite apart from the complementary fact that some homes were unsuitable as foster-homes.

The billeting breakdowns arising in these ways quickly degenerated into cases of antisocial behaviour. A child who did not do well in a billet either went home and to danger, or else changed billet; several changes of billet indicated a degenerating situation, and tended to be the prelude to some antisocial act. It was at this stage that public opinion became an important factor in the situation: on the one hand there was public alarm, and the activities of courts which represented the usual attitudes towards delinquency, while on the other there was the organising concern of the Ministry of Health, with the developing local interest in providing, for these children, an alternative management designed to prevent their reaching the courts.

The symptoms, in the evacuation breakdown cases, were of all kinds. Bed-wetting and faecal incontinence had first place, but every possible kind of difficulty was encountered, including stealing in gangs, burning of hay-ricks, train wrecking, truancy from school and from billet, and consorting with soldiers. There were also, of course, the more obvious evidences of anxiety, as well as maniacal outbursts, depressive phases, sulky moods, odd and insane behaviour, and deterioration of personality with lack of interest in clothes and cleanliness.

It was quickly discovered that the symptom-pictures were diagnostically useless, and were merely evidence of distress as a result of ecological failure in the new foster-home. Psychological illness, in the sense of deep endopsychic disturbance apparently unrelated to the current environment, could hardly be recognised as such in the abnormal conditions of evacuation. This situation was complicated by the natural process of mutual choice which led psychologically healthy children to find the good billets.

The initial reaction of the authorities to the emergence of a problem-group of children was to give such children individual psychological treatment, and to provide facilities where they could be placed while receiving treatment. Gradually, however, it became clear that success in providing accommodation of this kind demanded residential management. It emerged, moreover, that such management in itself constituted a therapy. Further, it was important that proper management, as a therapy, should be practical; for it had to be given by relatively unskilled persons—that is, by wardens untrained in psychotherapy, but informed, guided, and supported by the psychiatric team.

As a basic provision, therefore, hostels became organised for residential care of difficult evacuated children. In our county a big disused institution was first used; but from the difficulties of this initial experience the local authority developed the idea of setting up several small hostels, to be run on personal lines,[2] while the appointment of a Psychiatric Social Worker (P.S.W.) who was to be resident in this county arose out of the need to co-ordinate the work of the several hostels, and to build up a body of experience by which the whole scheme could benefit.

In the early stages it was thought that treatment could be given which would enable each child to be re-billeted in a foster-home, but experience showed that this idea was based on an underestimate of the gravity of the trouble. It was, indeed, the psychiatrist's task to direct attention to the fact that these children were seriously affected by evacuation and that nearly all had personal reasons why they could not find good billets to be good; to show, in fact, that these evacuation breakdowns occurred for the most part in children who had originally come from unsettled homes, or in children who had never had in their own homes an example of a good environment.

Therapy by management in residential hostels necessitated a long-stay policy, and the original intentions in regard to hostels had to be modified to allow children to stay for indefinite periods, up to two, three, or four years. In the majority of cases children who were difficult to billet had no satisfactory home of their own, or had experienced the break-up of home, or, just before evacuation, had to bear the burden of a home in danger of breaking up. What they needed, therefore, was not so much substitutes for their own homes as *primary home experiences* of a satisfactory kind.

By a primary home experience is meant experience of an environment adapted to the special needs of the infant and the little child, without which the foundations of mental health cannot be laid down. Without someone specifically orientated to his needs the infant cannot find a working relation to external reality. Without someone to give satisfactory instinctual gratifications the infant cannot find his body, nor can he develop an integrated personality. Without one person to love and to hate he cannot come to know that it is the same person that he loves and hates, and so cannot find his sense of guilt, and his desire to repair and restore. Without a limited human and physical environment that he can know he cannot find out the extent to which his aggressive ideas actually fail to destroy, and so cannot sort out the difference between fantasy and fact. Without a father and mother who are together, and who take joint responsibility for him, he cannot find and express his urge to separate them, nor experience relief at failing to do so. The emotional development of the first years is complex and cannot be skipped over, and every infant absolutely needs a certain degree of favourable environment if he is to negotiate the essential first stages of this development.

To be of value these primary home experiences belatedly provided in the hostels had to be stable over a period measured in years and not in months; and it can be well understood that the results could never be as good as the ordinary results of good primary homes would have been. Success in hostel work, therefore, is to be thought of in terms of lessening the failure of the child's own home.

A corollary of this is that good hostel work must make use of every ounce of value that may still remain in the child's own home.

The Task

There are various ways of describing the actual problem:

(1) The protection of the public from the 'nuisance' of children who were difficult to billet.
(2) The resolution of conflicting public feelings of irritation and of concern.
(3) The attempt to prevent delinquency.
(4) The attempt to treat and cure these 'nuisance' children, on the basis of their being ill.
(5) The attempt to help the children on the basis of their hidden suffering.
(6) The attempt to discover the best form of management and treatment for this type of psychiatric case, apart from the specific war emergency.

It will be seen that these various ways of stating the task have to be considered when the question is asked: What were the results? In reply, we might say, in respect to these different formulations of the task:

(1) As far as diminishing the 'nuisance' of difficult children was concerned, 285 children were housed and managed in hostels; and this was a success except in the case of about a dozen who ran away.
(2) With regard to public irritation, many people felt frustrated at times by the fact that 'offences' of the children were treated as distress signals, instead of indications for punishment; for example, a farmer whose rick had been burnt down would complain that the culprits seemed to have gained rather than lost by their antisocial act. As to public concern, a great many people who were genuinely concerned by the state of affairs that had developed were relieved by the knowledge that the problem was being tackled. The work of the hostels developed news-value.

(3) Delinquency, in a proportion of cases, was definitely prevented; as when a child obviously bound for the Juvenile Court before admission into the scheme was seen through to adolescence and a job, without major incident and without Home Office control. In other words, the difficulty was dealt with as a matter of individual and social health, and not merely as a matter of (unconscious) public revenge: the potential delinquency was treated, as it should be, as an illness.
(4) If we regard the problem as one of illness, a small proportion of the children were restored to health, and a fair proportion were brought to a much improved psychological condition.
(5) From the child-patients' point of view, intense suffering was discovered in many of them, as well as hidden or, indeed, open madness; and in the course of the routine work a great deal of suffering was shared and to some extent relieved. In a few cases personal psychotherapy could be added, but only enough to show the great need (on the basis of actual suffering) for more personal therapy than can ever be available.
(6) From the sociological angle, the working of the whole scheme gave an indication of the way to deal with potentially antisocial children and insane[3] children, suffering from disorders not produced by war, though evacuation made public the fact of their existence.

The Scheme Grows

Thus the scheme grew out of the acute local needs, and out of the wartime feeling that any cost could be borne, provided the working of the scheme solved the problem in hand. Because of the war, houses could be requisitioned; and in a few months there were five hostels in the group, as well as friendly relations with many others. 'Sick bays' for treatment of physically ill evacuees had, of course, been provided, even in excess of need, and these were available for some of the psychologically ill among the child population of the hostels.

The arrangement was as follows:

The national authority, the Ministry of Health, gave 100 per cent grant to the County Council—that is, accepted full financial responsibility—for this work. The County Council appointed a committee of county residents of standing (with a Deputy Clerk to the Council as Secretary) which was empowered to act as well as to report and recommend to its parent body. A full-time P.S.W. was appointed to work with the visiting psychiatrist, who paid a weekly visit to the county. From then on, the small psychiatric team could undertake to pay that attention to personal matters which is essential in this work; and at the same time, through the regular meetings of the committee, could retain contact with the broad administrative aspect of the situation. In fact, when this stage was reached, the central wide vision of the Ministry became focused on detail.

When this arrangement is examined it will be seen that a circle had been established.

The problem children, because of their nuisance value, had produced a public opinion that would support provision for them which, in fact, catered for their needs.

It would be wrong to say that demand produces supply in human affairs. Children's needs do not produce good treatment, and now the war is over it is very difficult to get such things as hostels for the same children whose needs were met in wartime. The fact is that in peacetime the nuisance value of the distressed children is lessened, and public opinion regains a sleepy indifference. In wartime, evacuation spread the problems of such children over the countryside; it also exaggerated them at a time when the general emotional tension of the community, and the shortage of goods and of manpower, made prevention of damage and theft imperative, and made extra police work unwelcome.

It was not that childhood distress produced child care, but rather that society's fear of the antisocial behaviour from which it suffered at an inopportune moment set in motion a train of events, events that could be used by those who knew of the children's suffering to provide therapy in the shape of long-term residential management, with personal care by an adequate and well-informed staff.

The Psychiatric Team

Because of the situation described, the task of the psychiatric team turned out to have two aspects: on the one hand, the will of the Ministry had to be implemented; and on the other, the needs of the children had to be met and studied. Fortunately, the direct responsibility of the team was to a committee which liked to be informed about all the details.

In this war experience the voluntary committee remained constant in membership and so developed with the scheme. By being itself stable the committee shared with the psychiatric team a gradual 'growth in the job', so that each success or failure helped to build up a body of experience which had general application and which benefited all the hostels.

To illustrate this, specific instances can be given, even although the main development was in a general way and not capable of illustration.

(1) Gradually, the idea of appointing joint married wardens was adopted. At first this was an experiment, which could only be

made in an atmosphere of mutual understanding, because of the complications arising out of the problems of the wardens' own family and its relation to the hostel children.
(2) The question of corporal punishment was brought up for discussion in the committee, at the appropriate moment, by means of a memorandum; and this led to the formulation of a definite policy.[4]
(3) The idea was put forward, and gradually adopted, that it was better to have one person (in this case the P.S.W.) in the centre of the whole scheme, rather than to have shared responsibility in the administrative office of the scheme, with consequent overlapping and waste of experience because it would not be integrated with total experience.
(4) The psychiatrist was originally appointed to give therapy. This was changed, and he was directed to classify cases before their admission, and to decide on the choice of hostel. Eventually he became the indirect therapist of the children through his regular discussions with the wardens and their staffs.

In these and countless other ways the committee, and the psychiatric team employed by them, retained flexibility and together developed an adaptation to the job.

The importance of this cannot be overestimated and can clearly be seen if we compare this situation with direct relation to a Ministry. In the British Civil Service it is essential that the officials get experience in each of the various departments of government. The consequence is, that if one enters into a personal and understanding relationship with the head of the appropriate department in a Ministry, when the inevitable reshuffles of training and promotion occur, one has to start again with another man. When this has happened several times one finds that whereas one has grown in the job oneself one can no longer feel that the head of the department has grown too; nor can one expect understanding of the details of the work. Since this situation must surely be accepted as an unavoidable phenomenon in large central organisations, one must look to such bodies to give general direction, but to abandon any attempts to keep in touch with detail. And yet in no work is detail more important than in work with children; and so there must always be a 'liaison' committee of interested people who represent the large parent body, and are yet able and willing to stoop to the detail which is the main preoccupation of the actual worker in the field.

It was important that the P.S.W. could take heavy responsibility, and this was made possible by her knowledge that she had the support of the clerk to the Council and the psychiatrist. The latter, by living away from the immediate problems, could discuss the local details without deep emotional involvement, and at the same time, being a medical man, he could accept responsibility for the risks that had to be taken if the best was to be done for the children.

Here is an example of the benefits of technical support and responsibility. A warden rings up the P.S.W. and says, 'A certain boy is on the roof, what shall I do?' He dare not take full responsibility as he is not psychiatrically trained, and he knows the boy has a suicidal tendency. The P.S.W. knows she has the psychiatrist's backing when she says, 'Ignore the boy and take the risk'. The warden knows this is the best treatment, but without backing would have had to give up whatever he was doing, ignore the needs of the other children, perhaps call the local fire brigade, and so do harm to the boy by putting the limelight on him and his escapade. In fact, the result of the advice given to the warden was that at the next meal-time the boy was in his place and no fuss had been made.

The P.S.W. and the visiting psychiatrist provided a psychiatric team that avoided clumsiness by being small, and yet could take responsibility over a wide field. Swift decisions could be made and action be taken within the framework of the powers of the committee by whom they were appointed, and to whom they were directly responsible.

Here are some further examples of detail which proved important:

(1) We found it necessary to take the trouble to gather together the fragments of each child's past history, and to let the child know that one person knew all about him.
(2) No member of the hostel staff could be unimportant. A child might be getting special help from his relationship to the gardener or to the cook. For this reason the staffing of the hostels was very much a matter of concern to us.
(3) It might happen that quite suddenly a warden could not tolerate a particular child any longer, and that the objective assessment of this problem required a very intimate knowledge of the situation. We acted on the principle that a warden should be able to express his feelings to someone who could, if necessary, take action, or who could prevent the matter from developing into an unnecessary crisis.

Classification for Placing

In different types of psychiatric work different ways of classifying patients are appropriate. For the purposes of placing these children satisfactorily in hostels, classification according to symptoms was useless, and was set aside. The following principles were developed and followed.

(1) In many cases no adequate diagnosis can usefully be made till a child has been watched, in a group, over a period of time.

In regard to the length of time needed a week is better than nothing, but three months is better than a week.

(2) If a history of the child's development can be obtained, the existence or non-existence of a fairly stable home is a fact of prime importance.

In the former case the child's experience of home can be used, and the hostel can remind the child of his own home and extend the existing home idea. In the latter case, the hostel has to provide a primary home, and the child's idea of his own home then gets mixed up with the ideal home of his dreams, compared with which the hostel is a pretty poor place.

(3) If a home of any kind does exist, then it is important to know of abnormalities there.

Examples of these are a parent who is a psychiatric case, certified or uncertifiable, or a dominating or antisocial brother or sister, or housing conditions that are in themselves a persecution. Hostel life can offer some correction of these abnormalities in the course of time and very gradually enable the child to view his own home objectively, and even sympathetically.

(4) If further details are available, it is of great importance to know whether the child did or did not have a satisfactory infant-mother relationship.

If there has been an experience of a good early relationship, even if this has been lost, it may be recovered in the personal relation of some member of the hostel staff to the child. If no such good start in fact existed it is beyond the scope of a hostel to create this, *ab initio*. The answer to this important question is often one of degree, but it is nevertheless worth seeking. In many cases a reliable early history is unobtainable, in which case the past has to be reconstructed through observation of the child in the hostel over a period of months.

(5) During the period of observation in the hostel there are certain specially valuable indications—ability to play, to persevere in constructive effort, and to make friends.

If a child can play, this is a very favourable sign. If constructive effort is enjoyed and persevered in without undue supervision and encouragement there is even greater hope of useful work being done through the hostel life. The ability to make a friend is a further valuable sign. Anxious children change friends frequently and too easily, and seriously disturbed children can only achieve membership of a gang—that is to say, a group whose cohesion depends on engineered persecution. A majority of the children drafted to evacuation hostels were at the outset incapable of play, or of sustained constructive effort, or of friendship.

(6) Mental defect has obvious importance, and in any group of hostels for difficult children there should be separate accommodation for children with low intelligence.

This is not only because they need special management and education, but also because they wear out the hostel staff to no purpose, and cause a feeling of hopelessness. In such difficult work as that with problem children, there must be some hope of reward, even if reward does not actually come.

(7) Bizarre or 'scatty' behaviour, and odd characteristics, distinguish some children who are on the whole unpromising material for therapy by hostel management.

Such children puzzle the hostel staff and make them feel mad themselves. In any case children of this kind need personal psychotherapy; although, even if it can be provided, their treatment is often beyond present-day understanding. They are, in fact, research cases for enterprising analysts, and there are but few satisfactory institutions for these children.

The classification outlined above formed the basis for placing; but the main consideration must always be: what can this hostel, these wardens, this group of children, stand at this particular moment? It was soon found to be a bad thing to decide to put a child in a hostel just because he was needing care and the hostel had a vacancy. Every new child, disturbed in the way that these billet-failures were disturbed, cannot help being, at first, a complication, and no asset to a hostel community. These children (except possibly in the first deceptive and unreal week or two) contribute nothing, and they absorb emotional energy. If they become accepted in the group they then start to be able to contribute to some extent, under supervision; but this is the result of hard work on the part of staff and the established children.

There is no one thing that is more helpful to the wardens of a hostel than this: that on introducing a new child one should present that child to the wardens before the issue of placing the child is settled. If this course is followed, a child is suggested for the hostel, but the wardens can accept or refuse. If the wardens think they can absorb this new child, then they have begun to want him. By the other method, of simply drafting children without prior consultation, wardens cannot help starting with negative feelings towards the child, and can only find other feelings in the course of time, and with luck. This joint consultation over admission to a particular hostel was very difficult to put into practice, but every effort was made to avoid exceptions to the rule, because of the vast practical difference between the two methods.

The Central Therapeutic Idea

The central idea of the scheme was to provide stability which the children could get to know, which they could test out, which they could gradually come to believe in, and around which they could play. This stability was essentially something that existed apart from the ability of the children, individually or collectively, to create or maintain it.[5]

The environmental stability was passed down, from the community in general, to the children. The Ministry provided the background, helped by the County Council. Against this background there was the committee, which in this scheme was, fortunately, made up of a group of experienced and responsible people who could be relied upon to continue to exist. Then there were the hostel staff, as well as the buildings and grounds, and the general emotional atmosphere. It was the task of the psychiatric team to translate the essential stability of the scheme into terms of emotional stability in the hostels. Only if the wardens are happy, and satisfied, and feeling stable, can the children benefit from their relations to them. Wardens in these hostels are in so difficult a position that understanding and support from someone is an absolute necessity for them. In the scheme we are describing it was the job of the psychiatric team to supply this support.

The most essential thing, then, was the provision of stability, and especially of emotional stability, in the hostel staff; although, of course, this could never be completely achieved. Nevertheless, work was done all the time with this aim. To help in the creation of a stable emotional background for the children the policy of employing married wardens— mentioned earlier—was recommended to the committee, and adopted. Joint married wardens may have children of their own, and then immense complications ensue. Nevertheless, these complications are outweighed by the enrichment of the hostel community through the existence of a real family within it.

It was once said in criticism, 'The hostel looks as if it were made for the staff'; but we felt that this was not a criticism. The staff must be living a satisfactory life, must be allowed time off, proper holidays, and, in peacetime, proper financial reward, if work with antisocial and mad children is to be done at all. It is not enough to provide a beautiful hostel with a nice staff. To do good by residential management the staff of the hostels must 'stay put' for a period of time—long enough for them to see children through to school-leaving age, and to the age of going to work; for the work of the staff is not finished until they have gradually launched the children into the world.

1

There is no particular training for hostel wardens, and even if there were, their selection as suitable people for the work would be of more importance than their training. We find it impossible to generalise about the type of person who makes a good warden. Our successful wardens have differed from each other widely in education, previous experience, and interests, and have been drawn from various walks of life. The following is a list of the previous occupations of some of them: elementary school teacher, social worker, trained church worker, commercial artist, instructor and matron in an approved school,[i] master and matron at a remand home, worker in a public assistance institution, prison welfare officer.

We find that the nature of previous training and experience matters little compared with the ability to assimilate experience, and to deal in a genuine, spontaneous way with the events and relationships of life. This is of the utmost importance, for only those who are confident enough to be themselves, and to act in a natural way, can act consistently day in and day out. Furthermore, wardens are put to such a severe test by the children coming into hostels that only those who are able to be themselves can stand the strain. We must point out, however, that there will be times when the warden will have to 'act naturally' in the sense that an actor acts naturally. This is particularly important with ill children. If a child comes and whines: 'I've cut my finger', just when the warden is in the middle of making Income Tax returns, if when the cook has given notice, he or she must act as though the child had not come in at such an awkward moment; for these children are often too ill or too anxious to be able to allow for the warden's own personal difficulties as well as their own.

We therefore try to choose as hostel wardens those who possess this ability to be consistently natural in their behaviour, for we regard it as essential to the work. We would count as important also the possession of some skill, such as music, painting, pottery, etc. Above and beyond all these things, however, it is, of course, vital that the wardens possess a genuine love of children, for only this will see them through the inevitable ups and downs of hostel life.

Brilliant people who organise one hostel well, and pass on to another to do the same there, would be better if they had never existed as far as the children

---

[i] Approved schools were residential homes for young offenders or those difficult to control within the parental home, first established in the UK in the early 1930s. See also the Introduction to Volume 2 and Winnicott's final report to the Q Camp committee [CW 2:3:1].

are concerned. It is the permanent nature of the home that makes it valuable, even more than the fact that the work is done intelligently.

We do not expect the wardens to carry out any prescribed type of regime, or even to carry out agreed plans. Wardens who have to be told what to do are of no use, because the important things have to be done on the spot in a way that is natural to the individual concerned. Only thus will the warden's relationship become real and therefore of importance to the child. Wardens are encouraged to build up a home and community life to the best of their ability, and it will be found that this is along the line of their own beliefs and way of life. No two hostels will therefore be alike.

We find that there are wardens who like organising large groups of children, and others who prefer to have intimate personal relationships with a few children. Some prefer abnormal children of one type or another, and some like true mental defectives.

The education of the wardens in the work is important, and has been discussed earlier as part of the work of the psychiatrist, and of the psychiatric social worker. This education is best done on the job, by the discussion of problems as they arise. It is a great help if wardens are confident enough in themselves to be able to think along psychological lines and discuss problems with other wardens and experienced people.

The staffing of hostels apart from the wardens presents peculiar difficulties especially where the children are rather antisocial. With normal children the assistants can be young people who are learning the job, practising taking responsibility and acting on their own initiative, with a view to becoming wardens themselves at a later date. Where the children are antisocial, however the management has to be strong, and cannot avoid being dictatorial, so that assistants have to be constantly carrying out orders from the warden when they would prefer to be working on their own initiative. They therefore become easily bored, or else they like being told what to do, in which case they are not much good. These problems are inherent in the work.

2

If it is recognised how intimately a child's sense of security is bound up with his relationship to his parents, it becomes obvious that no other people can give him so much. Every child has the right to his own good home in which to grow, and it is nothing but a misfortune that deprives him of it.

In our hostel work, therefore, we recognise that we cannot give to the children anything so good as their own good home would have been. We can only offer a substitute home.

Each hostel tries to reproduce as nearly as possible a home environment for each child in it. This means first of all the provision of positive things: a building, food, clothing, human love and understanding; a timetable, schooling; apparatus and ideas leading to rich play and constructive work. The hostel also provides substitute parents and other human relationships. And then, these things being provided, each child, according to the degree of his distrust, and according to the degree of his hopelessness about the loss of his own home (and sometimes his recognition of the inadequacies of that home while it lasted), is all the time testing the hostel staff as he would test his own parents. Sometimes he does this directly, but most of the time he is content to let another child do the testing for him. An important thing about this testing is that it is not something that can be achieved and done with. Always somebody has to be a nuisance. Often one of the staff will say: 'We'd be all right if it weren't for Tommy . . .', but in point of fact the others can only afford to be 'all right' because Tommy is being a nuisance, and is proving to them that the home can stand up to Tommy's testing, and could therefore presumably stand up to their own.

The usual response of a child who is placed in a good hostel can be described as having three phases. For the first short phase the child is remarkably 'normal' (it will be a long time before he is so normal again); he has new hope, he scarcely sees people as they are, and the staff and the other children have not yet had any reason to begin to disillusion him. Almost every child goes through a short period of good behaviour when he first comes to a hostel. It is a dangerous stage, because what he sees and responds to in the warden and his staff is his ideal of what a good father and mother would be like. Grown-ups are inclined to think, 'This child sees we are nice, and easily trusts us'. But he does not see they are nice; he does not see them at all; he just imagines they are nice. It is a symptom of illness to believe that anything can be 100 per cent good, and the child starts off with an ideal which is destined to be shattered.

The child sooner or later enters into the second phase, the breaking down of his ideal. He sets about this first by testing the building and the people physically. He wants to know what damage he can do, and how much he can do with impunity. Then if he finds that he can be physically managed, that is, that the place and the people in it have nothing to fear from him physically, he starts to test by subtlety, putting one member of the staff against another, trying to make people quarrel, trying to make people give each other away, and doing all he can to get favoured himself. When a hostel is being managed unsatisfactorily it is this second phase which becomes almost a constant feature.

If the hostel withstands these tests the child enters on the third phase, settles down with a sigh of relief, and joins in the life of the group as an ordinary member. It should be borne in mind that his first real contacts with the other children will probably be in the shape of a fight or some kind of attack, and we have noticed that often the first child to be attacked by a new child will later become that child's first friend.

In short, the hostels provide positive good things, and give opportunities for their value and reality to be tested continuously by the children. Sentimentality has no place in the management of children, and no ultimate good can come from offering children artificial conditions of indulgence; by carefully administered justice they must gradually be brought up against the consequences of their own destructive actions. Each child will be able to stand this in so far as he has been able to get some positive good out of hostel life, that is, in so far as he has found people who are truly reliable, and has begun to build up belief in them and in himself.

It must be remembered that the preservation of law and order is necessary to the children, and will be a relief to them, for it means that the hostel life and the good things for which the hostel stands will be preserved in spite of all that they can do.

The immense strain of the twenty-four-hour care of these children is not easily recognised in high quarters, and in fact any one who is only visiting a hostel, and who is not emotionally involved, can easily forget this fact. It might be asked why the wardens should let themselves get emotionally involved. The answer is that these children, who are seeking a primary home experience, do not get anywhere unless someone does, in fact, get emotionally involved with them. To get under someone's skin is the first thing these children do, when they begin to get hope. The experience subsequent to this state forms the essence of hostel therapeutics.

It follows, therefore, that hostels must be small. Moreover, wardens must not be burdened with one more child than they can emotionally stand at any given moment: for if one too many is put in a warden's care he is forced to protect himself, by ousting from 'under his skin' someone who is not ready for this. There is a limit to the number of people that a human being can be seriously concerned with at one time, and if this fact is ignored the warden is forced to do superficial and useless work, and to substitute dictatorial management for the healthy mixture of love and strength which he would prefer to show. Alternatively, and this is common, he breaks down, and the work he has done is undone. For every change of wardens produces casualties among the children, and interrupts the natural therapeutics of hostel work.

Notes

1. It could be said that the Ministry of Health threw a task at a county, watched results, and acted accordingly—a situation which recalls the principle of leaderless groups' tasks employed in British Army Officer Selection.
2. Cf. the Curtis Report on the Care of Children (1946), H.M.S.O., London.
3. The word insane is here used deliberately, for no other word is correct, and the official word 'maladjusted' begs the whole question.

4. Author's note—With regard to corporal punishment, the ruling was that the committee trusted the warden who was appointed, and left to him the right to give corporal punishment. If the committee did not like the way a warden worked the remedy was to get a new warden, and not to interfere directly. A restriction on corporal punishment is quickly found out by the children, and in practice it is a severe handicap to a warden to be curbed by the committee.

   In one case, when the committee had doubts, a warden was told to enter each such punishment in a book, which was inspected weekly.

   Along with this general policy, there was a drive towards the education of the staff, so that corporal punishment was avoided as much as possible. Through an understanding of the personal difficulties of each child, punishable outbreaks could often be prevented, and in some groups over long periods of time corporal punishment was, in fact, rare.
5. Surely, experiments in getting children to create their own central government should always be made first, if they have to be made, with those who have had a good early home experience? With these deprived children it seems to be cruel to make them do the very thing they feel hopeless about.

4

Further Thoughts on Babies as Persons

> Originally published in *New Era in Home and School*, 1947, 28(10), 179, as 'Babies are persons'. Also published in *The child and the outside world: Studies in developing relationships* (pp. 134–140). London: Tavistock, 1957; and *The child, the family, and the outside world* (pp. 85–92). Harmondsworth, UK: Penguin, 1964.

The human being's development is a continuous process. As in the development of the body, so in the development of the personality and in the development of the capacity for relationships. No stage can be missed or marred without ill-effect.

Health is maturity, maturity appropriate to the age. If certain accidental diseases are ignored this is obviously true of the body, and in matters of psychology there are practically no reasons why health and maturity should not mean the same thing. In other words, in the emotional development of a human being, if there are no hitches or distortions in the developmental process, there is health.

This means, if I am right, that all the care that a mother and father take of their infant is not just a pleasure to them and to the infant, it is also absolutely necessary, and without it the baby cannot easily grow up into a healthy or valuable adult.

In matters of the body it is possible to make mistakes, even to allow rickets, and yet rear a child with nothing worse than bow-legs. But on the psychological side, a baby deprived of some quite ordinary but necessary thing, such as affectionate contact, is bound, to some extent, to be disturbed in emotional development, and this will show in a personal difficulty as the young person grows up. Put the other way round; as a child grows and passes from stage to stage of complex internal development and eventually achieves a capacity for relationships, the parents can know that their good care has been an essential ingredient. This has a meaning for us all, for it follows that, in so far as we are reasonably mature or healthy as adults, each one of us must recognize that a good start to one's life was provided by someone. It is this good start—this basis for child care—that I try to describe.

The story of a human being does not start at five years or two, or at six months, but starts at birth—and before birth if you like; and each baby is from the start a person, and needs to be known by someone. No one can get to know a baby as well as the baby's own mother can.

These two statements take us a long way, but now, how to proceed? Can psychology tell anyone how to be a mother or father? I think this is the wrong way round. Let us, instead, study some of the things mothers and fathers naturally do, and try to show them a little why they do them, so that they may feel strengthened.

I will take an example.

Here is a mother with her baby girl. What does she do when she picks her up? Does she catch hold of her foot and drag her out of her pram and swing her up? Does she hold a cigarette with one hand and grab her with the other? No. She has quite a different way of going at it. I think she tends to give the infant warning of her approach, she puts her hands round her to gather her together before she moves her; in fact she gains the baby's cooperation before she lifts her; and then she lifts her from one place to another, from cot to shoulder. Does she not then put the baby up against her with her head snuggled in her neck, so that the baby may begin to feel her as a person?

Here is a mother with her baby boy. How does she bath him? Does she just put him in the electric washer and let the cleaning process happen mechanically? Not at all. She knows of bath-time as a special time both for her and for the baby. She prepares to enjoy it. She does all the mechanical part properly, testing the heat of the water with her elbow and not letting the baby slip through her fingers when he is soapy, but on top of this she allows the bathing to be an enjoyed experience which enriches the growing relationship, not only of herself to the baby, but of him to her.

Why does she take all this trouble? Can we not say quite simply, and without being sentimental, that it is because of love; that it is because maternal feelings have developed in her; because of the deep understanding of her baby's needs that comes from her devotion?

Let us go back to the business of picking a baby up. Can we not say that, without conscious effort, the mother did what she did in stages. She made being picked up acceptable to her little girl by:

(1) giving the infant warning;
(2) gaining her cooperation;
(3) gathering her together;
(4) taking her from one place to another and with a simple purpose that she can understand.

The mother also refrains from shocking her baby with cold hands, or from pricking him or her when she pins up the napkin.

The mother does not involve her baby in all her personal experiences and feelings. Sometimes her baby yells and yells until she feels like murder, yet she lifts the baby up with just the same care, without revenge—or not very much. She avoids making the baby the victim of her own impulsiveness. Infant care, like doctoring, is a test of personal reliability.

Today may be one of those days when everything goes wrong. The laundryman calls before the list is ready; the frontdoor bell rings, and someone else comes to the back door. But a mother waits till she has recovered her poise before she takes up her baby, which she does with the usual gentle technique that the baby comes to know as an important part of her. Her technique is highly personal, and is looked for and recognized, like her mouth, and her eyes, her colouring, and her smell. Over and over again a mother deals with her own moods, anxieties, and excitements in her own private life, reserving for her baby what belongs to the baby. This gives a foundation on which the human infant can start to build an understanding of the extremely complex thing that is a relationship between two human beings.

Can we not say that the mother *adapts herself* to what the baby can understand, actively adapts to needs? This active adaptation is just what is essential for the infant's emotional growth, and the mother adapts herself to the baby's needs especially at the beginning, at a time when only the simplest possible circumstances can be appreciated.

I must try to explain a little why it is that a mother takes all this trouble, and so much more than I can include in this brief description. One reason why I must do this is that there are some who honestly believe and who teach that in the first six months the mother does not matter. In the first six months (it is said) only technique counts, and a good technique can be provided in a hospital or a home, by trained workers.

For my part I am sure that while mothercraft may be taught and even read about in books, *the mothering of one's own baby is entirely personal, a job that no one else could take over and do as well as oneself.* While the scientists are at the problem, seeking proofs as they must do before believing, mothers will do well to insist that they themselves are needed from the start. This opinion, I may as well add, is not based on hearing mothers talk, on guess-work, or on pure intuition; it is the conclusion I feel I have been forced to draw after long research.

The mother takes trouble because she feels (and I find she is correct in this feeling), that if the human baby is to develop well and to develop richly there should be personal mothering from the start, if possible by the very person who has conceived and carried that baby, the one who has a very deeply rooted interest in allowing for that baby's point of view, and who loves to let herself be the baby's whole world.

This does not mean that a baby of a few weeks knows the mother as at six months or a year. In the very first days it is the pattern and technique of mothering that is perceived, and so also the detail of her nipples, the shape of her ear, the quality of her smile, the warmth and smell of her breath. Quite early an infant may have a rudimentary idea of a kind of wholeness of the mother at certain special moments. Apart from what can be perceived, however, the infant needs the mother to be continuously there as a whole person, for only as a whole and mature human being can she have the love and character required for the task.

I once risked the remark, 'There is no such thing as a baby'—meaning that if you set out to describe a baby, you will find you are describing a *baby and someone*. A baby cannot exist alone, but is essentially part of a relationship.

The mother, too, has to be considered. If the continuity of her relationship to her own baby is broken something is lost that cannot be regained. It shows incredible lack of understanding of the mother's role to take away her baby for a few weeks, then to hand the baby back, and expect the mother to continue just where she left off.

I will try to classify some ways in which a mother is needed.

(a) First I want to say that the mother is needed as a live person. Her baby must be able to feel the warmth of her skin and breath, and to taste and see. This is vitally important. There must be full access to the mother's live body. Without the mother's live presence the most learned mothercraft is wasted. It is the same with doctors. The value of a general practitioner in a village is largely that he is alive, that he is there and available. People know the number of his car, and the back view of his hat. It takes years to learn to be a doctor, the training may absorb all of a father's capital; but in the end the really important thing is not the doctor's learning and skill, but the fact that the village knows and feels that he is alive and available. The doctor's physical presence meets an emotional need. As with doctor so with mother, only much more so.

Psychology and physical care join here. During the war I was with a group of people who were discussing the future of the war-stricken children of Europe. They asked me for my opinion as to the most important *psychological* things to be done for these children at the end of the war. I found myself saying, 'Give them food'. Someone said, 'We don't mean physical things, we mean psychological things'. I still felt that the giving of food at the right moment would be catering for psychological need. Fundamentally, love expresses itself in physical terms.

Of course if physical care means having a baby vaccinated this has nothing to do with psychology. A baby cannot appreciate your concern lest smallpox should become rampant in the community—though the doctor's attack on his skin may of course produce crying. But if physical care means the right kind of meal at the right temperature at the right time (right from the baby's point of view, I mean), then this is psychological care too. I think this is a useful rule. The care that a baby can appreciate is fulfilling psychological and emotional needs, however much it may seem to be related simply to physical needs.

In this first way of looking at things the mother's aliveness and physical management provide an essential psychological and emotional milieu, essential for the baby's early emotional growth.

(b) Secondly, the mother is needed to present the world to the baby. Through the techniques of the person or the techniques of the people who are doing the minding comes the baby's introduction to external reality, to the world around. There will continue a struggle with this difficult matter all through life, but help is needed here especially at the start. I will explain what I mean with some care, because many mothers may never have thought of infant feeding in this way; certainly doctors and nurses seldom seem to consider this aspect of the feeding act. This is what I mean.

Imagine a baby who has never had a feed. Hunger turns up, and the baby is ready to conceive of something; out of need the baby is ready to create a source of satisfaction, but there is no previous experience to show the baby what there is to expect. If at this moment the mother places her breast where the baby is ready to expect something, and if plenty of time is allowed for the infant to feel round, with mouth and hands, and perhaps with a sense of smell, the baby 'creates' just what is there to be found. The baby eventually gets the illusion that this real breast is exactly the thing that was created out of need, greed, and the first impulses of primitive loving. Sight, smell, and taste register somewhere, and after a while the baby may be creating something like the very breast that mother has to offer. A thousand times before weaning a baby may be given just this particular introduction to external reality by one woman, the mother. A thousand times the feeling has existed that what was wanted was created, and was found to be there. From this develops a belief that the world can contain what is wanted and needed, with the result that the baby has hope that there is a live relationship between inner reality and external reality, between innate primary creativity and the world at large which is shared by all.

Successful infant feeding, therefore, is an essential part of the infant's education. In the same way, but I will not try to develop the theme here, the infant needs the mother's way of receiving the excretions. The infant needs the mother's acceptance of a relationship expressed in excretion terms, a relationship that is in full swing long before the infant can contribute by conscious effort, and before the infant can (perhaps at three, four, or six months) start to wish to give to the mother out of a sense of guilt; that is to say, to make reparation for greedy attack.

(c) Out of all that could be said I will add a third way in which the mother is needed, the mother herself, and not a team of excellent minders.

I refer to the mother's job of *disillusioning*. When she has given her baby the illusion that the world can be created out of need and imagination (which of course in one sense it cannot be, but we can leave this to the philosopher), when she has established the belief in things and people that I have described as a healthy basis for development, she will then have to take the child through the process of disillusionment, which is a wider aspect of weaning. The nearest that can be offered to the child is the grown-ups' *wish* to make the demands of reality bearable until the full blast of disillusionment can be borne, and until creativity can develop through mature skill into a true contribution to society.

The 'shades of the prison house' seems to me to be the poet's description of the disillusioning process, and its essential painfulness.[i] Gradually the mother enables the child to allow that though the world *can* provide something like what is needed and wanted, and what could therefore be created, it will not do so automatically, nor at the very moment the mood arises or the wish is felt.

Do you notice how I am gradually switching from the idea of need to that of a wish or desire? The change indicates a growing up, and an acceptance of external reality with a consequent weakening of instinctual imperative.

Temporarily the mother has put herself out for the child, she has at the beginning put herself in the child's pocket. But, eventually, this child becomes able to leave the dependence that belongs to the earliest stage when the environment must adapt itself, and can accept two coexisting points of view—the mother's as well as the baby's. But the mother cannot deprive the child of herself (weaning, disillusionment) unless she has first meant everything to the child.

It is not my intention to say that the baby's whole life is wrecked if there has been a failure actually at the *breast*. Of course a baby can thrive physically on the bottle given with reasonable skill, and a mother whose breast milk fails can do almost all that is needed in the course of bottle-feeding. Nevertheless, the principle holds that a baby's emotional development at the start is only to be built well on a relationship with one person, who should, ideally, be the mother. Who else will both feel and supply what is needed?

---

[i] Shades of the prison house begin to close
    Upon the growing Boy.

W. Wordsworth (1807). *Ode: Intimations of Immortality*, V.

5

The Child and Sex

Originally published in *The Practitioner*, 1947, 158. Also published in *The child and the outside world: Studies in developing relationships* (pp. 153–166). London: Tavistock, 1957; and *The child, the family, and the outside world* (pp. 147–160). Harmondsworth, UK: Penguin, 1964.

Only a little while ago it was thought bad to link sex with childhood 'innocence'. At the present time the need is for accurate description. As so much is as yet unknown the student is recommended to carry out research in his own way, and if he must read instead of making observations let him read descriptions by many different writers, not looking to one or another as the purveyor of the truth. This chapter is not the retailing of a set of theories bought wholesale, it is an attempt to put in a few words one person's description of childhood sexuality, based on his training and experience as a paediatrician and psychoanalyst. The subject is vast, and cannot be confined to the limits of a chapter without suffering distortion.

In considering any aspect of child psychology it is useful to remember that everyone has been a child. In each adult observer there is the whole memory of his infancy and childhood, both the fantasy and the reality, in so far as it was appreciated at the time. Much is forgotten but nothing is lost. What better example could direct attention to the vast resources of the unconscious!

In oneself, it is possible to sort out from the vast unconscious the repressed unconscious, and this will include some sexual elements. If special difficulty is found in allowing even for the possibility of childhood sexuality, it is better to turn one's attention to another subject. On the other hand, the observer who is reasonably free to find what is to be observed, not having to guard too much (for personal reasons) against finding whatever is to be found, can choose from many different methods for objective study! The most fruitful, and therefore the one necessary for anyone who intends to make psychology his life work, is personal analysis, in which (if it is successful) he not only loses the active repressions, but also discovers through memory, and by reliving, the feelings and essential conflicts of his own early life.

Freud, who was responsible for drawing attention to the importance of childhood sexuality, arrived at his conclusions through the analysis of adults. The analyst has a unique experience every time he conducts a successful analysis, in that he sees unfolding before him the patient's childhood and infancy as it appeared to the patient. He has the repeated experience of getting to see the natural history of a psychological disorder, with all the interweaving of the psychological and the physical, of the personal and the environmental, of the tactual and the imagined, of what has been conscious to the patient and what has been under repression.

In analysis of adults Freud found that the foundations of their sex life and sex difficulties went back to adolescence, and back to childhood, especially to the two- to five-year-old period.

He found that there was a triangular situation which could not be described except by saying that the little boy was in love with his mother, and was in conflict with his father as a sexual rival. The sexual element was proved by the fact that it was not just in fantasy that these things were happening; there were physical accompaniments, erections, excitement phases with climax, murderous impulses, and a specific fear—fear of castration. This central theme was picked out and called the Oedipus complex, and it remains today a central fact, infinitely elaborated and modified, but inescapable. Psychology built on a hushing up of this central theme would have been doomed to failure, and therefore one cannot help being grateful to Freud for going ahead and stating what he repeatedly found, bearing the brunt of public reaction.

In using the term 'Oedipus complex' Freud paid tribute to the intuitive understanding of childhood which is independent of psychoanalysis. The Oedipus myth really shows that what Freud wanted to describe has always been known.

A tremendous development of theory has taken place round the nucleus of the Oedipus complex, and much of the criticism of the idea would have been justified if the theory had been put forward as an artist's intuitive understanding of the whole of childhood sexuality or of psychology. But the concept was like a rung in a ladder of scientific procedure. As a concept it had the great merit that it dealt with both the physical and the imaginative. Here was a psychology in which the body and the mind were simply two aspects of one person, essentially related and not to be examined separately without loss of value.

If the central fact of the Oedipus complex is accepted it is immediately possible and desirable to examine the ways in which the concept is inadequate or inaccurate as a clue to child psychology.

The first objection comes from direct observation of little boys. Some boys do express in so many words and quite openly their in-love feeling for their mother and their wish to marry her, and even to give her children, and their consequent hate of father; but many do not express themselves in this way at all, and in fact seem to have more love feeling towards father than towards mother; and in any case brothers and sisters, nurses, and aunts and uncles, easily take the place of the parents. Direct observation does not confirm the degree of importance given to the Oedipus complex by the psychoanalyst. Nevertheless, the psychoanalyst must stick to his guns, because in analysis he regularly finds it, and regularly finds it to be important, and often he finds it severely repressed and only emerging after most careful and prolonged analysis. If, in the observation of children, their games are intimately examined, sexual themes and the Oedipus theme will be regularly found among all the others; but again, the intimate examination of children's games is difficult, and is best done in the course of analysis if it is carried out for research purposes.

The fact seems to be that the full Oedipus situation is but seldom enacted openly in real life. Intimations of it there certainly are, but the tremendously intense feelings associated with periods of instinctual excitement are largely in the child's unconscious or quickly become repressed, being nonetheless real for all that; temper attacks and the common nightmares that occur normally in the three-year-old cannot be understood except in terms of firm attachment to persons, with periodically rising instinctual tension, and acute exacerbation of conflict in the mind arising out of hate and fear clashing with love.

A modification of the original idea (one made by Freud himself) is that the very intense and highly coloured sex situations that an adult in analysis recovers from his own childhood are not necessarily episodes that could have been observed as such by his parents, but nevertheless are true reconstructions based on unconscious feelings and ideas belonging to childhood.

This brings up another point, what about little girls? The first assumption was that they fall in love with their fathers, and hate and fear their mothers. Here again is a truth, and here again the main part is likely to be unconscious, not something that the little girl would admit, except in very special circumstances of trust.

Many girls, however, do not get so far in their emotional development as to become attached to father, and to take the very great risks inherent in being in conflict with mother. Alternatively, an attachment to father is formed, but regression (as it is called) occurs back from a weakly acquired relation to father. The risks inherent in conflict with mother are great indeed, for with the idea of mother (in unconscious fantasy) is associated the idea of loving care, good food, the stability of the earth, and the world in general; and a conflict with mother necessarily involves a feeling of insecurity, and dreaming of the ground opening, or worse. The little girl, then, has a special problem, if only because when she comes to love her father her rivalry is with her mother, who is her first love in a more primitive way.

The little girl, like the little boy, has physical sex feelings appropriate to the type of fantasy. It might usefully be said that whereas a boy at the height of his sex wave (at the toddler age and at puberty) is especially afraid of castration, in a girl at a corresponding stage the trouble is a conflict in her relation to the physical world brought about by her rivalry with her mother, who was originally for the child the physical world itself. At the same time the little girl suffers fears in regard to her body, fears of castration like those of a boy, and fears that her body will be attacked by hostile mother figures, in retaliation for her wish to steal her mother's babies, and much else.

This description is obviously defective in respect of bi-sexuality. At the same time in a child's life that the ordinary heterosexual relationship is vitally important the homosexual relationship always exists, and can be relatively more important than the other. Another way of putting this is to say that a child normally becomes identified with each parent, but at any one moment principally with one parent; and this parent need not be the one of the child's sex. In all cases there is a capacity for identification with the parent of the other sex, so that in the sum total of a child's fantasy life (if search be made) there can be found the whole range of relationships, regardless of the actual sex of the child. It is convenient, naturally, when the main identification is with the parent of the same sex, but in psychiatric examination of a child it would be wrong to jump to a diagnosis of abnormality if the finding is that the child is mainly wanting to be like the parent of the other sex. Such can be the child's natural adaptation to special circumstances. In certain cases cross-identifications can, of course, be a basis for later homosexual tendencies of abnormal quality. In the 'latency' period, between the first sexual period and adolescence, cross-identifications are especially important.

A principle is being taken for granted in this description which perhaps ought to be deliberately formulated. The basis of sexual health is laid down in childhood, and in the reduplication of early childhood development that takes place at puberty. The corollary is equally true, that sexual aberrations and abnormalities of adult life are laid down in early childhood. Further, the basis of the whole of mental health is laid in early childhood and in infancy.

Ordinarily a child's play is greatly enriched by sexual ideas and sexual symbolism, and if there is strong sex-inhibition a play-inhibition follows. There is a possible confusion here arising out of the lack of clear definition of sex play. Sexual excitement is one thing, and the acting out of sex fantasy is another. Sex play with bodily excitement is a special case, and in childhood the outcome is liable to be difficult. The climax or detumescence is often represented more by the aggressive outburst that follows frustration than by a true relief of instinctual tension such as can be obtained by an older person after the onset of puberty. In sleep the dream life rises at times to excited states, and at the climax the body commonly finds some substitute for full sexual orgasm, such as wetting, or waking in nightmare. Sexual orgasm is not likely to be as satisfactory, as such, in the little boy as it can be after puberty, with emission added; perhaps it is more easily got by the little girl who has nothing to add as she matures, except being penetrated. These times of recurring instinctual tension must be expected in childhood, and substitute climaxes have to be provided—notably meals—but also parties, outings, special moments.

Parents know well enough that they often have to step in and induce a climax by a show of strength, even a smack producing tears. Mercifully, children get tired in the end, and go to bed and sleep. Even so, the delayed climax may disturb the calm of night, as the child wakes in a night-terror, and mother or father is needed immediately if the child is to regain a relation to external reality, and the relief that comes from an appreciation of what is stable in the real world.

All physical excitements have ideational accompaniments, or (the other way round) ideas are themselves the accompaniment of physical experience. Mental pleasure, as well as gratification and relief from tension, comes from the common playing of childhood which is the acting out of fantasy apart from physical excitement. Much of the normal and healthy play of childhood is concerned with sexual ideas and symbolism; this is not saying that children who are playing are always sexually excited. Children, when playing, may get excited in a general way, and periodically the excitement can become localized and therefore obviously sexual, or urinary, or greedy, or something else based on the capacity of tissues for excitement. Excitement calls for climax. The obvious way out for a child is the game with climax, in which excitement leads to something, 'a chopper to chop off your head', a forfeit, a prize, someone is caught or killed, someone has won, and so on.

Innumerable examples could be given of sex fantasy acted out, but not necessarily accompanied by bodily excitement. It is well known that a big proportion of little girls and some little boys like to play with dolls and to act towards the dolls as mothers do towards babies. They not only do as mother did, thereby complimenting her, but also they do as mother ought to have done, thereby reproaching her. The identification with a mother can be very complete and detailed. As in all these matters, there is a physical side of the experience along with the fantasy that is being acted out, and pains in the belly and sickness can be due to the mother game. Boys as well as girls stick their bellies out for fun, imitating pregnant women, and it is not very uncommon for a child to be brought to the doctor for enlarged belly when the trouble is a secret imitation of a pregnant woman, whose condition is supposed to have been unnoticed. As a matter of fact children are always looking out for swellings, and however successfully sex information is withheld from them they are unlikely to miss spotting a pregnancy. They may, however, keep the information in a compartment of the mind, unassimilated, because of the parents' prudery, or their own sense of guilt.

Children the world over have a game called 'Fathers and Mothers', which becomes enriched by an infinite quantity of imaginative material, and the pattern each group of children evolves tells a good deal about the children, and especially about the dominant personality in the group.

Children do often act out the adult type of sexual relationship in relation to each other, but usually this is done secretly and is not therefore recorded by people who are making deliberate observations. Naturally, children easily feel guilty in so playing and also they cannot help being affected by the fact that such play comes under a social ban. It could not be said that these sexual incidents are harmful, but if they are accompanied by a feeling of severe guilt and become repressed, unavailable to the child's consciousness, then harm has been done. This harm can be undone by the recovery of the memory of the incident, and it can sometimes be said that such an incident easily remembered has its value as a stepping-stone in the long and difficult journey from immaturity to maturity.

There are many other sex games which are related less directly to sexual fantasy. No claim is made here that children think only of sex: however, a sex-inhibited child is a poor companion, and is impoverished, like a sex-inhibited adult.

The subject of childhood sexuality simply does not allow itself to be confined rigidly to the excitement of sex organs and the fantasy that belongs to such excitement. In studying childhood sexuality it is possible to see the way in which the more specific excitement is built up out of bodily excitements of all types, reaching forward to the more mature feelings and ideas easily recognized as sexual; the more mature develops from the more primitive, the sexual from (for instance) the cannibalistic instinctual urges.

It can be said that a capacity for sexual excitement, in either sex, is present from birth, but the primary capacity of parts of the body for excitement has limited significance until the child's personality has become integrated and it can be said that it is the child as a whole person who is excited in that specific way. As the infant develops, the sexual type of excitement gradually acquires importance relative to the other types of excitement (urethral, anal, skin, oral), and at the age of three, four, or five years (as also at puberty) becomes capable, in healthy development, of dominating over other functions in appropriate circumstances.

This is another way of saying that all the innumerable accompaniments of sex in adult behaviour derive from early childhood, and it would be an abnormality and an impoverishment if an adult could not naturally and unselfconsciously employ all manner of infantile or 'pregenital' techniques in sex play. Nevertheless, the compulsion to employ a pregenital *instead of* genital technique in sex experience constitutes perversion, and has its origin in a hold-up of emotional development in early childhood. In analysis of a case of perversion there can always be found both a fear in regard to forward development to mature sex, and a special capacity to get satisfaction in more primitive ways. Sometimes there are actual experiences enticing the child back to infantile types of experience (as when an infant has become excited at introduction of a suppository, or has reacted with excitement to being tightly bound by a nurse, and so on).

The story of the building up of the mature child from the immature infant is long and complex, also it is vitally important for the understanding of the psychology of the adult human being. To develop naturally, the infant and child need a relatively stable environment.

Roots of Female Sexuality. The roots of a little girl's sexuality go right down to her early greedy feelings in relation to her mother. There is a gradation from her hungry attack on her mother's body to the mature wish to be like mother. Her love of her father can be as much determined by his being stolen (so to speak) from mother as by his actually being especially loving to her; indeed, when a father is away over the period of a girl's infancy so that she does not really know him, her choice of him as a love object may be entirely due to the fact that he is mother's man. For these reasons there is a close association between stealing and sex desire, and the wish to have a baby.

The consequence of this is that when a woman becomes pregnant and has a baby she has to be able to deal with the feeling, somewhere in her, that the baby was stolen from inside her mother's body. If she cannot feel this, as well as knowing the facts, she loses something of the gratification that pregnancy can bring, and she loses much of the special joy of presenting her own mother with a grandchild. This idea of theft can cause guilt after conception, and can cause miscarriage.

It is especially important to know of this guilt potential in the practical matter of management of the period immediately after childbirth. A mother is at that time very sensitive to the type of woman in charge of her and her baby. She needs help, but because of these ideas derived from early childhood she can only believe in a very friendly or a very hostile mother-figure at that time; and a mother having her first baby, even if she is healthy-minded, is very liable to feel persecuted by her nurse. The reason for this and other phenomena characteristic of the state of motherhood must be sought in the early roots of the little girl's relation to mother, including her primitive wish to gain womanliness by tearing it from her mother's body.

Here is another principle that is worth formulating: in psychiatry every abnormality is a disturbance of emotional development. In treatment, a cure is brought about by enabling the patient's emotional development to go ahead where it was held up. To get to this point where it is held up the patient must always get back to early childhood or infancy, and this fact ought to be of extreme importance to the paediatrician.

Psychosomatic Disorders. There is one way in which childhood sexuality is of direct importance to the practising paediatrician: that is, the transformation of sexual excitement into symptoms and physiological changes that resemble the symptoms and changes brought about by physical diseases. These symptoms, which are called psychosomatic, are exceedingly common in all medical practice, and it is from them that the general practitioner weeds out the occasional textbook diseases for the expert attention of the specialist in physical disease.

These psychosomatic disorders are not seasonal or epidemic; in any one child, however, they show a periodicity, albeit an irregular one. This periodicity is simply an indication of the underlying recurring instinctual tension.

Partly because of internal reasons and partly because of environmental exciting factors, every now and again a child becomes an excitable being. The phrase 'all dressed up and nowhere to go' might have been designed to describe this state. A study of what happens to this excitement is almost a study of childhood, and of the child's problem: how to retain the capacity for eagerness and excitement without experiencing too much painful frustration through lack of satisfactory climax. The main methods by which children cope with this difficulty are:

(a) Loss of capacity for eagerness; but this carries with it a loss of sense of body, and much else that is disadvantageous.
(b) Employment of some sort of reliable climax, either eating or drinking or masturbation, or excited urination or defecation, or a temper tantrum, or a fight.
(c) The perversion of the body functions in a way that enables a spurious climax to be reached—vomiting and diarrhoea, a bilious attack, exaggeration of a catarrhal infection, complaint of aches and pains that would otherwise be unnoticed.
(d) A general muddle of all these, with a period of unwellness, perhaps with headache and loss of appetite, a period of general irritability, or a tendency of certain tissues to be excitable (for instance, all the phenomena clumped together, in present-day nomenclature, under the word 'allergic').
(e) An organization of excitement into a chronic 'nerviness' which may remain constant over a long period ('common anxious restlessness', perhaps the most common disorder of childhood).

The bodily symptoms and changes related to emotional states and disorders of emotional development form a large and important subject for the attention of the paediatrician.

In a description of childhood sexuality, mention must be made of masturbation. Here again is a vast subject for study. Masturbation is either normal or healthy or else it is a symptom of a disorder of emotional development.

Compulsive masturbation, just like compulsive thigh-rubbing, nail-biting, rocking, head-banging, head-swaying or rolling, thumb-sucking, and the like, is evidence of anxiety of one kind or another. If severely compulsive it is being employed by the child in his effort to deal with anxiety of more primitive or psychotic type, such as fear of disintegration of personality, or fear of loss of sense of the body, or fear of loss of touch with external reality.

Perhaps the most common disorder of masturbation is its suppression, or its disappearance from a child's repertoire of self-managed defences against intolerable anxiety or sense of deprivation or loss. An infant starts life with the capacity to handle his mouth and to suck his fist, and indeed he needs this ability to comfort himself. He needs his hand to his mouth even if he has what is best for him, a right to his mother's breast when he feels hungry. How much more does he need it when he is regimented. All through infancy he needs whatever satisfaction he can get from his body, from fist-sucking, from passing water, from defecation, and from holding his penis. The little girl has corresponding satisfactions.

Ordinary masturbation is no more than an employment of natural resources for satisfaction as an insurance against frustration and consequent anger, hate, and fear. Compulsive masturbation simply implies that the underlying anxieties to be dealt with are excessive. Perhaps the infant needs feeding at shorter intervals, or he needs more mothering; or he needs to be able to know that someone is always near at hand, or his mother is so anxious that she ought to allow him more quiet lying in a pram, and less contact with her. It is logical to try to deal with the underlying anxiety when masturbation is a symptom, but illogical to try to stop the masturbation. It must be recognized, however, that in rare cases compulsive masturbation is continuous and is so exhausting that it has to be stopped by repressive measures, simply in order to give the child some relief from his or her own symptom. When relief is obtained in this way new difficulties must appear in the child's adolescence, but the need for immediate relief can be so great that troubles a few years ahead seem relatively unimportant.

When all goes well, masturbation accompanying sexual ideas happens without being much noticed, or is only recognized through a child's breathing changes, or because of a sweating head. Trouble follows, however, when there is a combination of compulsion to masturbate with inhibition of sex feeling. In this case the child becomes exhausted by his efforts to produce the satisfaction and climax that he cannot easily attain. To give up involves a loss of sense of reality, or loss of the sense of value. To persist, however, leads eventually to physical debility, and the notorious rings under the eyes which indicate conflict, and which are commonly ascribed wrongly to masturbation itself. Sometimes it is kind to help a child out of this impasse by paternal strictness.

Psychoanalytic study of children (as of adults) shows that the male genital is valued much more highly in the unconscious than would appear from direct observation, although of course many children do express their interest in the penis openly, if they are allowed. Little boys value their genitalia just as they value their toes and other parts of their bodies, but in so far as they experience sexual excitement they know the penis has special importance. Erection associated with love feelings determines castration fears. The penis excitement of a boy infant has its fantasy parallel, and a great deal depends upon the type of fantasy that goes with the early erections.

The onset of genital excitement is variable. Genital excitement may be almost absent in early infancy or, alternatively, erections may be almost constantly present from birth. Naturally, no good can come from artificial awakening of penis excitement. It seems likely that the dressings after circumcision frequently stimulate erections and cause an unnecessary association of erection with pain, this being one of several reasons why circumcision should almost never be performed (except on religious grounds). It is convenient when genital excitement is not a marked feature before the other parts of the body have become established as having an importance of their own, and certainly any artificial stimulation of the genitals of infants (either by post-operative procedure or by the desire of uneducated nannies to produce soothing sleep) is a complication; and the process of the child's emotional development is complex enough inherently.

To the little girl the visible and palpable boy's genitalia (scrotum included) are very liable to become an object of envy, but especially in respect of her attachment to her mother developing along identification-with-man lines. However, the matter is not as simple as this, and no doubt a large proportion of little girls are quite contented to have their own more hidden but just as important genitalia, and to allow boys their more vulnerable male appendages. In time a girl learns to evaluate the breasts. These become almost as important to her as the penis is to the boy, and when a girl knows she has the capacity, which a boy has not, to carry and produce as well as to feed babies, she knows she has nothing to envy. Nevertheless, she must envy the boy if she is driven by anxiety back from ordinary heterosexual development to what is called a fixation to her mother, or a mother-figure, with a consequent need to be like a man. Naturally, if a little girl is not allowed or does not allow herself to know she has an exciting and important part of her body in her genitalia, or is not allowed to refer to it, her tendency to penis envy is increased.

Clitoris excitement is closely associated with urinary erotism, which lends itself more to the kind of fantasy that goes with identification with the male. Through clitoris erotism the girl knows what it would feel like to be a boy with penis erotism. Similarly, a boy can experience in the skin of the perineum feelings that correspond to those that belong to the vulva of a girl.

This is quite separate from the anal erotism which is normally a feature in either sex, and provides, along with oral, urethral, muscle, and skin erotism, an early root of sex.

There is no lack of evidence in sociology and folk lore and in the myths and legends of primitive peoples of the paternal or ancestral penis, worshipped in symbolic form and exerting immense influence. In the modern home these things are as important as ever, although they are hidden; but their importance appears when a child's home breaks up, and he suddenly loses the symbols on which he had come to rely, so that he is at sea without a compass, and he is in distress.

A child is so much more than sex. In the same way your favourite flower is so much more than water; yet a botanist would fail in his job if in describing a plant he forgot to mention water, of which it is chiefly composed. In psychology fifty years ago there really was a danger that the sex part of child life might have been left out because of the taboo on childhood sexuality.

The sexual instinct gathers together in childhood, in a highly complex way, out of all its components, and exists as something that enriches and complicates the whole life of the healthy child. Many of the fears of childhood are associated with sexual ideas and excitements, and with the consequent conscious and unconscious mental conflicts. Difficulties of the sexual life of the child account for many psychosomatic disorders, especially those of recurring type.

The basis for adolescent and adult sexuality is laid down in childhood, and also the roots of all sexual perversions and difficulties.

The prevention of adult sexual disorders, as well as the prevention of all but the purely hereditary aspects of mental and psychosomatic illness, is in the province of those who care for infants and children.

6

Letter to the *British Medical Journal*

BATTLE NEUROSIS TREATED
WITH LEUCOTOMY

Originally published in *British Medical Journal*, 13 December 1947, 2(4536), 973.

SIR: I was glad to see the article by Drs William Sargant and C. M. Stewart (Nov. 29, p. 866) reporting a case of such battle neurosis treated by leucotomy. Sincere clinical reports, however inadequate they may be from the psychologist's viewpoint, are much needed. In the final comment it is said that the case is reported partly to encourage patients and relations to agree to this form of treatment when it is recommended. It must be agreed that in the matter of leucotomy the final decision must come from the good sense of the lay public, doctors being perhaps less able than other people are to see wider issues than the immediate relief of an individual's symptoms and distress.

There is still one doctor, however, who hopes that the public that clamours for whatever is on tap at the moment will stop short of asking to be leucotomized. He has lost hope that those who in their distress cry out even for a mutilating operation may be refused what they ask by the doctors themselves.—He is, etc.,

London. W.1.   D. W. WINNICOTT

PART 3

1948

PART V

BOOK

Reparation in Respect of Mother's Organized Defence Against Depression

Originally published in *Collected papers: Through paediatrics to psycho-analysis* (pp. 91–96). London: Tavistock, 1958.

Read before the British Psycho-Analytical Society, 7 January 1948. Revised August 1954.

The concept of the depressive position is generally accepted as a valuable one for use in actual analytic work as well as in the attempt to describe the progress of normal emotional development. In the analyses that we do we can reach the guilt in its relation to aggressive and destructive impulses and ideas, and we can watch the urge to make reparation appear as the patient becomes able to account for, tolerate, and hold the guilt feeling. There are other roots for creativeness, but reparation provides an important link between the creative impulse and the life the patient leads. The attainment of a capacity for making reparation in respect of personal guilt is one of the most important steps in the development of the healthy human being, and we now wonder how we did analytic work before we consciously made use of this simple truth.

Clinically however we meet with a false reparation which is not specifically related to the patient's own guilt, and it is to this that I wish to refer. This false reparation appears through the patient's identification with the mother and the dominating factor is not the patient's own guilt but the mother's organized defence against depression and unconscious guilt.

It may be that by expanding my title in this way I have said enough: certainly I do not feel that the idea is original or that it needs laborious development. Nevertheless, I shall attempt to illustrate my meaning briefly.

For 25 years a pageant of clinical material has been passing in front of me in my hospital Out-Patients Department. In the course of the years there is not much change in the general pattern. One type of child I remember well from the beginning. This child is particularly delightful and often talented above the average. If a girl, she is sure to be attractively dressed and clean. The point about her is a vivacity which immediately contributes something to one's mood, so that one feels lighter. One is not surprised to learn that she is a dancer or to find that she draws and paints and writes poetry. She may write a poem or two while waiting her turn to see me. When she draws me a picture I know there will be gay colours and interesting detail and the figures will have a certain sprightliness, seeming to be alive, moving. There may easily be a strong humorous element also.

The mother brings the child because at home she is irritable, moody, at times defiant, or frankly depressed. Perhaps many doctors have failed to believe that the child is anything but delightful. The mother tells me about various aches and pains of which the child complains and which at one time or another have been diagnosed by doctors as rheumatic, but which are really hypochondriacal.

Early in my career a little boy came to hospital by himself and said to me, 'Please, Doctor, mother complains of a pain in my stomach', and this drew my attention usefully to the part mother can play. Also it is a fact that the child who is supposed to have a pain has often not yet decided where the pain is. If one can catch him before his mother has indicated what she is expecting, one can find him bewildered and simply wanting to say that the pain is 'inside'. What is meant is that there is a feeling that something is wrong, or that there ought to be.

Probably I get a specially clear view of this problem in a children's out-patient department because such a department is really a *clinic for the management of hypochondria in mothers*. There is no sharp dividing line between the frank hypochondria of a depressed woman and a mother's genuine concern for her child. A mother must be able to be hypochondriacal if she is to be able to notice the symptoms in her child that the doctors are always asking for in their attempt to catch disease early. A doctor who knows nothing of psychiatry or knows nothing of the contra-depressive defences, and who does not know that children get depressed, is liable to tell a mother off when she worries about a child's symptom, and to fail to see the very real psychiatric problems that exist. On the other hand, a psycho-analyst fresh from newly discovered understanding of childhood depression could easily fail to notice when it is the mother who is more ill than the child. Watching many of these cases continuously over periods of ten or even twenty years I have been able to see that the depression of the child can be the mother's depression in reflection. The child uses the mother's depression as an escape from his or her own; this provides a false restitution and reparation in relation to the mother, and this hampers the development of a personal restitution capacity because the restitution does not relate to the child's own guilt sense. Of any series of promising students a proportion fail to reach the top because of the fact that reparation is being made in respect of the mother's depression rather than in respect of depression that is personal. When there seems to be special talent and even an initial success there remains an instability associated with dependence of the child on the mother. A homosexual overlay may or may not develop. Somewhere in a book on ballet, Arnold Haskell says: 'It should be remembered that every ballet dancer has a mother'. These children I am describing certainly have their mothers and their fathers. It is of course not always the mother. Many adolescent boys and girls seeming to have a capacity for successful work unexpectedly break down when their success in work is stolen by the needs of one or other parent or both. In the attempt of the adolescent to establish a personal identity the only solution then is through failure, and this especially applies to the case of the boy who is expected to follow exactly in his father's footsteps, and who yet never will be able to challenge the father's assumption of control.

It will be seen that these children in extreme cases have a task which can never be accomplished. Their task is first to deal with mother's mood. If they succeed in the immediate task, they do no more than succeed in creating an atmosphere in which they can *start on their own lives*. It can be readily understood that this situation can be exploited by the individual as a flight from that acceptance of personal responsibility which is an essential part of individual development. Where the child has the chance to dig down to personal guilt through analysis, then the mother's (or father's) mood is also there to be dealt with. The analyst must either recognize when the signs of this appear in the transference, or the analysis must fail, because of its success. I am describing a rather obvious phenomenon.

The usual observation is that the child's mother (or father) has a dominating personality. As analysts I think we shall want to say that the child lives within the circle of the parent's personality and that this circle has pathological features. In the typical case of the delightful girl I have described, the mother's need for help in respect of the deadness and blackness in her inner world finds a response in the child's liveliness and colour.

In a large number of these cases there is not an extreme of this condition, so that the child's reparation activities *can* be personal although there is a constant threat that the mother will steal the child's success and, therefore, the underlying guilt. In such cases it is not difficult to get astonishing clinical successes by actively displacing the parent in the early part of a psychotherapy of the child. In a favourable case it is possible to take the child's side against the parents and *at the same time* to gain and keep the parents' confidence.

> I was called in by a Teachers' Training College to see a student who was under threat of expulsion. She had suddenly kicked a fellow student on the ankle. I found a girl who had had a mother's depression to bear all her life, and who, at the end of her student career, had at last reached the problem—her own life

or mother's? I managed to get the mother to believe in me while I actually got in between her and her daughter. The latter was accepted back to the College, finished well, and set out on a series of jobs away from home. She has done very well and is now a senior teacher. This was a borderline case, and without my intervention she would have had to fail and break down, or else to have staged a false success, after giving up all hope of ever achieving an existence independent of her widow-mother's heavily organized mood.

One's most spectacular successes in professional work have been in this type of work. From this there is a lesson for the psycho-analyst who at the beginning of his career can easily be deceived into thinking that early success in a treatment is due to the interpretations, when really the important thing is that he has displaced a good but depressed parent. In spite of early success, the ordinary difficulties lie ahead, including the patient's discovery of his own guilt feeling. Initially the important thing is that the analyst is not depressed and the patient finds himself because the analyst is not needing the patient to be good or clean or compliant and is not even needing to be able to teach the patient anything. The patient can proceed at his own pace. He can fail if he wishes, and he is given time and a sort of local security. These external details of management are the prerequisites for the patient's discovery of his own love with the inevitable complication of aggression and guilt, that which alone makes sense of reparation and restitution. In the extreme case, the patient will come to analysis hardly having started on the task of coping with his own guilt, or not yet having reached his own aggression belonging to primitive love, and this in spite of the fact that the world has thought well of him.

Those who work with groups are much concerned with this relationship of the patient to an environmental mood. In some cases a useful comparison can be made between the group's mood, over which the patient has some control, and the mood of his mother when he was an infant, over which he had no control; as an infant he could only accept the fact of the mother's mood, and get caught in with the mother's contra-depressive defences. In other cases, the group mood cannot be entered into by the one member because of his having too strong a need to defend or fight for his own individuality.

The group can be a family. I would say that it is clearly of great value to family life when the depressive position has been reached securely enough on a personal basis by the individuals, so that the family mood is able also to have its place, being a common factor in the lives of the individual members. This is the same as any sharing of a culture. It is obviously pathological, or an impoverishment of the family or group, if an individual member cannot share in the reparation activities of a group. And, per contra, it is a serious impoverishment of the member's life if he can only take part in activities that are quite specifically group-activities. In the former case, when he cannot share, the individual must establish his own individual approach before sharing. In the latter case, where a group is necessary, he seems at first to be a useful co-operator, but eventually his co-operation breaks down; he remains to some degree in the position of the child caught up in mother's inner world, with consequent loss of personal responsibility.

It seems to me that there is a practical application of these ideas in the Psycho-Analytical Society. I refer particularly to the opinion expressed by Glover (1945, 1949). He feels that certain analysts (Melanie Klein and her pupils) are describing certain fantasies as if they were fantasies of their patients when probably these fantasies were those of the analysts themselves. Every analyst is aware of the task of disentangling his own fantasies from those of his patients, but it is generally reckoned that it is the psycho-analysts who are best able to be clear about this sort of thing. It is very difficult for me to believe that ideas that regularly appear in both my analytic and non-analytic work are subjective. Nevertheless I recognize that unless ideas can be subjective they cannot be objectively observed (cf. Whitehead, 1933: 'The material and conditions out of which the clinical investigator has to forge ordered knowledge are a constant challenge to his capacity for conceptual thinking as well as to his powers of observation'). It is important, however, to find out what prompts the remark, such as that of Glover, that the fantasies that we report are subjective, and not truly to be found in our patients. First, the question must be asked: has the analysis of the depressive position been put forward badly, in such a way that the ideas are unacceptable on account of the way they have been presented? (Cf. Brierley, 1951). For instance, has due recognition been given to the need for everything to be discovered afresh by every individual analyst? At any rate there must be kept clear the distinction between the value of ideas and the feeling about them roused by the way they have been presented.

Be this as it may, there remains a need to consider the problem along with the idea put forward in this paper.

It is legitimate to demand of me that if I claim to describe the fantasy of my patients, I know that patients at times do produce *the sort of things they feel I like getting*. This is the more true the more my expectations are unconscious. A patient, recently, was quite convinced that I liked anal material, and of course produced plenty for my benefit; it was some time before this came into the open, and before he reached his own true anal feeling. In the same way patients produce, and also hide, fantasy relating to the inner world because they feel a need to relieve my supposed depression, or to make it worse. In the transference a parental depression has been revived. I must be able to recognize this. When I claim to be truly objective about ideas that patients have about their insides, and about the contending of good and bad objects or forces within, I must be able to distinguish between that which is produced for me, and that which is truly personal to the patient. I believe that

Jungian analysts tend to receive 'Jungian type' dreams, and Freudians but seldom receive these elaborate mystical formations.

In this scientific group we have a common pool of theory, and we offer a group or setting for reparation activity in respect of a common pool of guilt. Each member becomes affected by the Society's mood, and is free to contribute to the group's restitution urge, which relates to the group's depressive anxieties. But always this restitution in the group must wait on the more important thing, that each individual shall reach to personal guilt, and to personal depressive anxieties. Each individual member of our Society must achieve his *own* growth at his *own* pace and develop his *own* sense of responsibility based truly on personal concern about his own love impulses and their consequences.

Summary

An individual's reparation urge may be related less to the personal guilt-sense than to the guilt-sense or depressed mood of a parent. The contribution of an individual to a group is affected by the relative success or failure of the individual in establishing personal rather than parental guilt as the root of reparation activities, and of constructive effort.

2

Paediatrics and Psychiatry

Originally published in *British Journal of Medical Psychology*, 1948, 21(4), 229–240. Also published in *Collected papers: Through paediatrics to psycho-analysis* (pp. 157–173). London: Tavistock, 1958.

Address from the Chair to the Medical Section of the British Psychological Society, 28 January 1948.

I have chosen the subject 'Paediatrics and Psychiatry' for my address because of the nature of my work. I am a paediatrician who has swung to psychiatry, and a psychiatrist who has clung to paediatrics. In an address from the Chair it is excusable, even usual, for the speaker to draw on experience that is peculiar to himself. My position, as I am a worker in two fields, ought to qualify me to communicate something that has interest for the children's doctor and also for the doctor whose work is concerned with the insane. It is, of course, inevitable that one who works in two subjects must sacrifice some degree of expertness in each.

The researches that more or less started with the pioneer work of Freud have established the fact that in the analysis of psychoneurosis the patient's childhood turns out to have harboured the intolerable conflicts which led to repression, and to the setting up of defences, and to the interruption in the emotional development of the individual, with formation of symptoms. Naturally, therefore, research became directed towards the emotional life of children. It was soon found that the reconstruction which adult patients gave of their childhood conflicts—conflicts associated with their instinctual ideas and experiences—could be seen in children, and seen clearly in the analytic treatment of children. It was not long before it began to be wondered whether the more psychotic illness of adults might not relate to the experiences of infants. Gradually a highly complex theory of the emotional development of the human being has been worked out, so that with all our terrible and at the same time exciting ignorance, we now have useful working hypotheses,

hypotheses, that is to say, that really work. There is now sufficient material available for attempts to be made to formulate things about infants which concern equally the psychiatrist and the children's physician, and I want to be one of those trying to say these things.

My thesis then is that the research worker in each of the two specialities has much to gain by meeting the research worker in the other. One assumption must be made; perhaps it will not be accepted. I assume a psychological basis for mental disorder. I assume that psychiatry can be studied in cases in which the health of the brain tissue is good. Naturally if a brain is diseased or physically disturbed, or cut about, mental changes must be expected. For myself I could learn but little from a study of the personality of an individual with a disordered brain, whereas there is so much that can be studied in the brain-intact individual—and so much remains to be understood about normal emotional development and its vagaries.

I hope it will not be thought that I am ignoring heredity or G.P.I. or senile dementia, injury, encephalitis, toxic delirium, or brain tumour, or even symptomatic improvement following the induction of fits.

Let me restate my idea, that it is possible to establish a clinical link between infant development and the psychiatric states, and likewise between infant care and the proper care of the mentally sick.

To do research one must have ideas, there is a subjective initiation of a line of inquiry. Objectivity comes later through planned work, and through comparison of the observations made from various angles. In justice to those who are doing research into this matter of the emotional development of the infant I will give a catalogue of the various methods of approach to any one detail that is being studied. The following types of approach provide observations that can be compared and correlated:

1. Through direct observation of the infant-mother relationship.

    An example of this is provided by Dr Middlemore's work (unfortunately cut short by her death) which is described in the book *The Nursing Couple*.
2. Direct periodical observation of an infant starting soon after birth and continuing over a period of years.

    In general practice and in a paediatric out-patient department of a hospital, parents attend when trouble arises or when they need advice.
3. Paediatric history-taking.

    In my own experience I have given a mother the opportunity of telling me what she knows of her infant's development in about 20,000 cases. There is always more to learn about history-taking, but with this sort of experience one becomes, I hope, more and more accurate in one's assessment of a mother's description.

4. Paediatric practice, typically the management of infant feeding and excretion.

    In the course of my paper I shall give an example of the psychological aspect of infant feeding problems. One could say that in the ordinary case where there is no disease process the work on the physical side has already been done by the physiologists and biochemists, and the practical problems are largely psychological.
5. Diagnostic interview with the child.

    In the first interview it is often possible, and not harmful, to do a sort of analytic treatment in miniature. If analysis is undertaken later it will regularly be found to take many months to cover the same amount of ground again. In these interviews the doctor is not so sure of his ground as he is in a long analysis, but, on the other hand, he gets a deep insight into a large number of cases, and this to some extent balances the restriction of numbers in his analytic experience. Incidentally, in psychiatry, a diagnostic interview is only fruitful if it is a therapeutic interview.
6. Actual psycho-analytic experience.

    This gives a different view of the patient's infancy according to whether the child is in the 2- to 4-year-old age group, or older, or near puberty, or in adolescence. For the analyst who is doing research on the earliest processes of emotional development, the analysis of fairly normal adults can be even more profitable than the analysis of children.
7. The observation in paediatric practice of psychotic regressions appearing as they commonly do in childhood and even in infancy.
8. Observation of children in homes adapted to cope with difficulties, whether these are antisocial behaviour, confusional states, maniacal episodes, relationships distorted by suspicion, or persecution, or mental defect, or fits.
9. The psycho-analysis of schizophrenics.

    This I am putting in a separate group because I think such analyses are for experienced analysts only. In my view the analysis of illness associated with depression and the defences against depression are now in the class of routine treatment and are not 'research cases'. This is also true of manic-depressive and even paranoid cases. Schizophrenics, however, are in a different class and their treatment is more of a pioneering venture.

At this point I have learned to expect a misunderstanding unless deliberate care is taken to avoid it. It has often been said to me: the idea that mad people are like babies, or small children, simply isn't true. Can I make it clear that I do not suggest that the insane are behaving like infants any more than that neurotics are just like older children. Ordinary healthy children are not neurotic (though they can be) and ordinary babies are not mad. The relationship between paediatrics and psychiatry is much more subtle than this.

The theory that I am putting forward is that in the emotional development of every infant complicated processes are involved, and that lack of forward movement or completeness of these processes predisposes to mental disorder or breakdown; the completion of these processes forms the basis of mental health.

The mental health of the human being is laid down in infancy by the mother, who provides an environment in which complex but essential processes in the infant's self can become completed. It would perhaps be a good initial study to describe the task of the ordinary good mother, in so far as we can see what is happening in this partnership. I will attempt this, but before doing so there is something that must be said about the *meaning* of the actual mother to the infant.

It is fully agreed that eventually the infant comes to feel himself as a whole person, and to hold his mother to be a whole person; soon after this stage is reached other people enter his life as people, but the complications that belong to this state of affairs need not be gone into here. There is not a general agreement as to the first age at which an infant feels mother to be a person, and so feels concerned as to the results of his real and imaginary attacks on her when under the sway of instinctual tension. This puzzle, fortunately, can be left unanswered, as at the moment we are considering a mother's care at the stage before the infant can feel concerned.

I think I see what Miss Anna Freud (1947, p. 200) is referring to when she states:

> This first 'Love' of the infant is selfish and material. Its life is governed by sensations of need and satisfaction, pleasure and discomfort. The mother, as an object, plays a part in this life so far as she brings satisfaction and removes discomfort. When the infant's needs are fulfilled, i.e. when it feels warm, comfortable, with pleasant gastric sensations, it withdraws interest from the object world and falls asleep. When it is hungry, cold and wet, or disturbed by intestinal sensations, it turns for help to the outside world. In this period the need for an object is inseparably bound up with the great body needs.
>
> From the fifth or sixth month onward the infant begins to pay attention to the mother also at times when it is not under the influence of bodily urges.

Dr Friedlander (1947, p. 23) wrote:

> ... during the first weeks and even months of life the relationship of the child to the mother is a rather simple one. The mother is the instrument

which satisfies the child's bodily needs. Anyone who fulfils this function will arouse the same response in the child....

However I think myself that by the seventh week or so a large proportion of infants show clearly that they have at times a contact with the woman who is their mother.

Let us attempt to study the mother's job. If the infant is to be able to start to develop into a being, and to start to find the world we know, to start to come together and to cohere, then the following things about a mother stand out as vitally important:

She exists, continues to exist, lives, smells, breathes, her heart beats. She is *there* to be sensed in all possible ways.

She loves in a physical way, provides contact, a body temperature, movement, and quiet according to the baby's needs.

She provides opportunity for the baby to make the transition between the quiet and the excited state, not suddenly coming at the child with a feed and demanding a response.

She provides suitable food at suitable times.

At first she lets the infant dominate, being willing (as the child is so nearly a part of herself) to hold herself in readiness to respond.

Gradually she introduces the external shared world, carefully grading this according to the child's needs which vary from day to day and hour to hour.

She protects the baby from coincidences and shocks (the door banging as the baby goes to the breast), trying to keep the physical and emotional situation simple enough for the infant to be able to understand, and yet rich enough according to the infant's growing capacity.

She provides continuity.

By believing in the infant as a human being in its own right she does not hurry his development and so enables him to catch hold of time, to get the feeling of an internal personal going along.

For the mother the child is a whole human being from the start, and this enables her to tolerate his lack of integration and his weak sense of living-in-the-body.

If I add that the mother continues to exist in spite of repeated attacks on her (made by the infant both in love and in anger), I am going too far ahead, reaching towards the functions of the mother relative to the infant who has instincts and the capacity to be concerned.

If we examine this admittedly incomplete description we can see that whereas some functions (such as the provision of suitable food) might be performed by anyone, much can only be done by someone who has a mother's interest; moreover, continuity cannot be well provided by a multiplicity of minders; and in any case there is the actual continuity of detail as observed by the infant, starting perhaps with the close-up of the nipple or of the face, and including the smell and the details of texture, and so on. Moreover, how can anyone who is not in the position of mother with a mother's love know the infant well enough to give well-graded enrichment, to give enough to foster growing capacity, yet not enough to engender confusion?

Here I think I come to the first statement of the paediatrician's clinical gain from psychiatric contact. If it be true or even possible that the mental health of every individual is founded by the mother in her living experience with her infant, doctors and nurses can make it their first duty not to interfere. Instead of trying to teach mothers how to do what in fact cannot be taught, paediatricians must come sooner or later to recognize a good mother when they see one and then make sure that she gets full opportunity to grow to her job; mistakes she may, and indeed will, make, but if by these she becomes able to do better in subsequent attempts there is in the end a gain.

Mothers cannot grow if they are frightened into doing as they are told. They must first find their feelings, and while doing so they need support— support against their own fears, their superstitions, their neighbours, and, of course, against physical accident and disease which can so largely be prevented or cured nowadays. I shall have more to say later about this support-without-interference, but if I were addressing a paediatric audience I could not too often mention the great danger to mental health that occurs when an infant is insulted by rude disruption of the delicate natural processes in the infant-mother partnership.

The environment is so vitally important at this early stage that one is driven to the unexpected conclusion that schizophrenia is a sort of environmental deficiency disease, since a perfect environment at the start can at least theoretically be expected to enable an infant to make the initial emotional or mental development which predisposes to further emotional development and so to mental health throughout life. An unfavourable environment later on is a different matter, being merely an additional adverse factor in the general aetiology of mental disorder.

Early Infancy

Now let me briefly indicate the task of the infant happily placed in the care of an ordinary good mother. It will be understood that the task which can be said to occupy the infant (at least from birth) is not ever a completed task, and the achievements of the first weeks and months must be many times lost and regained according to the turns of fortune.

It is not difficult to see that in the case of every infant at least these three things have to happen:

1. The infant has to make contact with reality.

2. The personality of the infant has to become integrated, and the integration has to gain stability.
3. The infant has to come to feel he lives in what we see so easily as the body of that infant, but which at first is not felt by the infant to be significant in the special way we know it is.

Three things: reality contact, integration, sense of body.

The psychiatrist will readily see in the nature of these tasks the reflection of symptoms that are his continual concern; loss of reality contact and of reality sense, disintegration and depersonalization.

In order to follow up one theme in some detail I must take only one of these three, leaving the others aside.

I have chosen to examine the matter of the establishment of reality contact, and even so I have to confine my attention to one example, the contact that arises out of that most primitive form of love, which is called greed, and which persists as cupboard-love. Equally significant is the reality contact in quiet periods between excitements, but I must not go too far from my subject.

As soon as an object relationship is possible it is immediately a matter of significance whether the object is outside or inside the child. I assume, however, that there is a stage prior to this at which there is no relationship at all. I would say that initially there is a condition which could be described at one and the same time as of *absolute independence* and *absolute dependence*. There is no feeling of dependence, and therefore that dependence must be absolute. Let us say that out of this state the infant is disturbed by instinct tension which is called hunger. I would say that the infant is ready to believe in something that could exist, i.e. there has developed in the infant a readiness to hallucinate an object; but that is rather a direction of expectancy than an object in itself. At this moment the mother comes along with her breast (I say breast for simplification of description), and places it so that the infant finds it. Here is another direction, this time towards instead of away from the infant. It is a tricky matter whether or no the mother and infant 'click'. At the start the mother allows the infant to dominate, and if she fails to do this the infant's subjective object will fail to have superimposed on it the objectively perceived breast. Ought we not to say that by fitting in with the infant's impulse the mother allows the baby the *illusion* that what is there is the thing created by the baby; as a result there is not only the physical experience of instinctual satisfaction, but also an emotional union, and the beginning of a belief in reality as something about which one can have illusions. Gradually, through the living experience of a relationship between the mother and the baby, the baby uses perceived detail in the creation of the object expected. In the course of breast feeding a mother may repeat this performance a thousand times. She may so successfully give her child the capacity for illusion that she has no difficulty in her next task, gradual disillusioning, this being the word for weaning in the primitive setting which is my interest in this paper.

It worries some people that there is no such thing in psychology as direct union, only an illusion of relationship; but I suppose psychiatrists are so used to patients' descriptions of loss of contact with reality that they will not be among those to object. Most of us are so good at using the objectively observed and expected that we manage without hallucinations, unless we are tired or weak from physical exhaustion. For the infant this clever use of shared reality which is another aspect of objectivity is by no means established, and everything depends on the mother at the beginning.

The mother does her job in this respect by simply being devoted, that is, provided she is allowed by doctors and nurses and helpful people generally to act as she loves to do.

This is where the paediatrician comes in—in clearing the way for the mother's native feeling towards her child. In accepting the psycho-analyst's help the paediatrician, incidentally, extends the usefulness of the analyst to a circle wider than that of his analytic practice. Doctors have made it very difficult for mothers to start off well in this function, one of the most important they have to perform. It is often very difficult for a woman, when preparing to have a baby, to be sure that she will be allowed to come to terms with her infant after birth in her own way, which is the infant's way. Let me quickly turn to an exception. Professor Spence[1] of Newcastle insists that each healthy baby in the maternity homes he supervises shall be in a cradle at the side of the mother. The mother has the skilled attention she so greatly needs, and she enjoys the confidence that is inspired by first-rate medical and nursing practice. At the same time she is expected to be the best judge of the feeding technique needed by her infant. There are no rules about regular feeding, and 'the nursing couples' (to use the late Dr Middlemore's term) usually find a convenient feeding rhythm sooner or later. Contrast this with the worst case, not difficult to find, of a maternity home in which the babies are kept in cots in a separate ward, even when healthy. At feed times they are wheeled in on a trolley, tightly wound round by a shawl, and at the right moment the nurse clocks in by thrusting the screaming infant's mouth at the breast of the bewildered, frustrated, often frightened mother.

This only refers to the initial stages of the feeding experience, and it will readily be seen that these ideas can be applied at all later stages. Nevertheless, if the beginning is bad the continuation is necessarily made more difficult. Moreover, clinically, serious feeding disturbances may start at the initial stage.

The paediatrician, taking careful histories of small children, cannot but be struck by the commonness of fairly or very severe feeding inhibitions.[2] He finds that there are certain critical moments that can be enumerated. (I had a severe case in a three-year-old in analysis, a little girl whose feeding inhibitions had started at twelve months on a definite day when she was sat up at table to eat with her father and mother, that is to say, all three together.) A common time for loss of zest for food would be the near arrival of a new baby. In many cases the loss of zest for food starts in infancy. There is the inhibition in respect of self-feeding, or there is a change from eagerness to refusal of food at the time of weaning from breast or bottle or from a special person, or at the introduction of solids, and even at the thickening of feeds. The arrival of teeth may be accompanied by refusal of feeds. Even in very young infants one finds the refusal of anything new, and sometimes, conversely, an interest only in the new.

Some of the inhibitions, however, start from the beginning. The infant and the mother just never 'click'. At this point the mother can be held theoretically responsible, though of course not to blame.

Ordinarily if breast feeding is difficult the baby is put on to a bottle, and there are all sorts of ways out of the difficulty when the breast milk does not come or suit. In a case of difficulty, to insist on the breast when a mother could easily feed her baby well by bottle is a mistake.

In these matters the infant's doctor is at a loss if he does not understand what is going on behind the scenes in the emotional development of the infant; and he needs, too, to know something about the psychology of nursing mothers.

It is relevant here to describe a common problem of infant feeding, as I see it. I mean as I see it *now*, for I have struggled through the phases all doctors experience, in the heartbreaking attempt to deal with feeding problems along physical lines, altering quantities, intervals, proportions of fat, protein, and carbohydrate and switching from one brand of milk to another. Well do I remember the day when I made it a rule to get a feeding going well *before* altering the brand of milk. It took me years to realize that a feeding difficulty could often be cured by advising the mother to fit in with the baby absolutely for a few days. I had to discover that this fitting in with the infant's needs is so pleasurable to the mother that she cannot do it without moral support. If I advise this I must ask my social worker to visit daily, else the mother will wilt under criticism and feel responsible for too much. Obeying a rule, she can blame others if things go wrong, but she is scared to do as she deeply wants to do. On the other hand, if all goes well she never forgets the fact that she had it in her to do the right thing for her baby, without help.

These are not clever things. They simply require an appreciation of what it is that the mother and the baby are doing together. With the human infant it is never adequate to think in terms of conditional reflexes.

I want to make it clear that I am describing the paediatrician's task in the management of infant feeding, suggesting that he works blindly unless he knows what is going on behind the scenes. There the processes of emotional development are dominant, and they are of a nature that can be found in a 'state of undoing' in schizophrenic illness.

It is here that something can be said about play. The first play at the breast is of great value in that it enables the baby to find the mother and to communicate with her so that she can be prepared to act in the right way. Without the chance of play, the baby and the mother remain strangers to each other. How important are the hands in this. At twelve weeks, an infant will sometimes feed his mother while at the breast, putting his finger in her mouth.

W. H. Davies in his poem 'Infancy' said:

> Born to the world with my hands clenched,
> I wept and shut my eyes;
> Into my mouth a breast was forced,
> To stop my bitter cries.
> I did not know—nor cared to know—
> A woman from a man;
> Until I saw a sudden light,
> And all my joys began.
>
> From that great hour my hands went forth,
> And I began to prove
> That many a thing my two eyes saw
> My hands had power to move:
> My fingers now began to work,
> And all my toes likewise;
> And reaching out with fingers stretched,
> I laughed, with open eyes.

Psychiatry and Infant Care

It is time I linked this with something of interest to the psychiatrist.

In the psycho-analysis of a woman (who had done well in life but who came for treatment because of an increasing dissatisfaction, and a growing feeling that nothing meant anything to her) the following happened. There was an hour in which the important thing was that I kept absolutely still and quiet and said nothing at all. The next hour the same was happening, but after a length of time I reached for a cigarette. The result of the tiny movement I made was nearly disastrous, and the situation was only saved by my patient's being able to see what was afoot. From what had gone before we both knew that she was right back in the infant-mother relationship. In the quiet my patient had been lying on her mother's lap. Just when I made the movement the patient was (in her mind) starting to reach up with her hand, and in doing so she would have found the breast, and in the course of time the mother would have responded, and the feed would have started. The two would have come to terms. It was for this very experience that this patient was unconsciously looking. As I moved, however, I broke the spell and suddenly became the nannie. (Historically she had had the breast for a period of one month and had then been handed over to a nannie and fed by bottle.) Now this meant a disruption of natural progress. The nannie, although in many ways a better mother than the real mother, because not depressed, nevertheless at the moment for a feed had to get up and fetch or even prepare the bottle, and by the time all was ready the infant had lost much of the ability to 'create' the bottle or the milk; it had become a thing coming at her, with which she had to try to come to terms.

This sort of case material leads me on to the description of other analytic studies. It is very difficult to convey to those (either paediatricians or psychiatrists) who are not doing psycho-analysis the feeling of conviction that one digs down to solid rock, by which I mean that one sees real things re-lived in this work. However, each one of us can only get a certain number of types of experience, and therefore each must inevitably rely on learning from the work of colleagues.

I have long struggled with a case which illustrates my point in that, to help this patient at all, I have had to be ready waiting when she comes. This woman is one of twins, and the different treatment afforded her as compared with her twin sister by her mother has always been a source of grievance with her. Her twin being the weak one was taken over by the mother and fed and cared for by her, and taken into the mother's bed, while my patient, being strong and large, was handed over to a nurse. This was the conscious reconstruction. Only gradually has the true early infantile situation come out in the transference. This patient comes to me from a mental hospital. She has a fairly severe degree of splitting of personality, and for the first two decades (apart from her infancy) she made an exceptionally good adjustment on a compliance basis. Then she broke down, and started on her long search for a chance to find her own self, and a relation to the world that she could feel to be real. Needless to say, she did not know what she was looking for, and at one stage, in despair, she developed rheumatoid arthritis with the unconscious aim of becoming bed-ridden and helpless, so getting her family to comply with her. Or, shall I say, she used her arthritis in that way.

Hope of getting what she needed from analysis brought with it the absolute need that I have mentioned for me to be ready for her. At one time I had to be at the front door myself, actually opening the door as the bell rang. It can be well imagined that there was an infinity of play round this detail of management. Sometimes she would telephone me on the way, otherwise not believing I existed at all. The reason why I had to take the trouble to do all this, which was very trying, was that otherwise it was no use seeing her at all; she would come, and talk and go, but would get no feeling of our having met. On the other hand, a long spell of my giving her direct access always brought its reward. In six years a great deal has happened but the basis of it all has been the provision of direct access. She is having an essential experience for the first time, although it belongs to infancy, and this fact comes out quite clearly in the detailed material that I have not time to reproduce here. In this case there is a strong regression element, the main trauma being related to early childhood rather than to infancy, namely a long period of rigid management by an almost insane nurse.

In case it should be thought that the analyst puts these ideas into the patient's head I would give a detail out of the treatment of a boy who was an apparent mental defective, but who was really a case of childhood schizophrenia, with regression to a powerfully controlled introversion. When the boy came to me at the age of five years he spent his time over a period of two or three months simply coming towards me and going away again, testing my ability to give direct access and egress.

Gradually this boy let himself sit on my lap, and go on to make affectionate contact. In the next phase he would get right inside my coat, and out of this developed a game of sliding out on to the floor head first from between my legs. During all this period I made very few verbal interpretations. In the next phase he had so strong a need for honey—it was wartime, and honey scarce— that he strained all resources until mercifully he became able to accept malt and oil instead, of which he ate voraciously. He now covered everything with saliva and became destructive with the honey-spoon. His saliva would form a pool on the doorstep if he was kept waiting. Out of all this there came a slow but steady development which had previously ceased and had become negative.

In this experience I seemed to see a child re-living early infantile experience and out of some need in himself correcting the faulty introduction to the world, being born again. I saw one environment supplanting another. After this, analysis by verbal interpretation became not only possible but acutely necessary. But in the phase I have described my job was to provide a certain type of environment, thereby allowing the boy to do the work.

There is a direct application of all this to the care of adolescents. Here is a typical adolescent case. A boy of sixteen at a public school tells his school doctor that he insists on seeing a psychiatrist. In the end he gets his own way and his parents bring him to me. I take a detailed history from the parents, and in the interview with the boy I find him depressed, and flabby. In about an hour I get nothing from him, and I do not make any effort to bring him out. As I find later, the important thing in that interview was the lack of any urge on my part to get him to respond. On parting I let him know that I was expecting to see him again sometime.

The next I hear is through the telephone. He rings me up from school and asks if I can see him tomorrow, a Saturday. I know that I must do this, as the gesture has come from him, and I put aside everything to fit in with him. On the phone I immediately say yes, before I have decided how to manage it.

These conditions bring a very different boy to my room. He makes very considerable use of me, and in an hour or two he has done an analysis in miniature. Considerable results follow this, more I think than would have been reached in weeks of a set analysis at this stage. In the next holidays I find the boy has left school on his own initiative, decided on a career, made arrangements to attend a university, and to live in London where he can have analysis over a proper period, whether from me or a colleague. I think that this is the right way for such an analysis to start, and that many treatments of schizoid types of adolescent fail because they are planned on a basis that ignores the child's ability to 'think up'—in a way, to *create*—an analyst, a role into which the real analyst can try to fit himself.

If this is true it follows that set techniques for interview defeat their aim, which, presumably, is to make a diagnosis and to initiate a therapeutic procedure. The set technique wastes the patient's ability to make one sort of contact, and with a case of schizoid type this waste of opportunity may act as a negative therapy, and may do harm.

In the analysis of a schizophrenic adolescent girl I had to adopt a procedure over a long period of time by which I saw her or dealt with analytic material over the telephone just exactly when she rang. Claustrophobia was activated if any sort of definite arrangement was made. With this proviso good analytic work was done. Eventually a regular time was achieved. If, however, I had forced a regular arrangement too early this patient would have been unable to have made a contact with me that meant anything to her. Over a long period we talked chiefly of infant management and infant feeding; as a matter of fact before coming to me this girl had been giving infants in her care just the management that she needed from me and that she failed to get from her mother. The mother had been excellent except for a tremendous need to get reassurance from her feeding activities. 'None of my children ever refused anything I offered them', she would say, and as she was a trained dietician they all waxed fat, especially my patient. But till she came to me this girl scarcely knew what it was to make contact with reality from her end.

I now wish to describe what I can see of the theoretical basis of all this. In the favourable case the expectation of the infant meets impinging reality, and at this point I would place the word 'Illusion'. In case this is not understood by someone the following story may help.

Recently, during a hot spell, an analyst had to do an extra analytic session in the lunch hour. He was tired and perhaps a little sleepy, and he had the following experience at the same time as being an ordinary competent analyst.

He could see out of his window, and on a roof some distance away he saw a man. This man was about 45 years old, and had a rather bald head. He had finished his sandwiches and had let his mid-day paper with its racing tips fall. Obviously he had allowed himself to drop off to sleep.

Dimly aware of all this the analyst would never have registered anything had it not been that there was a sequel. We all know the way in which a continuous noise may be unnoticed until it stops. Well, in this case the disturbing thing was that the man made no movement at all. After half an hour the analyst definitely registered the fact that the man ought to have woken up, and then suddenly: pop! the man's head swelled to the size of the rather large stone spherical ornament that it had been all the time. The sight of the man going to sleep was no more than an indication that my friend wanted to go to sleep himself. He had failed to confine his hallucinations to situations that could absorb them.

To return, in the favourable case impulse or expectation of the infant meets impinging reality.

What are the consequences of failure in the introduction of the shared world to the infant?[3] In the extreme of failure these two lines in a diagram would be parallel. The infant creates out of his native poverty, and the world impinges in vain. The lines never meet. In such a hypothetical case there must be mental defect even if there is normal brain capacity. Commonly there is some degree of this splitting at the earliest level, and the basis is thereby laid for the infant to have a relationship unshared by us with a self-created world, in which magic holds sway, and alongside this a compliance with mundane management from outside, convenient because life-giving, but unsatisfactory in the extreme to the infant. Later on in childhood or adult life the compliance breaks down, if it is too isolated from the other trend which contains all the child's spontaneity. These parallel paths regularly appear in our analytic work, illustrated at the simplest by the patient who said that his analytic sessions were in duplicate, a rather dull one actually with the analyst, and the operative one afterwards in relation to an imagined analyst.

Paediatrician and Psychiatrist

The main point about this is that in investigating the phenomena of human contact and communication, the paediatrician and the psychiatrist badly need each other's help. For instance very few psychiatrists can take a reliable history from a mother about early feeding details. Yet no history of a psychotic case is complete unless the last ounce of detail of the early nursing couple experience has been obtained, if it is available to skilled inquiry. Also, the paediatrician needs the psychiatrist. On his own he will fail to recognize the psychiatrically-ill infant, for such an infant may be in bursting physical health, never defiant or difficult, indeed most delightfully acquiescent. The ill baby may in fact be especially all the time good, 'we never knew we had him, doctor', able to be left on the arm of the chair with no danger of wriggling off, and so on. Healthy babies cry, do not by any means always take willingly, they have wills of their own, they are in fact a trouble. To their own mothers healthy babies are of course more rewarding than ill babies ever can be, because along with their nuisance value they also show spontaneous love feelings, so much more encouraging than the negative virtues.

In the matter of practical management I feel that those who care for infants (I mean mothers and nursery nurses) can teach something to those who manage the schizoid regressions and confusion states of people of any age. The provision of a stable though personal environment, warmth, protection from the unexpected and unpredictable, and the serving of food in a reliable way and accurately on time (or even following the whims of the patient), these things might help the nursing of schizoid cases.

The important thing for the psychiatrist, at the moment, however, is not practice but theory. I am saying that the proper place to study schizophrenia and manic depression and melancholia is the nursery, and if this be true then some modern trends in psychiatry are like barking up the wrong tree.

It may be asked, what do ordinary people do about this matter of contact with reality? Of course as development proceeds a great deal happens that seems to get round the difficulty, for enrichment by incorporation of objects is a psychical as well as a physical phenomenon, and the same can be said of being incorporated, including the eventual contribution to the world's fertility which is the privilege of even the least of us. And especially the sexual life offers a way round, with the conception of infants, a true physical mingling of two individuals. Nevertheless, while we have life, each one of us feels the matter of crude reality-contact to be a vital one, and we deal with it according to the way in which we have had reality introduced to us at the beginning. In some of us the ability to use the objectively verifiable, to objectify the subjective, is so easy that the fundamental problem of illusion tends to get lost. Unless they are ill or tired people do not know that there is a problem of relationship with reality, or a universal liability to hallucination, and they feel that mad people must be made of different stuff from themselves. Some of us, on the other hand, are aware of a tendency in ourselves towards the subjective, which we feel to be more significant than the world's affairs, and for such the sane may seem rather dull folk, and the common round seems mundane.

One of the ways out is the dreaming of dreams, and the remembering of them. In sleep we dream all the time and when we wake we need to carry something forward from the dream world into real life, just as we need to recognize everyday affairs turning up and weaving themselves into the dreams. Apart from this, is it not largely through artistic creation and artistic experience that we maintain the necessary bridges between the subjective and the objective? It is for this reason, I suggest, that we value tremendously the lone struggle of the creator in any art form. For us all, as for himself, the artist is repeatedly winning brilliant battles in a war to which, however, there is no final outcome. A final outcome would be finding what is not true, namely, that what the world offers is identical with what the individual creates.

I will end with an illustration which broadens the subject a little. A man dreamed he was driving a car up the curve of a hill when he saw a larger car coming at him down the curve of the hill, at speed. It was a flash dream. He swerved to the left, but he knew that if he had not wakened there would have been a terrific crash. It was a satisfactory dream, and he woke to the memory of banging his head on a pillar when walking with his mother as a little boy. This was an easy memory, an incident, never forgotten. Suddenly it occurred to him that the memory was a false one. He had been walking with his mother and it was *another* boy walking with his mother who had absent-mindedly crashed into the post and had badly hurt his head, producing a copious flow of blood.

The fact was that, because of analysis in respect of reality-contact, he had become able to understand that he envied the boy who crashed into the post. I mean, this crash seemed ever so real to him at the time it occurred, contrasting with his own growing and distressing inhibition and lack of reality-sense in his contact with his mother, secondary to the repression of his Oedipus wishes.

From this step forward in his analysis he got a new feeling about children's love of the awful phenomena of gangster films, and of crashing Spitfires and bombers, and the like.[4] I, too, realized more clearly than previously that in trying to unravel all the complex psychology of childhood behaviour it would be unwise to neglect the threat of feelings of unreality and loss of contact. I need hardly add to an audience of psychiatrists that the same applies to the study of adults.

It is those who feel that external reality lacks meaning whenever routine holds sway who need the refreshment of music or painting absolutely. Someone I know who is recovering from a long phase of loss of contact found the colour in van Gogh's pictures *painfully* real. The colour came at her as the car did in the man's dream. The colour was too much for her in a physical sense, and she had to go away and come back another day to complete the visit to the picture gallery.

In the management of children comparable happenings can be observed. Unreality feelings show as a craving for the new. This turns up in early feeding management, in the problem of the baby who is put on one food after another, and who does well for a few days on each, and then loses interest. But the new can also hurt. It would be wise to keep in mind that for the infant the new, whether in taste, texture, sight, or sound, can come at the infant as the colour did to my friend, and physically hurt. An ordinary good mother is sparing with new things, and yet provides them according to the infant's ability to come to terms with them. In psychiatric practice, as I have already suggested, there could perhaps be room for the attempt to coax back a withdrawn person by the provision of an extremely simplified bit of the world, a world into which the patient could gradually come back without suffering painful impressions. In the analysis of borderline cases some such provision is made in the limited setting of the analytic session, and such provision is a prerequisite for the work based on the verbal interpretation.

Summary

I have tried to focus attention on one process, that of the individual's contact with shared reality, and the development of this from the start of the infant's life. I have hoped to encourage a co-operation between the children's doctor and the psychiatrist in arriving at descriptive terms that have clinical meaning to each. I have made an attempt to do this in an examination of the normal establishment of reality-contact.

It was difficult to cast aside psychosomatic disorders, to turn a deaf ear to the common anxiety states, and a blind eye to depression, hypochondria, and persecution delusions. All these disorders affect the day-by-day work of the paediatrician. It was difficult to steer my course away from the pathological psychotic regressions and psychotic distortions which are much commoner in childhood than is generally supposed. Also it was difficult to choose the one process, and to ignore those of integration and body sense. However, as it is, I have had more to convey than can easily be listened to at one sitting, and I console myself that it is better to convey the idea that a thing is complex, if it is so, than to give a false impression of simplicity.

These things have been argued about by philosophers and psychologists, and psychopathologists of all schools have made their own attempts to state what they feel they see. Here is my statement, forged out of clinical work and a psycho-analytic training.

Notes

1. Later Professor Sir James Spence.
2. See 'Appetite and Emotional Disorder'.
3. For a clearer description see 'Primitive Emotional Development' [CW 2:7:8], 'Reality Adaptation'.
4. Today I would add horror comics (1957).

3

Letter to the *British Medical Journal*
'PATHIES IN A STATE SERVICE

Originally published in *British Medical Journal*, 14 February 1948, 1(4545), 313–314.

Sir: In a letter dated Aug. 21, 1943 (p. 243), I tried to draw attention to the danger that a whole-time State medical service could be forced by Parliament to accept osteopathy, homoeopathy, and other practices not accepted by the profession on scientific grounds. I have seen no satisfactory reply to this, which is a good example of the way in which loss of the non-State half of the medical profession would weaken it as a whole. Perhaps a majority of members of Parliament have direct or indirect evidence of the symptom-removing power of the magician where medical science has failed. We can hardly blame the layman for thinking that removal of symptoms is the whole thing and acting on his beliefs. Is it not the profession alone that should be in a position to decide what its ranks include and exclude? The profession must actively support the right of the unqualified practitioner to practise, on his own responsibility, at the same time absolutely protecting itself from the possibility of having its beliefs warped by political pressure. Letters to the Press have substantiated my belief that this threat is not to be lightly dismissed—witness *The Times* of Jan. 31:

> Another point which concerns me closely is the position of homoeopathy. Over a million people in this country prefer to be treated by homoeopathic practitioners, and this has so far been largely denied them by the medical profession which is hostile to this method. Will a National Health Service take steps to secure for this very large number of people the qualification and training of enough doctors to satisfy their needs? (From J. R. Sandy, Romford.)

Perhaps there is an official B.M.A. attitude to this matter.—I am, etc.,

London. W.1.   D. W. Winnicott

4

The Gwrw Tree

Dated 1 July 1948.

Once upon a time there was a tree, and it was called a Gwrw tree because it grew and grew, and in fact did practically nothing else. But who called it a Gwrw tree? Who was there about the place who would give a tree such a name. Ah, you have a cwlw? Yes, the man or woman who called that tree a Gwrw was not a Welsh man or woman, but he was an English man (or she was an English woman) who knew just enough about the Welsh language to use a 'w' to write 'oo', as in cwm for coombe. So here we have a tree and—well I'll tell you it was a man, and that'll save a lot of saying: 'man or woman as the case may be'. Because I know it's a man I'm talking about. How shouldn't I, especially as I'm the one that's making up the story?

I can't think what's going to happen, can you?

Well here was the Gwrw tree, growing and growing, and the man just getting more and more mazed. That's not amazed you know. Mazed means sort of dazed. You see, the tree had nothing else to do except grow, and so it went on and on getting taller and thicker, and the man soon wondered if he'd dislocate his neck watching it. Not that it grew fast. You know, trees don't. They grow ever so slowly, so slowly that you can't notice them changing till you suddenly notice they've changed. Like midday changing into teatime, which you wouldn't know except for the first wind on a hot still day. And the Venetian blinds flap against the window frames. And then there are strawberries and cream, or perhaps raspberries, on the lawn. Only there's no cream any more, more's the pity.

Well while I was saying all that a lot of time passed, and in about that time the tree had grown quite a lot, and the Englishman who knew just enough about Welsh to be able to use it wrong, fairly sweated. He wiped his brow, and breathed hard. What will that Gwrw tree do next? he murmured to himself, not expecting an answer; and in any case he knew, for the only thing the tree could do was to go on growing.

Now there's something awful about things that don't start and after a time finish. It's so natural when there's a jolly good working up to something and then everyone knows it's goodbye, see you again next time. Take a football match, or a piece of music or a film. But when a thing just goes on and on and . . . well the man felt quite upset about it, and he thought to himself, I must end this thing. If it won't end what it's doing of itself, I shall myself do it in in the end.

But he felt sad nevertheless, because somehow the Gwrw tree had almost become part of himself. Without it growing there in front of him he would feel personally hurt and humbled.

It was a long time that he watched the Gwrw tree as it grew and grew, perhaps hours, perhaps days, months or years. But in the end the whole thing got the better of him and he acted. Besides, he began to feel so small with the tree so big.

What would you do if you were worried to death by a Gwrw tree? Perhaps you'd do just as this man did.

He took a hose pipe and fixed one end of it to the garden tap, and then he pointed it at the tree, and then he turned on the tap. Now that was a terrible thing to do, a proper insult to a tree which likes a nice even dampness in the subsoil, or rain from heaven, but not a squirting up from below by some inferior human. Inferior, from the tree's point of view, I mean.

You may be sure that ended the Gwrw tree's little game of just going on growing. As the water reached the tree the very opposite started to happen, opposite to what had been all the time happening. The tree began to ungrow, and to dwindle and to diminish, and all the time just as slowly and deliberately and secretly as it formerly grew. All of which was very annoying to the man, who had longed somehow to produce some sort of relief.

Now the man had a new fear—the tree would dwindle and diminish to nothing. Then he would never be able to tell whether there really had been a Gwrw tree or whether he had just dreamed it. So he got into a panic, a veritable stew he got into, all worked up, and on edge! Edge, yes that word made him think of a hatchet, and of Jack and the bean-stalk, and other people who had cut off the heads of giants, criminals and snakes.

There he was, standing, red in the face, puffing and panting, holding the hatchet in the ready position over his right shoulder, waiting to stop the complete bedwindlement of the tree by cutting it down. You see there was an exact moment. Before this the tree was too big to be cut at all, let alone by one bold stroke, and as the bedwindlement was developing speed as it got nearer to its end, there would be precious little time after the exact moment, between it and there being nothing there at all to hack at. And then what would the man have to show people when they asked what had he been doing there all afternoon, with a hatchet too? It might be thought he had wanted to kill a man, and he might have been convicted in the High Court and himself beheaded.

You can be sure, that with all these thoughts in his head he wasn't going to easily miss his chance, and so miss his head and the thoughts in it, so he brought down his hatchet at exactly the right moment and cut the stem of the tree, and there lay the tree in two parts, and there was no more of growth or of bedwindlement.

And when some Welsh people came by the Englishman, who knew just enough Welsh to make an ass of himself with it, said nôs da, pronouncing it to rhyme with 'cross papa', which is wrong. He said nothing about the tree being a Gwrw tree because it no longer grew and grew, and the really Welsh people who were passing would have taken a poor view of all that. Englishmen should keep their little jokes to themselves.

5

Letter to Anna Freud

Originally published in Rodman, F. R. (Ed.), *The spontaneous gesture. Selected letters of D. W. Winnicott* (Letter 8, pp. 10–12). Cambridge, MA: Harvard University Press, 1987.

Anna Freud (1895–1982), the daughter of Sigmund Freud, was one of the founders of child psychoanalysis. After moving to London in 1938, she founded the Hampstead War Nurseries as well as the Hampstead Child Therapy Course and Clinic (now the Anna Freud Centre). She was also a co-editor of *The Psychoanalytic Study of the Child*.

6 July 1948

Dear Miss Freud:

One cannot help thinking about this horrible Mental Health Conference, and your task.[i] As one who was perhaps chiefly responsible for this programme of the Child Section, I feel concerned that one of the aims shall be fulfilled, namely that the work done specifically in Great Britain in the last 25 years, be put forward by whoever is representing Great Britain. For in my opinion, in the natural development of psycho-analysis, it has fallen to the lot of psycho-analysts in this country to bring the aggressive impulses and ideas into their proper place in psycho-analytic theory and practice. Particularly important

---

[i] The International Congress on Mental Health was held at the Central Hall, Westminster, London, 11–21 August 1948. The Congress was organised by the National Association for Mental Health and consisted of three separate International Conferences, on Child Psychiatry, Medical Psychotherapy, and Mental Hygiene. Some 2,000 delegates registered for the Congress from nearly 50 different countries; about 900 delegates came from abroad.

Anna Freud delivered the keynote paper in the Child Psychiatry Section, which Winnicott had helped to organise: 'Aggression in Relation to Emotional Development: Normal and Pathological'. Papers were also given by Wilfred Bion, Margaret Mead, Franz Alexander, John Rickman, and J. C. Flügel. In the end Winnicott did not present a paper.

has been the study of the relation of aggression, guilt and depression, and reparation to each other.

I am rather surprised to find that I owe you a letter on this subject. When I sent you my paper on Aggression (R.S.M.[ii]) you wrote and asked me for a summary.[iii] It is really awfully difficult to give a summary of so condensed a paper. Either the general tendency and the work it is based on is known and understood, or else (I should say) no summary is of the slightest use. Nevertheless I would say the following:—

(a) In this Congress the important thing to get across is that the world's troubles are not due to man's aggression, but are due to repressed aggression in individual man.

(b) Following this, the remedy is not education of children in ways of managing and controlling their aggression, but is to provide for the maximum number of infants and children such steady and reliable conditions (of emotional environment) that they, each one of them, may come to know and to tolerate as part of themselves the whole of their aggression (primitive greedy love, destructiveness, capacity for hate, etc).

(c) To enable human beings (infants, children or adults) to tolerate and accept their own aggression, respect for guilt and depression is needed, and full recognition of reparative tendencies when they exist.

(d) It is also important to state clearly that in this matter of aggression and its origins in human development there is a great deal that is not yet known.

These themes are developed in my paper.

You will understand that I for one am vitally interested in what you are intending to read in August, and it would give a great relief if you could let those of us who care a lot see what you have prepared in good time, so that discussion of it will be possible.

With good wishes,
Yours very sincerely,
D. W. Winnicott

[ii] Royal Society of Medicine.

[iii] Anna Freud's keynote paper for the Mental Health Congress was first given to a meeting of the Royal Society of Medicine, Section of Psychiatry, London, 9 December 1947. Winnicott had also written a contribution to this meeting, and it is probable that this is a version of what he had sent to Anna Freud. The alterations between Winnicott's contribution to the Royal Society of Medicine symposium in 1947 and the paper he published in 1958 ('Aggression in Relation to Emotional Development' [CW 3:5:2]) can be found in the editorial annotations to that paper.

6

Review: *The Psychology of the Unwanted Child*
BY AGATHA H. BOWLEY, FOREWORD BY S. CLEMENT BROWN (EDINBURGH: E. AND S. LIVINGSTONE, 1947)

Review originally published in *British Medical Journal*, 10 July, 1948, 2(4566), 78.

There is general agreement in the books appearing in the wake of the Curtis Report that a substitute home must supply 'affection and personal interest... stability... opportunity... and a share in the common life of a small group in a homely environment'. The difference between the books lies in the method and the clarity of presentation. The author of this book uses simple, clear, and in the main non-technical language, when jargon appears it often spoils by being inaccurate. For instance, in a helpful last chapter there appears the following comment on swearing and the use of vulgar language: 'It is a form of *oral* aggression, just as soiling was a form of *anal* aggression'. Surely such information is of no use whatever for ordinary people, and for the psychologist there is no reason why swearing should be oral rather than anal. If theory must be introduced, then the concept of the unconscious must come in with it, and much more should be made of the relation of fantasy to the unconscious instinctual life.

In Miss Bowley's practical work as a psychologist she has made considerable use of Raven's controlled projection test, in which the interview with the child is systematized without being made inhuman. While the child is drawing he is asked to help tell a story, and in this way he expresses his conscious joys, fears, hopes, imaginings, and his remembered dreams. Those in charge of a group of children who read this book may wonder at the relatively superficial picture that tests give, and the author might have included an explanation that psychologists do tests for the purposes of research and teaching and the presentation of material, and that these things have value as well as the actual care of the children. The glossary needs to be rewritten. For example: 'Guilt feeling—a technical psychological term indicating a sense of shame which is largely repressed'. Either guilt feeling means something quite evident, or else it means repressed guilt, or guilt in respect of repressed ideas or feelings. The word shame simply waters the concept down without adding anything useful. Again: 'Psychiatric, the art of healing the mind', and 'Prophylactic—preventative'. If preventative (or preferably preventive) is clearer, why not use it in the text? 'Oral—relating to the mouth, anal—relating to the anus'. This explanation is quite useless unless the whole theory of erogenous zones is presented. And so on. Such criticisms do not, however, detract from the value of this and all books written to gather together and present the results of a piece of field work.

Review: *Parents' Questions*

BY THE STAFF OF THE CHILD STUDY ASSOCIATION OF AMERICA, REVISED EDITION (LONDON: GOLLANCZ, 1947)

Review originally published in *British Medical Journal*, 31 July 1948, 2(4569), 257.

This book is to be welcomed. It can be given to parents and it will not worry them or tie them up in knots over psychological theory. It will be kept lying around or at the bedside, being picked up at odd times, being read at random. Gradually the answers given in 230 questions will be getting known. There is no doubt that the questions are exactly the ones that parents in Britain ask. 'Should you punish a child when he admits he has disobeyed you and says he is sorry?' 'We are getting a divorce . . . I don't know how to explain it to our son'. 'My fifteen-year-old daughter dresses in the most outlandish way. Is there anything we mothers can do. . .?' 'My boy and girl quarrel constantly. Do you think I ought to interfere or let them fight it out?' 'Can we prevent our children from using slang?' 'My six-months-old baby wakes up and cries at night for no apparent reason. How can I train her to have good sleeping nights?' These are random samples.

Each answer takes up a page or two, and the writers show tact and judgment and deep knowledge, and at the same time they avoid making the parent feel frightened or ashamed. They really do give advice, and parents welcome this if it is done with due recognition of the difficulties inherent in any situation where things have gone wrong. An analyst could say that here is the right complement to the analytic treatment of individual children. As the great majority of children who are emotionally disturbed have no access to psycho-analysis, it is fortunate that the authors make but sparing reference to the value that might come from such treatment if it were available. This is a revised version of a book first published in 1936, and would seem to justify its publication in Britain by being written in the kind of English we understand and by being concerned with the problems that beset us here, and perhaps others the world over.

8

Disorders of Childhood

Originally published in *Journal of the Royal Institute of Public Health and Hygiene*, 1948, 11(7), 244.

A version, shortened by Winnicott, of his lecture to the Institute of Public Health and Hygiene.

It is not easy, looking at medical practice as a whole, to see what it is all about. Adult patients come to the doctor for troubles that are due to the rough and tumble of life, and besides, the degenerative processes soon begin to cause casualties. In the attempt to see medical practice and what it is about the pediatrician has the best chance. The study of the disorders of childhood has much to teach the profession.

Text books mostly deal with diseases. Medical students have to be taught about the anatomy and physiology of the body, diseases, and disturbances of physical function. Examinations have to be about disease entities, and their prevention and treatment. It is becoming well-known, however, that the practice of medicine, except for the specialist, is not a simple matter of concern with disease entities. In fact, in pediatrics a curious state of affairs arises: the physically sick are collected together in centres where pediatrics is taught, and the young pediatricians are sent out into a world where there is not enough disease of the kind they know so much about to keep them occupied. Every children's doctor in private practice must encounter psychology, whether he acknowledges it or not. There is plenty of illness but it is not all physical disease.

The general practitioner knows that a number of children have to be passing through a department for the teaching type of case to be reliably included. If the children's doctor looks at his medical out-patient department where he teaches students, he will find that a great deal that he hands over to his assistant is very interesting material, but no good for teaching. He is passing on the emotional disorders. In other words, he is not coming to grips with the problem of his department; to do so he would have to add to his vast knowledge of the physical, a corresponding knowledge in respect of the psychological.

He may well claim that he has not time for this. But then he should surely let a psychologist-pediatrician do his sorting out for him: he can be the physician to whom the physical case is referred.

Let the doctor doing medical out-patients in a children's hospital think of his work in this way: his main function lies in the fact that he can be relied on to be there and to be interviewed during the whole period of any one patient's childhood, from birth to adolescence. In the course of this dozen odd years all manner of troubles will turn up, and it is of immense value to the parents if they know all the time that they can see the doctor they know by just turning up on his day, and waiting their turn.

What do the parents need?

They want advice about physical management, and about psychological management. They want an objective or a scientific examination of disorders of all kinds. They want education in the prevention of disorder and help with treatment. They want the doctor to take over responsibility at the critical moments of ill-health, just as they need to retain responsibility apart from such critical times. They want, off and on, an objective view of their children's condition, because they themselves are too close to the problem and too much involved emotionally, to sort out their own worries from the things that ought to be worried about. The clinician should be ready to act in these ways.

Now let the doctor look back on the notes of a child brought to him from time to time from birth to adolescence. He will find records of diseases, catarrhal attacks, infectious fevers, acute surgical episodes; he will find periods recorded in which the main trouble was some housing difficulty, or a home disturbance causing instability in the child's background; he will find the child has been through times of special personal trial; he will find he has been consulted when the child has had a feeding inhibition, urinary or bowel incontinence, night-mares, depressive phases, psychotic episodes, behaviour disorders, school troubles, and a number of other common disorders. If the whole medical practice in respect of one child is considered, then and then only do the physical diseases suitable for the teaching of medical students appear in proper proportions. Post-graduate doctors, who have had general medical experience, naturally feel disappointment and disillusionment if on returning for a refresher course, they still find themselves being taught on cases of florid rickets, Pink's Disease, Juvenile G.P.I., Mongolism and mitral stenosis.

The problem is indeed difficult because there is so much to learn. The specialist in child psychiatry must lose contact with the modern treatment of infantile dehydration by biochemically controlled intravenous drips. Similarly the full-term in-patient pediatrician cannot be asked to learn how to do the psycho-analysis of a child, or even come to understand what a psycho-analyst does. Nevertheless it would be disastrous if the teachers in each speciality were to teach without interdependence. Those who are out in the world practising medicine undoubtedly have to deal with a vast quantity of disorder which is best not labelled physical or psychological, but which is part of the natural process of the individual establishing his or her own identity while at the same time gaining introduction to external reality, and a relation to home and later to society.

In this personal struggle of every child the body and feelings and the personality and intelligence are all involved. Disorders of childhood include all the disorders inherent in this struggle, and the pediatrician must therefore concern himself with more than the body and its diseases.

(Dr Winnicott illustrated his lecture at its conclusion with a number of drawings done by children at his medical out-patient department, showing their emotional conflicts and fears.)

9

Review: *The Psychoanalytic Study of the Child, Volume 2*

EDITED BY ANNA FREUD, WILLIE HOFFER, EDWARD GLOVER, *ET AL.* (LONDON: IMAGO, 1946)

Review originally published in *British Medical Journal*, 21 August 1948, 2(4572), 389.

The Psychoanalytic Study of the Child was initiated as an Anglo-American venture in 1945 by a group of British and American analysts and collaborators of Anna Freud. Winnicott reviewed many of the volumes.

It is impossible to do justice to this volume in a short review, so that the reader is advised to get hold of a copy if his interest is in child psychiatry or in psychological theory. Much that is both interesting and clinically important is discussed, and the continued work of the Imago Publishing Company is justified by it. 'Problems of Child Development' includes a theoretical study of psychic structure, a study of laughter, a further contribution from Mrs Burlingham on twins, and a study of the pre-oedipal development of the male child. 'Clinical Problems' includes articles on feeding disturbances by Anna Freud, the psychogeneses of tic and of reading disabilities, the analysis of a child with night terrors, and clinical observation of enuretics, a valuable description of psychosis in childhood by Elizabeth Galeerd, and comments on the diaries of schizophrenics by Willie Hoffer. 'Guidance Work' and 'Problems of Education and Sociology' are other headings to sections, and there is a historical note on J. B. Felix Descuret (1795–1872).

Only one article can be picked out for detailed comment; that by Rene A. Spitz on what he calls anaclitic depression is chosen, because it involves consideration of Melanie Klein's concept of the depressive position in emotional development. Spitz makes a special point of disclaiming acceptance of this concept. The material of the article is excellent. The infants in an institution who had all been (unavoidably) separated from their mothers at the age of 6–8 months were found to become depressed at 8–11 months. The author gives interesting clinical details.

Klein uses the term depressive position to describe an achievement of the human infant. If all goes well with the emotional development of any infant a stage is reached at which the infant recognizes the results of erotic and aggressive impulses and ideas, so that henceforth he is concerned, is able to feel responsibility and guilt. Only if this stage is achieved is deprivation liable to cause depression or, in the simplest case, mourning. Failure to arrive at, or regression from, this stage indicates a severe (psychotic) disturbance of emotional development, and results in the infant's showing the more primitive defences such as a disintegration of the personality, depersonalization, and loss of contact with reality. But Spitz writes: 'Klein assumes that human beings are born with a finished and complete psychic structure'. In fact, she does not.

It could be said of the depression observed and described by Spitz that these infants, through early contact with their own mothers and through their subsequent management in the institute, had gone forward in development sufficiently to be capable of becoming depressed, this being an indication of health; more seriously disturbed infants would have failed to achieve this clear depressive mood in reaction to loss. On the basis of an understanding of Klein's theory the author's observation that depression occurred only at 8–10 months is a useful contribution to the discussion of the theory; without such understanding his good clinical, observations are wasted. It would be a pity if subsequent volumes must be marred by further uninformed references to Klein. The first volume contained a serious attack on Klein which was too biased to have an effect on scientific thought, but this article loses value through lack of understanding. It is urgently necessary that Klein's critics get to know what she is in fact saying.

Review: *The Personality of the Preschool Child: The Child's Search for His Self*

BY PROFESSOR WERNER WOLFF (LONDON: WILLIAM HEINEMANN MEDICAL BOOKS, 1947)

Review originally published in *British Medical Journal*, 23 October 1948, 2(4581), 747.

Intelligence tests are not altogether holding their own. Clinicians trust the results of routine tests on children only in so far as they are carried out by mature and understanding psychologists who make a good guess intuitively after adequate human contact. Tests of children under six are particularly suspected, and perhaps ought to be thought of as research. This study of the pre-school child is very interesting, is in many respects original, and is successful in getting behind the objections to the testing with which we are more familiar. The author's aim is to study the child and not to churn out quotients. He discusses the 'rhythm quotient', which serves to introduce organized comment on and evaluation of the drawings of children who have not learnt to draw and who draw subjectively rather than objectively. The book is profusely illustrated by children's conversations and drawings, and these ensure that the reader is kept in touch with the child that is being studied and is not lost in theory. The reader is free to see more than the author sees or to disagree with the author's drawings and comments.

The psycho-analyst, who concerns himself specifically with the dynamic aspect, who sees a need in therapeutics for resolving the repressed unconscious, will welcome this alternative non-therapeutic approach which enriches his perception of the young child's way of life and natural organization. For the educational psychologist the work described in this book would seem to offer a most welcome opening out of the subject and an escape from the psychologist's dilemma—his being employed more for his comments on cases, based on guesswork, than for actual results of tests performed. No doubt much that is published by Wolff as original is a development of ideas already suggested by other workers, but if this is so the author is exonerated by his providing an extensive bibliography of 622 relevant books and papers.

Obituary: Susan Isaacs

Originally published in *Nature*, 1948, 162(4127), 881. Also published in C. Winnicott, R. Shepherd, & M. Davis (Eds.), *Psycho-analytic explorations* (pp. 385–387). Cambridge, MA: Harvard University Press, 1989.

Susan Isaacs died on October 12 at the age of 63. Few can have had a greater influence in our time on the upbringing and education of children; indeed, the modern trend towards full recognition of the human aspect of nursery school and subsequent education owes much to her work.

Dr Isaacs was the daughter of William Fairhurst, of Bolton, Lancashire, and of Miriam Sutherland. Educated at Bolton Secondary School and at the Universities of Manchester and Cambridge, she became a research student at Cambridge in the Psychological Laboratory in 1912, and then lecturer in psychology at Darlington Training College. In 1924 she was invited to become principal of the Malting House School at Cambridge. It was during the following three years that she gathered the comprehensive data of children's behaviour, thoughts and feelings which she presented brilliantly in her two books *Intellectual Growth in Young Children* (1930) and *Social Development in Young Children* (1933).

In 1933 she was made head of the new Department of Child Development of the University of London, at the Institute of Education. She held this post with outstanding success for ten years. In the course of that time a large number of experienced teachers and educationists were enriched by the wide and deep new knowledge which she was able to impart, and above all by her vivid sense of every child as a full, living personality, needing to be imaginatively realised and understood in his own right.

Dr Isaacs turned to the new insight offered by Freudian psycho-analysis as soon as this work became generally known in England, and joined the British Psycho-Analytical Society in 1921. She was appointed a psychologist on the staff of the London Clinic of Psycho-Analysis in the year 1931. She remained on the staff of the Clinic until her death, and contributed signally in a great number of ways to the scientific work of the Society and to the practical work of the Institute. She was a valued member of the Training Committee and of the Council.

Dr Isaacs was a clear writer as well as teacher and lecturer; her books and scientific papers are well known to students of psychology to-day. Her small handbook for mothers and teachers, *The Nursery Years*, written in 1929, is known all over the world; it was awarded the *Parents' Magazine* Medal in the United States. *The Children We Teach* is another little book which is widely popular. One of the two books published just before her death is *Childhood and After*, containing essays and clinical psychological studies which belong to the later period of her life. A chapter in it called 'Children in Institutions', originally a memorandum presented to the Home Office Care of Children Committee, known as the Curtis Committee, in 1945, was probably the most important single document consulted by that Committee.

Dr Isaacs' gifts were based on a combination of intellectual and emotional factors. Her passionate interest in the conditions, first, of young children's education, and, secondly, of their general upbringing in the home, arose out of her own experiences. Her mother's death when she was just 6, terminating a fatal and incapacitating illness which started when Susan was barely 4, led her to find in her first elementary school in a Lancashire town in the 1880s a refuge and solace from the tragedy at home, but also to become very quickly a rebel against its manifold constraints and inadequacies. This disappointed eagerness and keen sense of what 'school' might have been like, but in fact was not, remained in the background of her mind throughout her growth and did much to shape her later life-work.

It became clear to her at an early stage in her development that mere criticism and mere abandonment of existing methods could bring no constructive results. She quickly assimilated and adopted the most advanced educational ideas current at the time, and her immediate response to the new teaching of psycho-analysis showed that no conventional opposition or resistances could stand in the way of her unhesitating acceptance of anything that offered her wider horizons and deeper understanding. In the same way, at a later stage, when Melanie Klein's ideas were first put forward in Great Britain, she was among the earliest to sense the further sources of knowledge which were now opening up. She saw how these new ideas could be developed to the general benefit of every child's upbringing, and from that moment she pursued that knowledge, and applied it untiringly up to the very last.

Her outstanding intellectual characteristic was an extremely rapid and comprehensive grasp of the matter in view and an ability to classify and summarize it, to present it with remarkable clarity, and to discuss it from various angles. Her exceptional capacity for instantly translating her thoughts and impressions into verbal expression served as a powerful instrument for all her other gifts.

It was characteristic of Susan Isaacs that when she found that there was a great deal which she had not yet encompassed, especially in the work of Melanie Klein, she decided (although she was already a member of the British Psycho-Analytical Society) to start again as a trainee and to go through the whole course. Thus she developed further, undergoing a second long personal analysis, and greatly enriched her own work and the contribution which she was eventually able to make to general psychoanalytic research. In her last years, she devoted herself almost entirely to actual analytic practice, and felt this to be the most satisfying of the various kinds of work she had done.

In her husband, Nathan Isaacs, she had a constant friend and supporter, and a constructive critic.

12

Primary Introduction to External Reality: The Early Stages

Originally published in R. Shepherd, J. Johns, & H. Taylor Robinson (Eds.), *Thinking about children* (pp. 21–28). London: Karnac, 1996.

This lecture was part of a series of talks given to students at the Institute of Education, University of London, in 1948.

We seem to have made a start in regard to the study of the development of the human being, and we are gradually, I hope, getting earlier in our study of the child and development. You may have the idea that a human being starts early and that development is in one long line in which there is no gap. Any gap means ill-health, and health really means things have gone on at their own pace and completed themselves and got as far as they could reasonably be expected to at the right time.

I was thinking how to illustrate why I am not talking about all the psychoanalytic theory of development. Partly it is because much is well known and you can read it, and partly because it does not affect your actual work. It is a bit more difficult to talk about normal psychology, and I was thinking of an illustration. Take the fact that certain people are preoccupied with ideas of beating. It comes into their lives a great deal, and some children have a preoccupation with such ideas mixed with masturbation. We have to be able to talk of these things in order to talk about punishment. A woman who has been bothered by these particular things eventually comes to psychoanalysis, an ill person who wants to do something about it. A great deal of work is done patiently over a long time. In the course of treatment these fantasies turn out to be where this patient has kept something from infancy which could not be integrated into her personality: the aggressive part of her relationship to the mother, to the breasts, and to the mother's body at the very beginning. These very aggressive excitement fantasies come along and destroy the quiet relationship to the mother's body. To make it clearer, this patient, in reliving these things in the specialized setting of analysis, found that she could not tolerate in her infancy the direct attack on something so beautiful that she felt was part of herself, the body she was in contact with, and nearly lost everything, but just held something, because, when frustrated, she could feel all the hate and destructiveness towards frustrating things—the buttons, fastenings, and delays. So two things were separated off, one the loving and the complying and the other the taking, taking of what was given. This eventually turned into the excitement about the beating etc., as when the infant is free and finding his mother's body and having instinctual tension and is suddenly overtaken by an overwhelming desire to have a go at it ruthlessly.

This is a difficult situation inherent in the development of every child which the child has to come to terms with, with the help of the mother and her loving experiences with the infant. A person's life can be disturbed for years and years from difficulties starting in these early times. Therefore, I have made a special point of the development of the capacity for concern, of the very big problems that it raises to do with the child's development of a sense of guilt, which is a big step forward.

We now come on to some of the earlier stages. I have said that a sort of psychoanalytic understanding is not what you want when looking after children in school and helping a child to continue his process of coping with his guilt feelings. There you are coming into it not so much by an intellectual understanding of his problem as by being an important person in his life. He has feelings of different kinds, and you are there and continue to exist and give him the chance to feel pleased and sorry and, if he wants, to have the opportunity to make up for the hurt he feels he has done. There is much more in it than is covered by the words 'you continue to exist over a period of time in a child's life'. You don't have to know all that is going on in the child. You know a great deal is going on and if you continue to exist he will be able to come through. It is not just that you continue to live. He gets to know you and to allow for you as a human being. Not in a good temper on Monday mornings, but nevertheless on Friday everything is all right. There is one thing implied in all this, which is that what starts in infancy is never finished then. With every child it is going on all the time, consolidating positions, which can always be lost and gained again. So if we can state something to do with infancy, we are talking about something which continues all the time. If we show why it is important for an infant to enjoy his bath, we are also showing why it is important that children bathe in the sea and why it is important to provide baths for them and to let them swim and dive and there should be soap for them etc. later on. It is not something new but something which joins on to the importance of bathing at the beginning. And if we have the idea of the importance for the infant to be seen naked, we also see it is important for children to be seen naked. Very often people rely on the doctor to see them. I was once horrified by a psychologist saying why he had taken up psychology: because, as he said, 'I can't bear children's bodies'. One of the difficulties about child guidance for me as a paediatrician is that I like seeing children's bodies and should lose this as a psychiatrist: and I should be handing over the children to a friend to examine. But also I should not like to be only examining their bodies and have nothing to do with their feelings and ideas. Therefore it suits me to have the child there, examining him all over. This is an advantage. For some children it is really important that one person sees the body and the psychology as one thing. It is very funny that sometimes as psychiatrists we want a grown-up patient examined by a doctor, and perhaps they don't get properly examined and come back. I remember a case of a hypochondriacal person. He always came with a report that the doctors could find nothing wrong. All perfect. But he could not get a doctor to undress him and see him as a whole person including his genitals. As these had not been examined, he was convinced all the trouble was there. As someone once said, 'At any rate osteopaths undress you!' It is important for people to be seen.

All this is really an apologia because I am talking about infantile needs and getting to earlier infancy when I am actually talking to persons who are dealing with children. Now for some more primitive things in human development, more the things you take for granted—for instance, that you the teacher comes on time or are always three minutes late and that you don't teach your children in the dark. If you started teaching children in the dark they would not know where you were, you would get all mixed up with the hallucinations. You could not introduce reality to them in the dark. It would be so complicated. If they were blind, then you could have special techniques to deal with the darkness. If we liked, we could look into all the things you do, into how important they all are, when we are talking in terms of the earlier stages of infant development.

Let us simplify the matter of primitive development and say there are three things which can be separated out. One is making contact with reality. Another is feeling that you live in your body, and the other is the integration of the personality. These things overlap, but give us tags to hang on to. Let us take the integration of the personality. I have spoken to you about the stage being arrived at at which a child can make a circle and say this is a person and mother is another person, a similar one. He can begin to know the inside world and the outside world and that there is something at the edge and this is himself. This line between inner and outer can also be very weak and hardly discernible, and at the beginning one could say there are all sorts of different things which Glover calls 'ego nuclei': all sorts of things which the child can use 'I' about and it is only a little bit of 'I' such as a toe seen, a finger moving, a hungry impulse, or the feeling of warmth from a hot-water bottle. This includes anything that impinges on the child and that the child is aware of, not at first separated out externally from the self, but only very gradually becoming separate. All these bits and pieces go to make the human being. How important it is at such a stage that the mother has the child in her mind as a whole person, because the child can then afford to be in pieces. No doubt, sometimes when babies are very hungry, all out in an attack, they come together and flow into something which becomes almost like a whole. Or, if they are very angry, things gather up into the anger and no doubt the bits come together.

In the quiet moments there is no line between inner or outer but just lots of things separated out, sky seen through trees, something to do with mother's eyes all going in and out, wandering around. There is a lack of any need for integration.

This is an extremely valuable thing to be able to retain: we miss something without it. It has something to do with being calm, restful, relaxed, and feeling one with people and things when no excitement is around.

For the world to flow in and out without hungry taking and angry giving, infants need very satisfactory management at the beginning and then they are able to manage this as well as the actually more exciting experiences. On the other hand, some children have not managed this, such as the patient I was telling you about. The aggressive attack was kept separate and developed into an organized beating fantasy. On the other hand, those who have a wonderful life built up on a quiet basis can identify with nature and people in a quiet way.

The integration of the personality is something which becomes an achievement through two sets of things. One is the times of keen feeling of one kind or another which makes the infant gather together and become one person, angry or hungry. The other is the management of the child. I try to think of it as what the mother does when she picks up her baby. She does not take him by the toe. She may make a little noise to give him time, folds him round, and somehow gathers him together. She does not assume he is an acrobat. She shows that she knows what is going on. Let us jump to a patient who throughout childhood had great difficulty in establishing her identity.

> She had to hide her identity from her powerful-minded father. She drew a picture of her father when he suddenly called her name. She drew a very meek little girl looking very good and absolutely nothing was there, but little bits of herself were rushing round trying to get there in time, bits from the dog where she had placed most of herself all rushing trying to catch up before she got to her father but they never did, and she was an ineffective bit of flesh. Anyway, she parked herself out in little boxes, behind things. (She was the patient up in the box at the top of a tree sometimes.)

This is to illustrate that we are not dealing with things only at the beginning, but we are saying that when you call a child, two children, in your classroom,

Introduction to External Reality: Early Stages

one is there, but the other you have to take as the infant all over the place who you have to collect into himself, to be there, and to be there at the right time. You can't be certain that one is better than the other. They are different types.

When you deal with children it is much like managing a baby. When collecting a child of 6, he may be a child specializing in being part of nature—a poet. He finds his life as an interchange with the world. He can't come immediately you call, he will be confused unless you really make him integrate and then he will suddenly come together. Therefore, you have two things making a child come together: one instinctual experience, and the other your management. You are giving children all sorts of satisfactions in giving them something with which to pull themselves together from within. You make what you are teaching interesting, and also you manage them in such a way as to keep the class-room somehow related to their bodies. I think architecture comes in here. I was helped one day by an architect. I said 'Why is it, although I did not know I liked the old Regent Street, I feel quite different about the new one?' He said: 'In the old Regent Street the proportions wherever you looked were similar to the proportions of the human being and therefore people felt they extended easily into the buildings, but the present buildings have no relation to the human being at all except by chance, therefore people feel like robots. They have to find other ways of getting into contact'.

Everybody has their own right to an opinion about the building we are in [Senate House, University of London]. It may be that some people love this building and I would hate to hurt their feelings, but when it comes to children it is different. Did you know that in the old days Dr Susan Isaacs had a nursery school here? I don't know what the children felt about the proportions, but I don't think it is the thing to ask little children to come into this huge building. By temperature, air, etc. you are managing children and creating conditions which they can identify with as human beings. I think many big buildings have no proportion to people; the building tends to be a sort of place where there are innumerable bits and you are one of the bits.

This subject is much like the subject of the child feeling he lives in his body because here there are two things, the child having experiences in which the whole body is involved, kicking, running around, eating, getting to know himself, as the place where he lives, and also the management from the outside. Don't take it for granted that people live in their bodies quite easily. Anyone, if very tired, could easily find themselves not exactly where they are, and as I have said before about Lawrence of Arabia, after five days on the camel he said he was about five yards up on the camel's right ear. This is how you get absent from your body and not know, therefore, where you begin and end. There is the complication that we have all had differences within ourselves. Take the example of the man who has lost a leg. It is all right when he is not tired, but if tired the memories of the other leg come back. In the same way, we are all very different, all sorts of differences inside ourselves, and if a person is very much reliving a childhood experience the body feels heavy and he doesn't know what to do with it. In this photo you see the child who left her body and did not come back for three years. She had never had a good contact with reality. She had a good brain but did not make use of it. Her head drooped and eventually she went away. She was the most flabby creature, except where she lived—in her eyelids and in her jaws. She was fed through the nose. Her eyelids were always closed, but it was possible to see that she sometimes opened them enough to see what was going on. At present she is coming round, walks, says things, and even laughs at jokes. This is an extreme case of what you can often find in normal children. A child has a bilious attack and becomes like death, flabby and absent. You put him to bed. It is very frightening, and just as suddenly he has recovered and is playing on his scooter. As long as we know, we shall not get alarmed but be able to allow for these things.

I would like to leave a bit of time for people to ask questions and leave contact with external reality. [Question on concentration]. Concentration has to some extent expressed a hate to external reality and some people are not wanting to risk an alteration of the environmental feeling sufficiently to concentrate. They would rather maintain the good relations to the world and to that extent deliberately sacrifice some of the concentration, and on the other hand they have the advantages of what they maintain in contact with the environment, and may have something to go back on.

13

Environmental Needs; the Early Stages; Total Dependence and Essential Independence

Originally published in R. Shepherd, J. Johns, & H. Taylor Robinson (Eds.), *Thinking about children* (pp. 29–36). London: Karnac, 1996.

This lecture was part of a series of talks given to students at the Institute of Education University of London, in 1948.

You have been listening to me now for a number of lectures. In what we have dealt with I have, as it were, tried to put up a building. I think that building (outside) is what lectures look like at the moment. I want to consider children in different phases of development. I was thinking we could compare the different phases now, taking the word morality. For children who have reached a certain stage, that of whole human beings, I would say morality is a matter of compromise. They have their own ideas of what they think is right and wrong, but you know they can see that the other person has a point of view, so, very often, the word compromise comes in. In the stage a bit earlier, morality seems to be represented by reparation in respect of guilt; this is the sense of guilt which is tolerable if something is being done about it. When we come to these more primitive things, morality has become a terrific and terrible thing. There is no compromise; it is life or death. If somebody has failed to complete something in these earlier stages then nothing can be done, they can't accept compromise, they may prefer to spend their lives in a mental hospital rather than give in. We can understand what that means when we take extreme cases in ourselves, or in children who are managing to have times when they must stand up for something, their own integrity, their own individuality, their own rights as individual human beings. At any rate, it seems to me there is something very fierce in the morality of the infant, and in all that which is in us which belongs to infancy, and to earlier infantile development.

I want to speak now about the introduction of external reality to the human infant, and I don't want to be misunderstood if I talk about a mother and her new-born infant when I say I know what happens in the case of a new-born infant. I would say that an infant comes into the world, and no doubt a great deal goes on which we are not talking about, but, at a certain moment, he begins to become interested in some outward thing; there is an outward turning of the personality towards something. He begins to get hungry. He is ready to accept something outside himself and he has no idea of what that is going to be, but here is that line towards something, the mother. Then there is the mother with her breast and she has got something to offer, too, and it seems so easy, if one has not thought it out. The baby looks, sees and feels whatever is there, and that stimulates the baby, who stimulates the breast, and all that is physiological, and it is quite true but not quite enough. We have to see that here we have a very tricky situation, one which makes me tremble when I think how doctors and nurses interfere so easily. Here is the baby's capacity to hallucinate something and here is the mother who has what she knows is good but the baby does not yet know, and the mother has to manage to place herself here so that what the baby is willing to find is actually herself. In that case we could say that she manages to give the baby the illusion that what he actually gets and takes and finds is what he created out of his own feelings, his own power to hallucinate. This, of course, is a matter of a living experience. The mother makes all sorts of arrangements about how to manage her contact with the baby. But it is a matter which goes on, and, in the ordinary case, the mother has many times placed herself in the right direction for the infant and he has come, gradually, to have material from the real experience to hallucinate with, so that he is managing to see the actual nipple and experience the details of the smell and the breast and everything, and gradually by a painful and long process he is able to imagine what is actually likely to come. It is something which is done, and when it is successfully done it has given the infant the basis for mental health which it is very difficult for the infant to lose. But it is never entirely successful, and we will now look and see what happens in the case of failure.

The words 'illusion' and 'reality' come into the writings of psychologists and philosophers, but it is something one can pinch, an idea. We may say they are talking about something like this, but we say to them, you are liable to miss out the basis of this thing, the experience between the mother and the infant at the beginning. This is not a theoretical concept. If we have no difficulties here, we owe something to someone. This is the external factor. It seems that one can say there is some degree of failure which must be very common, and then, sometimes, one has a complete failure.

Here is a splitting of the personality at a very early level, which is one of the meanings of the word schizophrenia. Here a child has two relations to external reality. In one there is compliance, the actual *taking* on a compliant basis, and then a purely imaginary experience with an imagined reality. In the extreme case, there is very little contact taking place, the child has nothing to imagine with except what is in himself, which is just a matter of something rather like thumb-sucking or rocking movements, something very poverty-stricken. On the other hand, *enough* of real contact and illusion can have taken place for an infant to have built up a world which has quite a lot in it that we could recognize has come from our shared reality. And in a case where this has become an important feature because of breakdown later on, and a child has gone back to a split, you can often have a child in a world which is extremely rich, and rich with things which we know about in our reality-shared world.

When you see children, you can see two relations to external reality. One seems sometimes to be very satisfactory in the sense that the child is, on the food basis, taking everything or, on the teaching basis, accepting everything and behaving well, but you feel all the time there is something lacking and you are not surprised to find, later on, a breakdown to this relationship which is not to external reality but to an inner world. I want to refer to a child who had been asleep for three years, who had really lived in this world for a long period of time and had regressed and retired into her world. When you meet a child who retires for minutes, weeks, or years, you will be interested to try and guess what in this inner-world experience there is of the external world that we know about.

If we talk about Shakespeare and being able to get into one's inner world, we can see that Shakespeare's inner world was as rich as the world we live in. Whatever came from him was something which could have been based on very acute observation of human beings in the real world. All that he felt and knew had gone in, and when he was able to bring it out we can recognize it and check up on it. We can look to Shakespeare to keep a sense of proportion on it. But if we take a musician, like Beethoven, we shall find, too, that all the human emotions and feelings and relationships are represented here, not in persons, but in terms of 'to and fro' of forces of spontaneity, without human beings being brought into it. But if you look at the 'turning in' activities of children in your care, some of them you will feel not too worried about because they have an inner world which is rich and has a relation to the external world, and their life is rich. But with another child, you feel their inner world is very poverty stricken, is so much cut off, that you recognize this as illness. Take two children, both preoccupied. One you do not worry about because you know he is full of richness, but the other you worry about because you know he is ill, his preoccupation has no richness. There has never been anyone at the beginning to give enough for this child to have an illusion about reality. Reality has remained something which can never be accepted in a whole way.

On another occasion I was bold enough to talk about the infancy of Juliet.[i] It so happens that Shakespeare took the trouble to say a great deal about Juliet's infancy. Perhaps this is not off the subject. The question is whether Shakespeare can be talked of in that way at all. Desmond McCarthy in the Sunday Times was very cross with a psychologist for having written a book on Hamlet. 'How could there be a childhood of somebody who had never lived?' He said the reason why Shakespeare made Hamlet have a conflict was because the play had to last two hours! But I do think that when we take somebody like Shakespeare, any little detail of the conversation has something to do with the main themes of his play. I don't believe he put the bit in about Juliet's infancy because on the first night he knew some midwives were coming. He tells us Juliet's mother was about 13 and the nurse 14, and the nurse's child died and she wet-nursed Juliet. He thereby gives us to understand that the nurse had a great deal of sweetness in her and knew the difference between wet-nursing someone else's child and her own. And Juliet had something like an adopted child's difficulties. The nurse could not wean her until she was nearly 3 and then only because Juliet had a rather fresh conversation with the nurse's husband the day before. The husband had made remarks when the child fell down. And when she weaned the child, she did it, not in the ordinary way, but by bitter aloes. She weaned the child in this indirect way. It seems to me Shakespeare was trying to show why Juliet had to have the split in her nature. The compliance to her mother and everybody is all right for this other thing, the extreme of romanticism, whereby the impossible is going to happen. She is going to have all the feelings of love in relation to somebody who is coming along, something which is actually doomed to end in death and actually by poisoning. A great deal is made of the poisoning being a breast experience, being good because it is bad. All this is Shakespeare's understanding of the need to go back to infancy to explain the later developments in a person's type of life. But the rich inner world of a person like Shakespeare makes bridges between the inner and outer worlds. He was describing somebody without any bridges between the inner world and external reality.

In coming to the business of guilt feelings and reparation, I said what a tremendous amount you as teachers provide when it comes to reparation in respect of guilt by being a person or a set-up in which a child can find, in course of time, the love and the aggression and the guilt and the opportunity to give. When you mention primitive things, you are talking about processes that are going on all the time. You do a great deal for a child because you can't just fit in for every child. You let him have some things, and not have others, but by being more or less there and reliable you give him an opportunity

---

[i] See 'The Infancy of Juliet' [CW 3:4:4].

to experience his love and hate. No child completes these experiences; they are going on in your school work, using you to reinforce the good start they have had.

In the case of treating patients, we get these things illustrated many times. I have told you before about this patient I am going to describe.

> For a long period this patient had no relation to me at all unless I turned up on the doorstep and was there inside the door as the patient came and rang the bell. I had to be there actually at the moment when this patient came, in a very, very real way. For quite a number of months I had to put aside everything for twenty minutes beforehand, because, if I did, the patient could come and we had a good session, but if anything went wrong there was no relationship. An ill person this, to illustrate the extreme. This patient came and she took two years to break down and be as ill as she had to be. When she came she was still apparently well. She had formed a very good relation to everybody and was called the little friend of all the world and everyone said, 'well, if anyone is sane, you are'. And then she broke down in the end by having a physical illness which turned out to be produced by herself in a certain way, but all this took a long time. In the beginning she had missed it. She had been one of twins and she had been handed over to other people. So I had to provide something which she had never had.

So with an ordinary patient or child, you are dealing with people who have had a good early position and you can slip in to that position and reinforce it into a position which other people have created, guiding and expanding and widening their growth. But if there has been failure at the start, you would have to be like doctors doing a difficult job and this would be impossible.

[Question: 'Is it then important that you stay in a school for a number of years?']

That is an interesting question. You get to know the children, it is wasted if you leave. There are always casualties when teacher leaves, and a sigh of relief from one or two. And then with these things there are phases the children have to go through. You will find that certain ones are using you at certain times for certain purposes. Some have finished with you for the time being. I think a lot of troubles are there whenever you leave. On the other hand that brings up the whole subject of whether you take your class on with you or not. Children who are adolescent are like small children, with instincts, tremendously important instincts carrying them away, and then there is something special about this need to find people to reinforce whatever is there in their experience.

> A typical case would be a boy of 17 recently who was in difficulties. He told his school he must see a psychologist. It upset the school, but his parents found me. He was dumb when he came and nothing happened at all, and

so I said, 'I will see you again some time'. And then, one day a telephone message came to say, 'Can I see you tomorrow?' I knew I had got to say 'Yes'. In that situation you have either to fail or do the right thing. Then I had to rearrange all my plans. I had to be like the mother with the tiny baby. Then he came, and we had an extremely rich hour and a half, did a tremendous lot of work which had a big effect. He took everything into his own hands, left school, got work in London in order to have a long treatment. It all depended on my doing every thing at that moment.

There must be moments like this for you, and other moments when you will feel it silly to give up things to meet the child's immediate need.

But if you look round you can see when children are depressed—they can't put it on. When they are ill you know that if you try to make contact with them you can't. You have to let them feel the urge and then be there for it.

Although you are employed to take the responsibility for the children, having a relationship to a child is much more difficult. Take being a doctor at a clinic. It seems as if the community is trying to find out whether he will be allowed to do this difficult thing, to be a good doctor. It is odd that the doctors are putting up any response at all. Why should they be expected to ask to be allowed to be called up in the middle of the night? They may perhaps hope to get something very important out of it, but if it is challenged they will give it up. The same with mothers. They will not choose to do the difficult thing, the responsibility for the infant's feeding and bringing up, if they are going to hand over to the state. The same with teachers; it is not all teachers who come to courses like this which makes their work more difficult. Perhaps some could think it will make work very easy, but in practice it either makes no difference or, as time goes on, you find yourself taking personal responsibility. Doing things. Living experiences with children in your care. Thinking things out, risking things which otherwise you would have let go or done by rule of thumb. By coming to this course, it means that you have thought these things out. If psychology is dynamic and making a difference, in a way it is making it more of a strain and making it much more difficult. The difficulty about psychology is that if you get off the academic rails, talking about feelings, this can't be done without disturbing oneself. This is why it would not be a good idea to force all teachers to come to psychology lectures, because it would reduce anger and hate and make people less good. Nor would it be good to make all mothers go to lectures on the psychology of infancy. And if you said to all artists, poets, 'you must come to a thing on psychology', you would come across terrific feelings, because the best artists loathe psychology.

PART 4

1949

1

Letter to Paul Federn

Originally published in Rodman, F. R. (Ed.), *The spontaneous gesture. Selected letters of D. W. Winnicott* (Letter 9, p. 12). Cambridge, MA: Harvard University Press, 1987.

Paul Federn (1871–1950) was a Viennese-born American psychologist.

3 January 1949

Dear Dr Federn,

I have only just read your lectures on Psychoanalysis of psychoses 1943[i] and I am writing to say that I have very much enjoyed them. The wealth of clinical experience behind them is so clear. I am very much wanting to have a copy of these for re-reading as the copy I read was a photostat belonging to the U.S. Army. If you happen to have a reprint I would be very grateful if you would send me one. Alternatively I can order a copy of the Psychiatric Quarterly from the publishers. In a week or two I hope to be able to send you a reprint of a lecture of my own on another aspect of the same subject.

You may remember me as the young analyst who never wrote to thank you for taking such a lot of trouble over an article I wrote a long time ago on play or some such subject. That article was written under the influence of Melitta Schmideberg when I was quite unready to write on the theme. The whole thing seemed to me rather unreal at the time and it took me many years to get it into perspective. When you came to England you said to me that this must represent a strong negative transference which had got caught on to yourself. I think this was not correct; there was another explanation, which was that

---

[i] Posthumously published as 'Ego Psychology and the Psychoses', edited by Eduardo Weiss, 1952.

I had been persuaded to do something which was not really part of me and which I really resented.

With good wishes,
Yours very sincerely,
D. W. Winnicott

Letter to the *British Medical Journal*

TAKING CHILDREN'S TEMPERATURES

Originally published in Rodman, F. R. (Ed.), *The spontaneous gesture. Selected letters of D. W. Winnicott* (Letter 10, pp. 13–14). Cambridge, MA: Harvard University Press, 1987.

This letter was not submitted for publication.

6 January 1949

Sir: My friend Dr Joan Malleson in her letter of December 18th 1948 invites comments from psychologists on the matter of taking the temperature of children by the rectum as advocated by Professor Moncrieff and Dr Hussey in an article in the previous number.

I hesitated before taking up this matter because my first reaction on reading the article was to feel glad that reference was made in it to the psychological side of the matter. Paediatrics is notoriously out of touch with psychology and here was an exception. Also an infant does not feel much from having a thermometer stuck in the rectum, so that the main trouble comes, if at all, from the interest in his rectum which the nurse must take by using this method. In the majority of cases I imagine there is no special difficulty here except where there has already been a good deal of rectal interference by soapsticks, enemas etc. which has roused resistance in the child to that sort of thing.

As Dr Malleson has raised the matter, however, I can say that I felt that the words 'possible difficulties from the point of view of the psychological trauma . . . are discussed', which occur in the summary of the article, seemed to promise more than actually appeared in the article itself, which really only dealt with what could be called the *human* aspect. We hope this is never missing in the management of children, whether by a physician or nurse.

The trouble is that if a matter like this is to be discussed psychologically, there must be a willingness on the part of all to give time to the discussion and to learn about the use of the techniques by which information can be collected. Even this relatively simple matter of the taking of temperatures by the rectum involves considerations that cannot be put in a letter. Dr Malleson raises wider issues and it can certainly be said that one cannot do justice to the subject of the effects of enemata for worms and for constipation and other gross anal manipulations except to a group of students who are willing to settle down to a series of 10 or 20 lectures. Even so these lectures would have to be spread over a period of time so that the students could gradually come to be able to get the feeling of the infantile situations, and also in order that they should have opportunity for various kinds of clinical approach to the problems raised in a more theoretical way in the lectures.

It can be said therefore that this subject is not one for treatment in a correspondence column; nevertheless it is only by such means that attention can be drawn to the need for doctors to be willing to treat psychology as a subject comparable to physiology and requiring of the student a hard discipline.

I am, etc.,
D. W. Winnicott, F.R.C.P.

3

Letter to Marjorie Stone

Originally published in Rodman, F. R. (Ed.), *The spontaneous gesture. Selected letters of D. W. Winnicott* (Letter 11, pp. 14–15) Cambridge, MA: Harvard University Press, 1987.

Marjorie Stone was a manufacturer of children's toys.

14 February 1949

Dear Mrs Stone:

Thank you for your letter in which you let me know that you are making dolls to a specification supplied by the Institute of Child Psychology.

I am sure that your motive in making these dolls is a good one, and probably you will be rather surprised to hear that actually I am not at all certain that the idea is sound. At any rate I would like you to know that if there were a public discussion on this matter and I had to take one side or the other, I should probably come down heavily on the side against the distribution of these dolls. You would probably expect a psycho-analyst to hold a different view.

My reasons for this view are more complex than could be stated in a letter. Whilst I appreciate that there are certain children at certain times who might get something out of dolls with sex organs shown, I feel very much more certain that to the vast majority of children it would be exceedingly muddling if they were to find themselves presented with dolls that had these characteristics. I feel that there is much more about a doll than that it is an unalive baby. In fact it is only to quite a small extent necessary that it should look like a baby. It seems to me that the logical conclusion would be to make a teddy bear which really bites if you tease it.

I would of course develop this theme if I felt you were interested, but I thought you would like to know in these few words that I feel that in spite of your good intention you are directing your energies in a direction which is not really desirable.

Yours truly,
D. W. Winnicott, F.R.C.P.

4

The Infancy of Juliet

Dated 1 March 1949. This is probably one of the lectures Winnicott delivered to students at the Institute of Education, University of London, in 1948 or 1949 (see also 'Primary Introduction to External Reality: The Early Stages; [CW 3:3:12] and 'Environmental Needs; The Early Stages; Total Dependence and Essential Independence' [CW 3:3:13]). Winnicott also delivered a lecture titled 'The Possible Significance of the Nurse Scene in *Romeo and Juliet*' at the University of London on 21 May 1966.

It happens that we know a good deal about Juliet's infancy. The question arises whether this is a matter of chance or whether in Shakespeare's amazing mind there was room for the recognition of infantile roots for adult patterns of behaviour.

The Main Theme of the Play

The theme that knits the play together is the feud between the two houses. It is this that stamps death's seal on the two lovers, it is this that makes the Friar's action sensible, for if he had not hoped to mend the feud by the marriage he could not have agreed to perform a secret marriage rite, being an honourable man and certainly not a conspirator.

> The fearful passage of their death-marked love,
> And the continuance of their parents' rage,
> Which, but their children's end, nought could remove.[i]

This theme dominates to the very end, when the feud does actually resolve by reason of the twin and tragic deaths.

---

[i] Prologue.

Romeo and Juliet took their life 'From forth the fatal loins' of two foes, and it would be profitable in another study to make a comparative study of the many famous feuds settled by intermarriage. In the minds of two lovers, what is the effect of this setting? On a conscious plane it should release love, for it is as far away as possible from incest. It is exogamy exactly. Yet at a deeper level, incest is implied by being reacted against or denied. But this is not the problem I wish to discuss here.

Internal Setting for the External Feud

It is worth considering whether we are not meant to go intuitively deeper, and to *feel* that Romeo and Juliet had within themselves a high degree of internal feud, the warring in each, even if in different ways, of mutually antagonistic 'internal' forces. Romeo is perhaps the more easy to understand of the two.

We know Romeo as an adolescent with good background and satisfactory emotional development, with a latent depressive mood, this mood being dispelled by his being 'in love'; that is to say, in him there is a preponderance of 'letting the loved one become a good object to fill an inner gap', over 'seeing the loved one as a person to be used in sensuous experience'. The friar had been chiding him about this, and no one is surprised to learn that the effect of this admonishing was weak.

Romeo knew he would be likely to get into trouble by going to the enemy's house for the feast and dance. At this point we are invited to think that for him some solution to internal difficulties would come through a love that would carry with it the death penalty, but this theme is common in literature and potential in the affairs of every full grown human being.

Can we find a way of stating the unconscious problem that was solved for Romeo by the tragedy? I would say that in the setting of the love affair the male enemy of fantasy was externalised for him and this allowed the reservoir of the incestuous basis of his externally directed loving to flow into his relationship with Juliet. Apart from this setting, his nature would have tended to have kept Juliet as an 'internal' idealised object, to be protected from instinct drives. By implication, Romeo is a well integrated adolescent, with unified personality, capable of bearing anxiety and of holding a depressed mood. Moreover his inner world is peopled with human beings, not populated by cardboard figures nor cluttered up with lifeless objects, nor made chaotic by the interaction of blind forces. This is a negative way of describing the maturity of his emotional development which we are meant to take for granted in our appreciation of his journey to death.

Juliet is not so easily measured. The suggestion made here is that Shakespeare took the trouble to weave the first and delightful nurse episode into the play to prepare us by the details given in it for Juliet's lovely personality and for her dreadful destiny.

Juliet's Early History

We are told that Juliet's mother was fourteen when she gave birth to her. She did not look after her, but handed her over to a wet nurse. This delightful person with so rich a personality was by then already a mature person, unlike Juliet's mother. She had nursed many babes. Being married she had had one of her own, but this infant, Susan, had died; 'She was too good for me'. The nurse, grieving her own beloved Susan, had taken on Juliet for wet-nursing, and as a solace.

Juliet was still at the breast at the age of three, perhaps a usual feature in those days, who can say? However, the nurse evidently had some difficulty over weaning the child, because she accomplished it by laying wormwood on her dug.

(In clinical practice I have found that weaning delays almost invariably reflect maternal depression.)

At the time of weaning Juliet was very much the child of the nurse and her husband, because just then her actual parents were away together at Mantua.

Now this decision on the part of the nurse to put the infant off, to make her 'fall out with the dug', did not come just then for nothing. At that time Juliet could walk 'high-lone', and not only that, but she had shown signs of becoming emotionally ripened, as she might well be at the age of three. On a certain day, Juliet had fallen and had hurt her head. The nurse's man was there, because we knew what he said. In analytic work we are familiar with the symbolic meaning of a girl of three falling in the presence of a man. We know it can mean that the little child is in love, is sexually attracted, perhaps is overwhelmed by unexpected orgasm.

Now the nurse's husband understood all this. He made a joke which the nurse would not forget, nor its sequel, 'An if I should live a thousand years'.

The man took up the child; 'Yea', quoth he, 'dost

> thou fall upon thy face?
> Thou wilt fall backward when thou hast more wit;
> Wilt thou not, Jule?' and, by my holidame,
> The pretty wretch left crying, and said 'Ay'.
> To see now, how a jest shall come about!
>   . . . 'Wilt thou not, Jule?'
> And, pretty fool, it stinted*, and said 'Ay'. [ii]

(*stinted - ceased, i.e. ceased crying.)

[ii] Act 1, Scene 3.

The nurse shows by going over and over the ground, till Juliet and her mother are exasperated, that the incident meant much to her.

And the next day she put wormwood to her dugs. We are invited by the poet to associate this event with big things. There was an earthquake at that moment.

> When it did taste the wormwood on the nipple
> Of my dug, and felt it bitter, pretty fool,
> To see it tetchy, and fall out with the dug;
> Shake, quoth the dove-house.[iii]

This would not be the first or last time that a poet used an earthquake as a portent.

It is not doing justice to Shakespeare if we fail to see that the nurse's breasts had gone bad (in her unconscious fantasy) *before* she put the wormwood on the nipples, because of the incest play of the previous day. She now had hate of the child in her, and she could no longer deny the child the right to grow up and to claim a place in the world of emotions.

It must be remembered, however, that Juliet could only arrive at this maturity in the adoptive home; her own home could not provide the required simple setting, and in any case the nurse it was who had personally nursed her and cared for her.

One more detail. As a result of the fall the child had a bump on the forehead. The nurse could not forbear to give this a sort of pregnancy of significance, 'at an oral level' (in the jargon used by psycho-analysts).

> And yet, I warrant, it had upon its brow
> A bump as big as a young cockerel's stone,
> perilous knock.[iv]

This, in the fantasy of the unconscious, implies that the child had become pregnant by oral incorporation of the husband's male genital.

The nurse is no prude, and a little later she interrupts the mother who is extolling the virtues of Paris, the chosen husband:

MOTHER: So shall you share all that he doth possess,By having him, making yourself no less.
NURSE: No less! nay, bigger! women grow by men.

Is it not astonishing that all this should be made plain, unless there is some light to be thrown on Juliet's personal problem through this knowledge?

[iii] Act 1, Scene 3.
[iv] Act 1, Scene 3.

One could say that Juliet had been well loved and well cared for, and that her nurse had plenty of riches to impart along with her dug-milk.

The problem was there, however, that the mother who devoted herself to her was not her own mother. She had two sets of parents, and the more natural and easy and mature and well matched were not the parents who conceived her.

The nurse was certainly (in her early relation to Juliet) a depressive, using Juliet as a good object with which to fill a hole in herself, the hole made by the death of her own Susan, and this links with what has been guessed about Romeo's nature.

Above all, there is the suggestion that Juliet was profoundly affected by being weaned because of having on the previous day turned to the nurse's husband.

In psychological terms, the infant had started to move from the stage in which oral erotism normally dominates to a stage in which genital erotism gradually claims attention, and this change was marked by a turning to the man. The nurse reacted to this change in the child. In the place of the simple relationship between herself and the child there had come the triangular relationship, herself, her man, and the child, this necessitating a reorientation for the nurse too.

Incidentally, by weaning the child because of her turning to the man, the nurse is suggesting that the child's desire of the man is oral in type. Here one is reminded of the metaphor used in the preface.

'And she steals love's sweet bait from fearful hooks'. This metaphor employs pregenital fantasy of oral type in description of intercourse.

It is a matter of emphasis, and I am not suggesting that anything pathological is meant. It is much more likely that the infancy details may give us the clue to the quality of Juliet's *healthiness*. It is this healthiness that enables us to let her be the lodging place of love which is at the same time the most beautiful and the most deeply in conflict.

It would be unwise to assume that in health there is anything easy. The essential difficulties of human existence are avoided or slurred over by most people, or are side-tracked by illness. Only the healthy (in a psychiatric sense) can know and feel the essential tug between the claims of external reality and internal or psychic reality. For this reason mature people do not always look as well as the immature or ill.

Inferences to Be Drawn

If it be accepted that these details of infancy are significant, what are we to learn from them?

It would be interesting to hear a discussion among psycho-analysts on the relative importance of the various factors, the double parentage, the depression of the wet-nurse, the trauma of the weaning on top of the sexual maturing of the three-year-old child, and the manner of the weaning.

The view put forward here is that the double parentage is the important thing; that is to say, the fact that Juliet had real parents and also what practically amounted to foster-parents, the real parents aloof, and the foster-parents crude, intimate and body-conscious. This gave Juliet a divided self in respect of marriage.

Juliet's attitude to her real parents' proposal that she should consider marriage in general and Paris in particular was that of compliance with the demands of duty. All is decorum itself.

> LADY CAPULET: Tell me, daughter Juliet,
>   How stands your disposition to be married?
> JULIET: It is an honour that I dream not of.
> NURSE: An honour! Were not I thine only nurse
>   I would say thou hadst suck'd wisdom from
>   thy teat.

The ordinary gulf between compliance and dream is here stated and emphasised. This is the problem of everyone, and Juliet is a young adolescent, at the very age when there is the greatest difficulty when the love dream is threatened with a reality test; and a prospect of marriage for life is the severest possible reality testing.

We are not shown Juliet's revolt against compliance. The only other words here are:

> JULIET: I'll look to like, if looking liking move;
>   But no more deep will I endart mine eye
>   Than your consent gives strength to make it fly.

Does this not mean: I will look to like, but not allow spontaneity to carry me away—only allow the strength supplied by the mother's wishes in the matter to darry the dart as far as the man? If so, Juliet is being dutiful in the extreme.

Juliet does not yet know of Romeo, but we may suppose she has had her dreams.

Instead of a revolt against her parents' management of her love affairs we are presented with the complete jump from Juliet's compliance to the romantic dream-come-true side of Juliet's nature. Her next words are spoken when she is with Romeo at the ball, and by this time she has endarted her eye without anyone's consent but her own.

At this moment both Romeo and Juliet are keyed for the acute event. Romeo was depressed, and his last words had been:

> ROMEO: My mind misgives
>   Some consequence, yet hanging in the stars,

> Shall bitterly begin his fearful date
> With this night's revels, and expire the term
> Of a despised life, closed in my breast,
> By some vile forfeit of untimely death;
> But He, that hath the steerage of my course,
> Direct my sail![v]

It seems likely that Shakespeare intended the audience to get the full sense of the two characters' readiness for something to happen.

In a trice the kiss has sealed the doom of both, and the rest follows as night the day.

It is perhaps worth noting the way the nurse plays two parts here. Her respectable self, the employee of the Capulets, interrupts the lovers with the words:

> NURSE: Madam, your mother craves a word with you.

But she is thoroughly excited by the romance and tickles it up a bit immediately in her own way!

> NURSE: I tell you, he that can lay hold of her
> Shall have the chinks.[vi]

This part of her nature takes her through the whole matter of 'jauncing up and down' and acting the go-between.

The double nature of the nurse helps Juliet's double nature now, and presumably has always been mixed in with the dichotomy in Juliet represented by compliance and romance, between obedience and spontaneity, the relation to real and foster-parents.

In Juliet from now on the spontaneity is pure; not alloyed by defiance. Because of the split in her nature we are enabled to see the young adolescent's personal love blossom and reach its flower and fruit.

There is a danger here in this part of the study of Juliet in that it will be thought by some that the intention is to draw attention to abnormalities. On the contrary, the contention is that there is a blossoming, flowering and fruiting in personal spontaneous love which is innate and inevitable, and which shows in Juliet's love of Romeo because of the elaborately conceived setting. In the ordinary case the sequence is spoiled or at any rate disturbed by the emotional immaturity of the adolescent lover, or through illness of the lover (in a psychiatric sense) or the confusion of the setting, and especially by the impurity of the romantic experience, this being, as has been already suggested, contaminated by defiance.

---

[v] Act 1, Scene 4.
[vi] Act 1, Scene 5.

Defiance in adolescence is only another aspect of compliance, and is notably absent in Juliet as we are shown her.

The essential basis for all this is Juliet's satisfactory emotional development in the infantile as well as in the early childhood stages, so that there is no suggestion of psychosis or neurosis. The split in her is an adjustment to the real split in her external environment.

In Juliet, as in Romeo, there is no lack of reality contact, there is a sense of body, and of living in the body, and integration of the personality can be taken for granted. There is no delusional system, with projection of persecutors. There is extreme richness of inner world, with an enviable ease of self-expression of sophisticated yet personal kind. There is no envy of the male sex. Moreover the girl is brave, and willing to take any risk that belongs to this unfolding of her life-story.

It seems that we are told about all this so that we shall not in any way feel that Juliet is a psychopathological case, or (to put it positively) so that the universal applicability of the tragedy shall be felt by every member of the audience.

It is not that every adolescent, if healthy, must meet tragedy. But, every adolescent, in to some extent complying, fitting in with what society expects, loses not only the full richness of love but also the fullness of tragedy, and this means a loss of the full feeling of living one's own life.

The gain from compliance is positive, but this depends, in adolescence, on the ability of the parents to come to meet the young person's spontaneity half way.

Juliet's parents could not do this as they were not in close enough touch with her. They never had been. The nurse and her man could not have done this for the parents because they had never been the actual mother and father.

It could be said in reverse, and for balance, that the adolescent is in a bad way who makes a too good adjustment on a compliance basis, sacrificing too much of the spontaneity with its realness, its richness and its tragedy. Such a boy or girl is liable to be welcomed by the world as an example of successful upbringing, of good adjustment, of sanity, of success. Everyone but the psycho-analyst is surprised when the protest suddenly comes in mental break-down, suicide, psycho-somatic disorder, or in political activity that is defiant and non-constructive in quality.

The value to the world of the play *Romeo and Juliet* is great. The mere existence of the play, however, is nothing. To have its effect it must be repeatedly acted, well acted, and acted without cuts. Audience after audience must get caught up in total effect of the play, not a line of which can be left out.

It is said that, in schools, the part in which the nurse described Juliet's infancy is sometimes omitted! This study is an attempt to show how great a loss can follow the omission of any part. Would anyone show Botticelli's

Venus rising from the waters, with a piece of plain paper pasted over, for instance, the head with distended cheeks, and the mouth that puffs?

The Final

Finally, there is the manner of Juliet's end. There is a great deal that is worth study in the details given.

This time Juliet looks to the kiss to poison her. Here the theme of the bad mother and the bad breast returns. The breast poisons both because it is hated on account of the weaning, and more fundamentally because in the primitive love impulse the breast is destroyed when loved.

Romeo has drunk all the poison, and only for this reason does Juliet not die by that means. Romeo has taken to himself the bad external breast (nipples with wormwood on them) and so Juliet is freed. She can now die in a more mature way, by stabbing herself. Here (for the unconscious) she is experiencing intercourse. She takes Romeo's dagger.

> O happy dagger!
> This is thy sheath; (stabs herself) there
> rust and let me die.[vii]

She falls on Romeo, and so her life ends, with a fall. According to the suggestion in this study it was a fall, the fall in front of the nurse's man, that started the story of the play, and that made the nurse wean the child with '. . . wormwood on the nipple of my dug'.

[vii] Act 5, Scene 3.

5

Letter to Roger Money-Kyrle

Roger Money-Kyrle (1898–1980) was a British psychoanalyst and follower of Melanie Klein.

22 March 1949

Dear Money-Kyrle,

Would you like to be one of several people I am sending this to for active participation?[i]

If you agree—just chew up the pages and send them back with comments, additions, suggestions, corrections, etc etc

I think it will go into *Human Relations*.

Yours
D. W. Winnicott
I shall be at this address till end of month.[ii]

---

[i] Winnicott enclosed a draft of 'Some Thoughts on the Meaning of the Word Democracy' [CW 3:5:17].

[ii] Winnicott gave his and Alice's home address in Hampstead, where they had lived since 1932. His change of address at the end of March signals their separation (see [CW 3:4:6]).

6

Letter to Roger Money-Kyrle

Roger Money-Kyrle (1898–1980) was a British psychoanalyst and follower of Melanie Klein.

31 March 1949

Dear Money-Kyrle,

My address for the next three weeks will be c/o Mrs Q. Henry, ..., Saxmundham.[i]

I wish to thank you very much indeed for your letter about the Democracy paper.[ii] The point is, would you care for us to write a joint paper with me incorporating your suggestions and then your working up any parts you wish to work up, eliminating what you do not like, or would you be content for me to use your suggestions with acknowledgements? I should be happy over either arrangement.

I want to get this finished by the end of April as it will then be printed somewhere about June.

The question I want to ask you is whether the value of the paper is lessened by all the part that I have written after the main part with the 'mathematics' in it? I think perhaps it would be better to make the paper into two parts indicating that the second was subsidiary in importance.

Do not let this bother you if you are busy, but I shall be able to find time to work over any suggestions you make while I am away.

With very good wishes,

Yours sincerely,
D. W. Winnicott

---

[i] Winnicott's change of address at the end of March signals his separation from his first wife, Alice.

[ii] Winnicott had sent Money-Kyrle a draft of his paper 'Some Thoughts on the Meaning of the Word Democracy' [CW 3:5:17].

7

Letter to Roger Money-Kyrle

Roger Money-Kyrle (1898–1980) was a British psychoanalyst and follower of Melanie Klein.

2 May 1949

Dear Money-Kyrle,

Many thanks for your Bulletin which I return herewith. I do not want to give this important reference. If you think my latest version of 'Democracy'[i] is clearer this is largely due to your constructive criticism and moral support.

With good wishes,
Yours sincerely,
D. W. Winnicott

---

[i] 'Some Thoughts on the Meaning of the Word Democracy' [CW 3:5:17].

8

Birth Memories, Birth Trauma, and Anxiety

Originally published in *Collected papers: Through paediatrics to psycho-analysis* (pp. 174–193). London: Tavistock, 1958.

Presented at a Scientific Meeting of the British Psychoanalytical Society on 18 May 1949. The discussion of this paper was continued on 15 June (see 'Notes on the Discussion' [CW 3:4:11]).

In this paper I wish to present certain clinical examples illustrating fantasies and possible memories of the birth experience.

In psycho-analytic theory there has been some confusion since Freud put forward the valuable idea that the symptomatology of anxiety may be related to birth trauma. It is not clear whether birth memories are individual or racial, whether birth can be normal or whether trauma is an inherent part of birth or a variable and chance accompaniment. Also, what exactly is the nature of the trauma in terms of ego psychology? There is therefore much left over for research, and perhaps the following collection of ideas may be useful in stimulating thought.

It is difficult to know how to quote Freud usefully at this point. To do Freud justice one would have to write a separate paper tracing the changes in his views on the relationship between anxiety and birth trauma. This would be an excellent exercise and it has already been done, notably by Greenacre.[1] In any case it is not necessary for me to try to do justice to Freud's views here. On re-reading many of his references to the subject since writing the main part of my paper, I think I can find everything that I have suggested somewhere in his writings. Perhaps I could best quote the sentence where he says: 'Now it would be very satisfactory if anxiety, as a symbol of separation, were to be repeated on every subsequent occasion on which a separation took place, but unfortunately we are prevented from making use of this correlation by the fact that birth is not experienced subjectively as a separation from the mother, since the foetus, being a completely narcissistic creature, is totally unaware of her existence as an object'. Again, comparing birth with weaning, he says, 'the traumatic situation of missing the mother differs in one important respect from the traumatic situation of birth. At birth no object existed and so no object could be missed. Anxiety was the only reaction that occurred' (Freud, 1926).

What interests me is precisely this subject of the foetus and the child who is being born, the 'completely narcissistic creature'; I want to know what is actually happening there. I like to think that Freud was feeling round this subject without coming to a final conclusion because of the fact that he lacked certain data which were essential to the understanding of the subject. In considering Freud's view therefore we have constantly to try to remember what he, a scientific worker in the field, would do if he were alive now and active in the psycho-analytic world, taking into consideration advances in our new understanding of infants.

The main thing really is that Freud believed in the significance of birth trauma as a scientific worker, and not only as an intuitive thinker. It is rare to find doctors who believe that the experience of birth is important to the baby, that it could have any significance in the emotional development of the individual, and that memory traces of the experience could persist and give rise to trouble even in the adult. Those who knew Freud, and I am not one of them, may have information as to his latter-day belief in the importance of the birth trauma. In *Group Psychology* Freud says: 'Thus by being born we have made the step from an absolutely self-sufficient narcissism to the perception of a changed outer world and to the beginnings of the discovery of objects'. He goes on to say '... and with this is associated the fact that we cannot endure the new state of things for long and that we periodically revert from it in our sleep to our former condition of absence of stimulation and avoidance of objects'. Here however he is introducing a new subject and I do not take for granted that sleep has a simple relation to intra-uterine existence. This subject needs separate discussion.

I had thought that Freud believed that in the history of every individual there were memory traces of the birth experience which determined the pattern anxiety would take throughout the life of the individual. Greenacre appears to think, however, that Freud linked anxiety with birth by a sort of collective unconscious theory, with birth as an archetypal experience. (I am using Jungian expressions here on purpose because they seem to apply.) But whatever Freud wrote or did not write he held the view that the personal experience of birth is also important to the individual if the following story is true: when he heard of an infant that was born by Caesarian section he remarked that it would be interesting to remember this fact, which might eventually be found to affect the pattern of anxiety in that individual.

Much of what I wish to contribute is already expressed by Greenacre (1945). She writes:

In summary, it seems that the general effect of birth is, by its enormous sensory stimulation, to organize and convert the fetal narcissism, producing or promoting a propulsive narcissistic drive over and above the type of more relaxed fetal maturation process that has been existent in utero. There is ordinarily a patterning of the aggressive-libidinization of certain body parts according to the areas of special stimulation. Specifically, birth stimulates the cerebrum to a degree promoting its development so that it may soon begin to take effective control of body affairs; it contributes to the organization of the anxiety pattern, thereby increasing the defense of the infant, and it leaves unique individual traces that are superimposed on the genetically determined anxiety and libidinal patterns of the given infant.

The matter needs study. Greenacre's two articles (1941) need much more attention than I have been able to give them so far. In the summary of the first of these two papers she says, 'The anxiety response which is genetically determined probably manifests itself first in an irritable responsiveness of the organism at a reflex level; this is apparent in intra-uterine life in a set of separate or loosely constellated reflexes which may become organized at birth into the anxiety reaction', and so on. It may be seen from this that she is asking for a reconstruction of the problem of the relation of anxiety to birth trauma in the light of the work that is being done on infant behaviour.

In the second article, which is more clinical, and more related to psycho-analytic work, Greenacre draws attention to the value to be got from correlating early infant histories with material elicited in the course of subsequent therapy. In her summary she says: 'It is clear that the consideration of these cases takes us back to the need for more observation with infants, work which appears to me the source of the richest material for psycho-analysis'. I expect she would agree, however, that there is no more important method of studying the birth trauma than the one which we have especially at our disposal, namely the psycho-analysis of adults and children. 'The other methods are also important and they include particularly the studies based on observations of infants at birth, before and immediately after birth, and also the type of investigation which can only be carried out by the neurological specialist'.

I would like to draw attention to Dr Grantly Dick Read's work (1942). He sees the birth process from the midwifery point of view, and much of his success in practice is due to the fact that he adds to his knowledge of the physical side of birth processes a belief in the importance of giving the mother confidence. He aims at preventing or overcoming the fear in the mother which he finds so seriously disturbing to her function at the time of parturition. He is sympathetic to psycho-analysis and psycho-analytic theory. Dr Read is quite willing to believe that the psychology of an individual is something which can be studied pre-natally and at the time of birth, and that the experiences at this early date are significant. In this I feel that he is ahead of many obstetricians and paediatricians.

The personal view that I am putting forward in this paper is based on analytic work.[2] My ideas fall into three groups.

The first point I want to make is that there are various types of material appearing in an analysis. When I add to them the birth trauma type of material I am not claiming that treatments can be done on birth material alone. The analyst must be prepared to expect whatever type of material turns up, *including birth material.*

The analyst must indeed expect environmental factors of all kinds. For instance, one needs to recognize and assess the type of environment that belongs to the intra-uterine experience, also the type of environment that belongs to the birth experience; likewise the mother's capacity for devotion in respect of the newborn infant, the capacity of the parental team for taking joint responsibility as the infant develops into a little child; and also the capacity of the social setting for allowing maternal devotion and parental co-operation to play their parts, and for continuing these functions and extending them, eventually enabling the individual to play his or her part in the creation and maintenance of the social setting.

In other words, no consideration of the birth trauma can have value unless a sense of proportion can be maintained. Nevertheless in a discussion of any one subject one should not be afraid *temporarily* to seem to over-estimate the importance of the subject under discussion.[3]

The second point that I want to make is that in common with other analysts I do find in my analytic and other work that there is evidence that the personal birth experience is significant, and is held as memory material. It is generally held that in psychotic states those very things are remembered that are unavailable to consciousness in more normal states. You will notice that in stating my second point I have used the word 'birth experience' instead of 'birth trauma' and I will return to this point, but first I wish to describe an episode in the analysis of an apparently defective boy whose defect was probably secondary to early psychosis, and not due to brain limitation.

> This boy, who was then five, spent a month or two of his analysis testing out my ability to accept his approaches without demanding anything, and actively to adapt to his needs in a way that his mother could not do. He repeatedly came towards me and went away again, testing out my ability to accept him. Eventually he came to sit on my lap. No words were spoken at all for the whole of this period. The further development of his relation to me took the following unexpected form. He would get inside my coat and turn upside down and slide down to the ground between my legs; this he repeated over and over again.

When he had thoroughly established this procedure which seemed to follow his decision that I could be used as the mother that he needed, he would get up from the floor and demand honey. I procured honey (and later cod-liver-oil and malt, which was easier to get during the war) and he would often scoop out as much as half a pound and eat it immediately with great relish. This was the beginning of a tremendous phase of oral activity with excessive salivation. He would make a pool on the doorstep with his saliva as he waited for me to open the door. Previously to this his oral desires only turned up as hallucinated objects (which he called Käfers) which appeared on the walls and of which he was very frightened. The interpretation which had made him able to lose these hallucinated insects was this: that they were his own *mouth*. In the next phase he became a Käfer himself and then he started on the phase of the analysis which I have described, in which he was testing me out as a mother who could actively adapt.

After this experience I was prepared to believe that memory traces of birth can persist. Of course the same thing in play has turned up in many analyses and on still more occasions in the play of normal children and in one's own play as a child.

The following case also presents certain features which help in the approach to the study of birth experience:

Miss H. is a nurse (50 years old). She had treatment from me when she was about 25, at a time when I was house physician at St Bartholomew's Hospital and had only read a book or two on psycho-analysis. This patient had a very severe neurosis, including constipation of a degree that I have never met before or since. She had been a shorthand-typist but after getting help from me she became a hospital nurse. Later on she specialized in the care of psychotic children. She has an unusual intuitive understanding of the needs of children who are in a state of regression.

In this patient's treatment, which was cathartic in quality, she would lie and sleep, and then suddenly wake in a nightmare. I would help her to wake by repeating over and over again the words that she had shouted out in the acute anxiety attack. By this means when she wakened I was able to keep her in touch with the anxiety situation and to get her to remember all sorts of traumatic incidents from her very eventful early childhood.

I never knew what to make of her reconstruction of her birth. Birth memories appeared with fantastic embellishments clearly derived from all stages of development and from the sophistication of the adolescent, if not of the adult. Nevertheless the effect seemed to me to be real in its terrific intensity. *While disbelieving the details described as memories I found myself prepared to believe in the accompanying affect.*

Recently this patient has been looking after a little girl of seven, a psychotic case (autistic) undergoing analysis. Miss H. suddenly was taken ill and without being able to let anybody know she simply did not turn up at her job, which was to take the child for treatment and to look after her during the day. I was able to visit her and found that she was just beginning to recover from an illness of a kind that was not new to her, but which had previously never been so acute. She had suddenly had to go to bed with what she called a 'blackout'. She had lain absolutely rigid and curled right up tight on her side, unable to do anything at all, and as near unconscious as may be. A doctor was called in who said he could find nothing wrong with her body. While she was in this condition she was unable to do anything about food at all. Gradually she became conscious, and allowed herself to be moved to a friendly place, and in the course of a week or ten days she was able to get about again. This nurse frequently keeps me in touch with the details of whatever case she is nursing, but previous to this occasion she had never once, since the time twenty years ago when I was treating her, asked me about herself. On this occasion, however, before going back to her job, she came to me and sat down and said, 'What about this blackout? What had it to do with?' I had no idea, and I told her so. Then she went on talking, and I gradually realized that although she was not expecting to be having a therapeutic session, nevertheless she was giving me from her unconscious the material which would enable me to explain her blackout.

I found that she had been living with this little girl of seven and had been identified extremely closely with the child as she always is with psychotic children in her charge. She told me that in order to understand the child's condition, she had been imitating her more and more, putting a hand here, and walking in this way, and that, and doing everything she saw the child do 'in order to get the feeling of the child's state of mind and body'. Now it so happened that this little girl was going through an acute anxiety state and had developed a very great fear of travelling in the Underground. Miss H. had been trying to take her in the Underground to distract her attention and to show her by experience that the Underground was not as bad as expected. A great deal of material of this kind suddenly showed me that I must say to Miss H. that she herself was reliving the birth experience along with the little girl. Here was no hysterical reconstruction. She had been actually having to re-experience the physical thing, which in her case had included a feeling of asphyxiation. Interpretation along these lines produced a most dramatic effect. Miss H. felt better, felt she understood what was going on, and went back confidently to her job. The doctor of the case said to me, 'Somehow or other Miss H. looks much better since her illness'. After this she continued to do good work with this little girl, and with a more objective understanding of the anxiety that is actually important in the little girl's case.

Hysterical patients make us feel that they are acting, but we know better than they can know that true affect is displayed and hidden in the hysterical manifestations.

In many child analyses birth play is important. In such play the material might have been derived from what has been found out by the patient about birth, through stories and direct information and observation. The feeling one gets is, however, that the child's body knows about being born.

I return to the fact that I used the words 'birth experience' instead of 'birth trauma'. This leads to the third point that I wish to make. I feel that Freud's remarks become very much more understandable when he separates birth experience from birth trauma. Greenacre emphasizes this. Possibly birth experience can be so smooth as to have relatively little significance. This is my own view at present. Contrariwise, birth experience that is abnormal over and above a certain limit becomes birth trauma, and is then immensely significant.

When there has been a normal birth experience, birth material is not likely to come into the analysis in a way that draws attention to itself. It will be there, but if the analyst does not easily think in birth terms the patient is not likely to force the issue in these terms. There will be more urgent and apposite settings for the anxiety which both patient and analyst are trying to reach.

When, however, birth experience has been traumatic it has set a pattern. This pattern appears in various details which will need to be interpreted and dealt with each in its own right, at the appropriate time.

I wish to emphasize, however, that interpretation in terms of birth trauma will not suddenly produce total and permanent relief. It is rather this, that since the birth trauma is real it is a pity to be blind to it, and in certain cases and at certain points the analysis absolutely needs acceptance of birth material in among all the other material.

It would be useful to give three categories of birth experience. The first is a normal, that is to say healthy, birth experience which is a valuable positive experience of limited significance; it provides a pattern of a natural way of life. This sense of a way of life can be strengthened by various kinds of subsequent normal experiences, and so the birth experience becomes one of a series of factors favourable to the development of confidence, sense of sequence, stability, and security, etc.

In the second category comes the common rather traumatic birth experience which gets mixed in with various subsequent traumatic environmental factors, strengthening them and being strengthened by them.

I refer at a later stage to the extreme of traumatic birth experience, which provides a third category or grade.

It will be seen that it is difficult for me to think that what happens in anxiety is determined by birth trauma, because that would mean that the individual who is born naturally has no anxiety or has no way to *show* that he is anxious. This would be absurd.

I would like to bring in at this point a discussion of the word 'anxious'. I cannot think of a baby as being anxious at birth, because there is no repression or repressed unconscious at this early date. If anxiety means something simple like fear or reactive irritability, all is well. It seems to me that the word 'anxious' is applicable when an individual is in the grips of physical experience (be it excitement, anger, fear, or anything else) which he can neither avoid nor understand; that is to say, he is unaware of the greater proportion of the reason for what is happening. By the word unaware I am referring to the repressed unconscious. Should he become rather more conscious of what is afoot, he will no longer be anxious, but instead he will be excited, afraid, angry, etc.

Freud in *Beyond the Pleasure Principle* states: '*Angst* denotes a certain condition as of expectation of danger and preparation for it, even though it be an unknown one'. But he does not seem here to express what I am trying to say, that the individual has to have reached a certain degree of maturity, with capacity for repression, before the word anxiety can be usefully applied. This is an example of the considerations which make me want to ask that the theory of a relationship between anxiety and birth trauma should be held in abeyance while work is being done on the psychology of the infant before, during, and after birth.

My present thesis is therefore a composite one, namely that the normal birth experiences are good, and can promote ego strength and stability.

I now wish to draw attention to the way in which birth trauma comes into the analytic situation, making it especially clear that talking with the patient about the birth trauma is something that is extremely likely to be sidetracking the main issue. I would doubt the value of an interpretation along birth trauma lines in the case of a patient who is not deeply regressed at the time in the analytic situation, and who is not clinically ill in the times between analytic sessions.

One of the difficulties of our psycho-analytic technique is to know at any one moment how old a patient is in the transference relationship. In some analyses the patient is most of the time his own age, and one can reach all that one needs of the childhood states by means of his memories and fantasies expressed in an adult way. In such analyses I think there will be no useful interpretation of birth trauma; or birth material will appear in dreams, which can be interpreted at all levels. An analysis, however, may be allowed to go deeper if necessary, and the patient does not have to be very ill to be at times an infant during an analytic session. At such a time there is a great deal that one has to understand without asking for an immediate description of what is happening in words.

I am referring to something which is more infantile than the behaviour of a child playing with toys. According to the predilections of the analyst and according to the diagnosis of the patient there will be variations in the wisdom or unwisdom of working with the patient on these terms. What I am trying to make clear is that if birth experiences are coming into the analytic situation there will certainly be a great deal of other evidence that the patient is in an extremely infantile state.

Birth Experience

It will be understood, Freud having pointed it out, that birth experience has nothing to do with any sort of an awareness of a separation from the mother's body. We can postulate a certain state of mind of the unborn. I think, we can say that things are going well if the personal development of the infant ego has been as undisturbed in its emotional as in its physical aspect. There is certainly before birth the beginning of an emotional development, and it is likely that there is before birth a capacity for false and unhealthy forward movement in emotional development; in health environmental disturbances of a certain degree are valuable stimuli, but beyond a certain degree these disturbances are unhelpful in that they bring about a *reaction*. At this very early stage of development there is not sufficient ego strength for there to be a reaction without loss of identity.

I am indebted to a patient for a way of putting this which came from an extremely deep-rooted appreciation of the position of the infant at an early stage. This patient had a depressed mother whose rigidity was marked and who continued after the child was born to hold the child always tightly for fear of dropping her. It is for this reason that the description is in terms of pressure. Together we worked out the following statement which eventually proved to be vitally important in that analysis. The understanding of this reached right down to the bottom of her difficulties and described accurately enough the extent of the regression which she had to make before starting to come forward again in her emotional development. This patient said: 'At the beginning the individual is like a bubble. If the pressure from outside actively adapts to the pressure within, then the bubble is the significant thing, that is to say the infant's self. If, however, the environmental pressure is greater or less than the pressure within the bubble, then it is not the bubble that is important but the environment. The bubble adapts to the outside pressure'. Along with the understanding of this the patient felt that for the first time, in the analysis, she was being held by a relaxed mother, that is to say, a mother alive, awake, and ready to make active adaptation through the quality of being devoted to her infant.

Before birth, and especially if there is delay, there can quite easily be repeated experiences for an infant in which, for the time being, the stress is on environment rather than on self, and it is likely that the unborn infant becomes more and more caught up in this sort of intercourse with the environment as the time for birth arrives. Thus, in the natural process *the birth experience is an exaggerated sample of something already known to the infant.* For the time being, during birth, the infant is a reactor and the important thing is the environment; and then after birth there is a return to a state of affairs in which the important thing is the infant, whatever that means. In health the infant is prepared before birth for some environmental impingement, and already has had the experience of a natural return from reacting to a state of not having to react, which is the only state in which the self can begin to be.

This is the simplest possible statement that I can make about the normal birth process. It is a temporary phase of reaction and therefore of loss of identity, a major example, for which the infant has already been prepared, of interference with the personal 'going along', not so powerful or so prolonged as to snap the thread of the infant's continuous personal process.

It will be noted that I do not at present hold that it is essentially traumatic to start breathing. The normal birth is non-traumatic by virtue of its non-significance. At the birth age an infant is not ready for prolonged environmental impingement.

It is precisely by reason of its being significant to the infant that experience of the birth trauma is psychologically traumatic. The individual's personal 'going along' is interrupted by reactions to prolonged impingements. When birth trauma is significant every detail of impingement and reaction is, as it were, etched on the patient's memory in the way to which we become accustomed when patients relive traumatic experiences of later life (the sort of experiences that are sometimes successfully recovered by abreaction or by hypnosis). In collecting together examples of impingement I will not attempt to preserve any order because I have not yet decided how to do this; in the study of an analytic patient, however, one meets an order of detail which cannot fail to impress.

It may be pointed out that the most important thing is the trauma represented by the need to react. Reacting at this stage of human development means a temporary loss of identity. This gives an extreme sense of insecurity, and lays the basis for an expectation of further examples of loss of continuity of self, and even a congenital (but not inherited) hopelessness in respect of the attainment of a personal life.

The repeated phases of unconsciousness (here the word is used in the physical sense) either due to brain changes or to the anaesthetic administered to the mother, are unlikely to prove significant. When the patient gives a clear picture of having become unconscious once or several times in this situation it is likely that what is being re-enacted is the snapping of the thread of continuity of the self due to the repeated phases of prolonged reaction to environmental impingements, such as pressure. Unconsciousness (as after concussion) is not remembered.

Among features typical of the true birth memory is the feeling of being in the grips of something external, so that one is helpless. You will note that I am not saying that the baby feels that the mother is gripping. This would not be talking in terms of a baby at this stage. The point is that the external impingements require the baby to adapt to them, whereas at the birth age the baby requires an active adaptation from the environment. The infant can stand having to react to impingement over a limited period of time. There is a very clear relation here between what the baby experiences and what the mother experiences in being confined, as it is called. There comes a state in the labour in which, in health, a mother has to be able to resign herself to a process almost exactly comparable to the infant's experience at the same time.[4]

Belonging to this feeling of helplessness is the intolerable nature of experiencing something without any knowledge whatever of when it will end. A prisoner-of-war may say that the worst part of the experience is that there is no knowing when the imprisonment will end; this makes three years worse at the time than a twenty years' sentence. It is for this reason fundamentally that form in music is so important. Through form, the end is in sight from the beginning. One could say that many babies could be helped if one could only convey to them during prolonged birth that the birth process would last only a certain limited length of time. However, the baby is unable to understand our language; moreover there is no precedent for the baby to use, no yardstick for measurement. The birth-age baby has a rudimentary knowledge of impingements which produce reaction, so that the ordinary birth process can be accepted by the infant as a further example of what has already happened; but a difficult birth goes far beyond any prenatal experience of impingement that produces reaction.

In the case of one patient in whose analysis there was a particularly good opportunity to watch the birth process, since it was relived repeatedly, I became able to detect each ego nucleus as it appeared in reaction appropriate to the type of impingement. To mention a few: urinary-tract nucleus, flatus nucleus, anal nucleus, faecal nucleus, skin nucleus, saliva nucleus, forehead nucleus, breathing nucleus, etc. Perhaps these considerations throw light on the difficulty we have in describing the weak ego of the immature individual knowing as we do how tremendously strong each ego nucleus is. What is weak is the integration of a total ego organization.

In the present context there is a great deal that can be said about what happens when, with extremely immature ego organization, an infant has to cope with an environment which insists on being important. There can be a false integration which involves some kind of abstract thinking which is unnatural. Here again there are two alternatives; in the one case there is a precocious intellectual development; in the other case there is a failure of intellectual development. Anything in between these two extremes is of no use. This intellectual development is a nuisance because it is derived from too early a stage in the history of the individual, so that it is pathologically unrelated to the body with its functions, and to the feelings and instincts and sensations of the total ego.[5]

Here it may be observed that the infant that is disturbed by being forced to react is disturbed out of a state of 'being'. This state of 'being' can obtain only under certain conditions. When reacting, an infant is not 'being'. The environment that impinges cannot yet be felt by the infant to be a projection of personal aggression, since the stage has not yet been reached at which this means anything. In my opinion a severe birth trauma (psychological) can cause a condition which I will call congenital, but not inherited, paranoia. Observation of many infants in my clinic gives me the impression that a severe paranoid basis can be present immediately after birth. I cannot better illustrate my meaning than by giving you a dream which a patient (woman, age 28, diagnosis: schizophrenia with paranoid features) dreamed in reaction to reading Rank's *Trauma of Birth*.

She dreamed that she was under a pile of gravel. Her whole body at the surface was extremely sensitive to a degree which it is hardly possible to imagine. Her skin was burned, which seemed to her to be her way of saying that it was extremely sensitive and vulnerable. She was burned all over. She knew that if anyone came and did anything at all to her, the pain would be just impossible to bear, both physical and mental pain. She knew of the danger that people would come and take the gravel off and do things to her in order to cure her, and the situation was intolerable. She emphasized that with this were intolerable feelings comparable to those which belonged to her suicide attempt. 'You just can't bear anything any longer. It's the awfulness of having a body at all, and the mind that's just had too much. It was the entirety of it, the completeness of the job that made it so impossible. If only people would leave me alone. If only people wouldn't keep getting at me'. However, what happened in the dream was that someone came and poured oil over the gravel with her inside it. The oil came through and came on to her skin, and covered her. Then she was left without any interference whatever for three weeks, at the end of which time the gravel could be removed without her suffering pain, and when it was taken away her skin had almost entirely healed. There was, however, a little sore patch between her breasts, a triangular area which the oil had not reached, from which there came something like a little penis or a cord. This had to be attended to, and of course it was slightly painful but quite bearable. This simply didn't matter, someone just pulled it off.

Here is much less of the sophisticated overlay than there was in the dreams of the patient Miss H., since the patient was not an hysteric, but was psychotic.

Hence the true affect is evident. The person who understood, and who poured oil over the patient was I, the analyst, and the dream indicated a degree of confidence gained through my handling of her case. However, the dream itself is a reaction to an impingement (the reading of Rank's book) and the analysis suffered a temporary set-back.

THE HEAD

In the ordinary birth the head of the infant is the forward point and does the work of dilating the maternal soft parts. There are several ways in which this is remembered. There may be retained as important a mode of progression which can be described by the word 'reptation'. This word appears in a book by Casteret called *My Caves*. The author is describing the way he gets through holes in deep cave exploration. The point about reptation is that the arms are not of any use, nor the hands. In fact the reason why there is any forward movement is not clearly known to the author. I suppose that in the memory trace of a normal birth there would be no sense of helplessness. The infant would feel that the swimming movements of which we know a foetus is capable, and the movements that I have referred to under the word reptation, produce the forward movement. The actual birth can easily be felt by the infant, in the normal case, to be a successful outcome of personal effort owing to the more or less accurate timing. I do not believe that the facts justify the theory that in the birth process itself there is *essentially* a condition in which the infant feels helpless. Very frequently, however, delay produces this very thing, helplessness, or sense of infinite delay.

There can very easily be delay at a time when there is constriction round the head, and it is my definite view that the type of headache which is clearly described as a band round the head is sometimes a direct derivative of birth sensations remembered in somatic form. In analytic work this band round the head can be found to be related to the experience of being caught up in an environmental impingement that has no predictable end. It is possible to conceive that there are all sorts of sensations not quite so clearly delineated, such as noises, blood rushing to the head, a feeling of congestion at the top, and the feeling 'that something gives way, as if blood is escaping'. These and other common head-symptoms in the psychosomatic field are related to the psychotic delusions in which there is a discharge through the top of the head, and I have known helmets and hoods to be important as providing reassurance that the self will not escape through the top of the head. Scalping has primary significance, and is not merely a castration displacement. Associated with this are all the variations on the theme of horns and unicorns which may derive an important root from the extension forward of the personality in this birth process whereby the body propels itself.

There is a basis here for a fantasy of re-entry into the mother head-first. This was brought out clearly in one analytic experience. The patient, the second of twins, had been unexpected and had been left for a long time after birth unattended. In the analysis there was a time when the patient's dilemma was whether to retain the relationship that was known or to become a separate entity with no external object presenting itself. The former alternative provided a false object relationship and was represented in the analysis at that time by a compulsion to have the hand over the forehead, the hand representing the mother's body. This easily got woven into a kind of false homosexuality in which the patient went into the woman head first. In this case the arms were notably useless. In the first dream she brought to me she was attempting to have intercourse without use of arms and she had developed rheumatoid arthritis confined at first to the elbows and wrists so that arms for which she had no fundamental use had virtually become eliminated. Needless to say, oral erotism was severely inhibited as part of the same complex, and she had already had all her teeth removed.

The identification of the whole body with the male genital often appears in psycho-analytic work. It should not be forgotten that there can be a basis for this in the birth experience in which the body acts as a whole, and without the arms and without oral or any other erotism (except that of the muscles employed in swimming or reptation movements). The body simply proceeds through a narrowed environment.

THE CHEST

The next in importance to the experiences of the head are those of the chest. This part of my description can be divided into three parts: first there is the memory of actual constricting bands at various levels around the chest. These constrictions can be desired, and we meet this especially in certain perversions, but also in the ordinary details of clothing. One could say that the individual with the strong memory trace of such a thing as a constriction round the chest would rather feel a constriction which is known and under control than continue to suffer from a delusion of a constriction based on memory traces of birth.

The second part of this description is in terms of function. I have found that the memory trace of restriction of chest expansion during traumatic birth process can be very strong, and an important thing about this is the contrast between reactive chest activity and the chest activity of true anger. During the birth process, in reaction to the construction of the maternal tissues, the infant has to make what would be (if there were any air available) an *inspiratory* movement. After birth, if all goes well, the cry establishes the expression of liveliness by *expiration*. This is an example in terms of physical function of the difference between reacting and simply going on 'being'. When there is delay and exceptional difficulty the changeover to normal crying is not definite enough and the individual is always left with some confusion about anger and its expression. Reactive anger detracts from ego establishment. Yet in the form of the cry anger can be ego-syntonic from very early, an expulsive function with clear aim, to live one's own way and not reactively.

The third thing about the chest and birth is the simple feeling of a lack of something, a lack which could be relieved if breathing could be freed. In a case with history of placenta praevia with very much delayed birth and marked asphyxiation, the patient when only six years old complained of a constant feeling of 'lack of oxygen'. She had known before then that the air seemed to lack something, and when she heard of oxygen she used the idea of it immediately. This feeling persisted as a very important symptom. The actual experience of breathing difficulty in the birth process must not be forgotten, in my opinion, when one is tracing out the various roots of breathing disturbances and the perversions that include breathing obstruction. The desire to be suffocated can be extremely strong and turns up as a masturbation fantasy, in the acting out of which many who had no suicidal intention have died. It is present in inverted suicide which is commonly called murder. By a reversal of roles, active suffocating can be a perverted kindness, the active person feeling that the passive one must be longing to be suffocated. There is something of all this, as of everything else, in the healthy passionate sexual relationship.

Study of the need to be able to do without breathing, a need that can be found in the mystical practices of various religions of the East, cannot be complete unless the individual's body-memory of his birth can be taken into consideration. There are of course other equally important things entering into the mystic's denial of the necessity to breathe, particularly his attempt to deny the difference between internal reality and external reality.

CONCLUSIONS

In order to preserve the personal way of life at the very beginning the individual needs a minimum of environmental impingements producing reaction. All individuals are really trying to find a new birth in which the line of their own life will not be disturbed by a quantity of reacting greater than that which can be experienced without a loss of the sense of continuity of personal existence. The mental health of the individual is laid down by the mother who, because she is devoted to her infant, is able to make active adaptation. This presupposes a basic state of relaxation in the mother, and also an understanding of the individual infant's way of life, which again arises out of her capacity for identification with her infant. This relationship between the mother and the infant starts before the infant is born and is continued in some cases through the birth process and after. As I see it, the trauma of birth is the break in the continuity of the infant's going on being, and when this break is significant the details of the way in which the impingements are sensed, and also of the infant's reaction to them, become in turn significant factors adverse to ego development. In the majority of cases the birth trauma is therefore mildly important and determines a good deal of the general urge towards rebirth. In some cases this adverse factor is so great that the individual has no chance (apart from rebirth in the course of analysis) of making a natural progress in emotional development, even if subsequent external factors are extremely good.

In consideration of the theoretical point of the origin of anxiety it would be a false step to link such a universal phenomenon as anxiety with a special case of birth, birth that is traumatic. It would be logical, however, to attempt to relate anxiety with the *normal* birth experience, but the suggestion is made in this paper that not enough is known yet about the normal birth experiences from the infant's point of view for us to be able to say that there is an intimate relationship between anxiety and normal untraumatic birth. Traumatic birth experience seems to me to determine not so much the pattern of subsequent anxiety as to determine the pattern of subsequent persecution.

Recapitulation

The study of birth trauma is an important study in its own right.

The clues to the understanding of infant psychology, including birth trauma, must come through psycho-analytic experience where regression is a feature. This takes priority over intuitive understanding and even over the objective study of infants and the infant-mother relationship in its early stages.

When birth material turns up in an analysis in a significant way the patient is certainly showing other signs of being in an extremely infantile state. A child may be playing games that contain birth symbolism, and in the same way an adult frequently reports fantasy related consciously or unconsciously to birth. This is *not* the same as the acting out of memory traces derived from birth experience, that which provides the material for study of birth trauma. It is psychotic patients who tend to relive such early infantile phenomena, bypassing fantasy which employs symbols.

I have postulated a *normal birth experience* which is non-traumatic. I have not been able to prove this. Nevertheless in order to clarify my ideas I have assumed the existence of a normal birth experience and have invented two grades of traumatic birth, the one being common, and largely annulled as to its effects by subsequent good management, and the other being definitely traumatic, difficult to counteract even by most careful nursing, and leaving its permanent mark on the individual.

If these assumptions should be found to be justified, there would seem to follow certain theoretical considerations.

Since anxiety is a universal phenomenon it cannot be directly correlated with a special case of birth, namely a traumatic birth.

Perhaps the clue to the well-known fact that there is a relation clinically between anxiety manifestations and the details of birth trauma may be that birth trauma determines the pattern of subsequent persecutions; in this way birth trauma determines *by indirect method* the way in which anxiety manifests itself in certain cases.

A by-product of this theory is that it provides a way of looking at the fairly common congenital, though not inherited, paranoia. The point that I am making is contained in the title of Greenacre's two articles as well as in her text. She writes of a predisposition to anxiety. She does not, however, exactly state that the traumatic birth experience determines the *pattern of expected persecution*. The suggestion is that a traumatic birth experience can determine the existence as well as the pattern of a paranoid disposition. In other words, if one accepts Melanie Klein's theory of paranoid anxiety, in which relief in analysis only comes from a full acceptance on the part of the patient of oral sadism and ambivalence towards the good object, one has to consider what one thinks about the fairly common cases in which the paranoid history dates from birth. My suggestion, which is based on psychoanalytic work, is that in certain cases in which the history goes back to birth, there is so strong a predisposition to ideas of persecution (as well as a set pattern for persecution) that probably the paranoia in such a case is not consequent on oral sadism. In other words, in my opinion there are certain cases of latent paranoia in which the analysis of the paranoia along the lines of recovering the full extent of the oral sadism does not bring about the complete resolution because there is needed in addition a reliving of the traumatic birth experience in the analytic setting. An environmental factor needs to be displaced.

May I be clearly understood? No paranoid case can be analysed by enabling the patient simply to relive the birth trauma. I am only suggesting that in a percentage of paranoid cases there is this additional fact that birth was traumatic, and placed a pattern on the infant of expected interference with basic 'being'. Probably with more experience one could sort these cases out from other paranoid cases according to their clinical picture as well as by very careful history-taking.

In another way I find a link between birth trauma and the psychosomatic disorders, notably certain headaches, and breathing disturbances of various kinds. In this case one could say that the birth trauma can influence the pattern of the hypochondria.

A positive statement can now be made. Freud recognizes a continuity between intra-uterine and extra-uterine life. I think we do not know how much Freud was able to support this intuitive flash from his analytic work. In the very close and detailed observation of one case I have been able to satisfy myself that *the patient was able to bring to the analytic hour, under certain very specialized conditions, a regression of part of the self to an intra-uterine state.* In such a case the to and fro from extra-uterine to intra-uterine existence and back involves experiences that belong to that individual's birth, and this has to be distinguished from the usually more important and more common movement *in fantasy* in and out of the mother's body and in and out of the patient's inner world.

One can certainly assume that from conception onwards the body and the psyche develop together, at first fused and gradually becoming distinguishable the one from the other. Certainly before birth it can be said of the psyche (apart from the soma) that there is a personal going-along, a continuity of experiencing. This continuity, which could be called the beginnings of the self, is periodically interrupted by phases of reaction to impingement. The self begins to include memories of limited phases in which reaction to impingement disturbs the continuity. By the time of birth the infant is prepared for such phases, and my suggestion is that *in the non-traumatic birth the reaction to impingement which birth entails does not exceed that for which the foetus is already prepared.*

It is generally assumed that the new experience of breathing must be traumatic. It is more likely that delay in breathing associated with prolonged birth provides the traumatic factor rather than the initiation of breathing. My psycho-analytic experience makes me think that it is not necessarily true in all cases that the initiation of breathing is significant.

It seems to me that *it is in relation to the border-line of intolerable reaction phases that the intellect begins to work as something distinct from the psyche.* It is as if the intellect collects together the impingements to which there had to be reaction, and holds them in exact detail and sequence, in this way protecting the psyche until there is a return of the continuing-to-exist state. In a rather more traumatic situation the intellect develops excessively and can even seem to become more important than the psyche, and subsequent to birth the intellect can continue to expect and even to go out to meet persecutions so as to collect them and hold them, still with the aim of preserving the psyche. The value of this defence is shown when the individual ultimately comes to analysis, for in the analytic setting we find that carefully collected primary persecutions can be remembered. Then, at long last, the patient can afford to forget them.

I am indebted to Dr Margaret Little for the observation that this may account for the way in which in paranoia scattered persecutions become integrated and organized as in the common clinical picture. The organizing is done by the intellect of the individual in defence of the psyche, and for this reason the organization of scattered persecutions itself is stoutly defended.

A corollary of this is that in some cases there is such a muddle of persecution that the intellect fails to bind and hold the sequence, and in that case instead of enhanced intellect one finds clinically an apparent mental defect, this in spite of the original normal brain tissue development.[6]

It would be possible to develop this subject by a description of the physical sensations belonging to birth trauma which appear in common psychosomatic symptomatology. The important thing, however, is that *for the individual patient the pattern is carefully set,* and also that in the reliving which can occur in the course of psycho-analytic work, a definite sequence in time is maintained. In any analysis of this kind of case one becomes familiar with the sensations and their sequence in so far as they belong to that particular patient.

An important practical point in this connection is the way in which *one thing at a time can be dealt with, whereas two or more factors spell confusion.* One of the main principles of the psycho-analytic technique is that a setting is provided in which the patient can deal with one thing at a time. There is nothing more important in our analytic work than that we try to see what the *one* thing is that the patient is bringing for interpretation or for reliving in any one particular hour. A good analyst confines his interpretations and his actions to the detail exactly presented by the patient. It is bad practice to interpret whatever one feels one understands, acting according to one's own needs, thus spoiling the patient's attempt to cope by dealing with one thing at a time. It seems that this is the more true the further back one gets. The integration of the immature psyche at the time of birth can be strengthened by one experience, even a reaction to impingement, provided it does not last too long. Two impingements, however, require two reactions, and these tear the psyche in half. The ego effort which I have described is an attempt to hold the impingements at bay by mental activity, so that the reactions to them can be allowed one at a time and without disruption of the psyche. All this can be very clearly demonstrated in psycho-analytic work provided one is able to follow the patient right back in emotional development as far as he needs to go, by regression to dependence, in order to get behind the period at which impingements became multiple and unmanageable.

Finally, I repeat that *there is no such thing as treatment by the analysis of birth trauma alone.* To arrive at these early stages one has to have shown to the patient one's competence in the whole range of the ordinary psycho-analytic understanding. Moreover, when the patient has been fully dependent and has started to come forward again, one will require a very sure understanding of the depressive position, and of the gradual development towards genital primacy, and of the dynamics of interpersonal relationships as well as of the urge to attain independence out of dependence.

Notes

1. This part has had to be re-written (1954) as I discovered Greenacre's work after writing and reading this contribution, although much of her work had been published and was available before the date of my contribution.
2. It will be observed that I am now leaving the work of other writers and am making an attempt to state my own position in my own words. I am only too happy when after making my own statement, I find that what I have said has been said previously by others. Often it has been said better, but not better for me.
3. For instance, when I write a paper for this Society on any subject I nearly always find myself dreaming dreams which belong to that subject.
4. I now call this special state of sensitivity in the mother 'Primary maternal preoccupation', 1957. (See 'Primary Maternal Preoccupation' [CW 5:2:16]).
5. Idea developed further in 'Mind and Its Relation to the Psyche-Soma' [CW 3:4:20].
6. See 'Mind and Its Relation to the Psyche-Soma' [CW 3:4:20].

9

Letter to Joan Riviere

Originally published in Rodman, F. R. *Winnicott: Life and work* (pp. 153–155). Cambridge, MA: Perseus, 2003.

Joan Riviere (1883–1962) was a psychoanalyst, supporter, and follower of Melanie Klein, and Winnicott's second analyst. She was a cofounder of the British Society and an early translator of the works of Freud.

19 May 1949

I am sending you a rather long paper at your request.[i] I was unable to get this paper down to proper proportions for reading at the Society, and although I chose from it as I went along, I had to leave the last few pages out, and I should think a fairly chaotic impression was given. At any rate it was decided to give me another chance in a few weeks' time, when I shall be able to pull together the threads of what I did manage to say and finish reading the paper. This should leave time for a long discussion, and I think that a lot of people are wanting to make comments.

The paper I am sending you contains a great deal that I did not read, nor did I intend to read; for instance, the episode of the dream of my own which I had when I was ill, in which the heart took over every other function . . .

At present I am very fit and I am keeping my life down to what I can do without rush and with nice intervals for sleep and wandering in the park.[ii] This I enjoy. It is something new for me to stay calm and be not rushed around. Unfortunately this last fortnight has been disturbed a little by the fact that we were suddenly told at Paddington Green that the hospital was to

---

[i] 'Birth Memories, Birth Trauma, and Anxiety' [CW 3:4:8], which was given to the British Psychoanalytical Society the previous evening, with the discussion continuing on 15 June.

[ii] Winnicott's health was a significant factor at this time: he had heart attacks in 1948 after his father's death, and again in 1949 and 1950.

be closed and reopened as an adult skin and throat hospital. I had to decide whether to fight for the existence of this hospital, which I consider to be a very valuable one to the local community, or to let it slip. I found that a great deal depended on me, and in fact I have had to attend about ten committee meetings dealing with the matter.

The reason why I am mentioning this is because my reading round the subject of this lecture was seriously interfered with by these committees, and I was especially sorry not to be able to make a fuller study of the work of Greenacre, whose three articles on this subject really contain everything that I want to say. The worst part of it was that the vital committee meeting at St Mary's Hospital was timed for 5 o'clock yesterday, and it was my business to represent the hospital, the only other possible person, the present chairman, being away on holiday. The meeting was very tense, and I am glad to say that we managed to get the matter referred back, which was all that we could get the committee to do at 7 o'clock. I had come very near to the end of the somewhat limited capacity of my heart, which is a maddening thing to have to take into consideration when I feel absolutely well. I was able to rest a little, but at the meeting I was all the time conscious of being near to the limit of my present capacity. This spoilt my enjoyment of the evening, and probably made me rather bad at choosing what to leave out.

However, I believe the Society somehow or other managed to get something out of what I said. I certainly got something out of it myself, and now feel that in a year's time, when I try to write this out as a paper with the co-operation of two patients who are too ill to co-operate at the moment, I shall start from a firmer foundation through having made this first attempt.

Letter to Roger Money-Kyrle

Roger Money-Kyrle (1898–1980) was a British psychoanalyst and follower of Melanie Klein. The six letters to Money-Kyrle in 1949 and 1950 [CW 3:4:10; CW 3:4:12; CW 3:4:13; CW 3:5:9; CW 3:5:11; CW 3:5:13] discuss the possibility of Winnicott preparing a paper for publication in Melanie Klein's 'birthday book', which became the *International Journal of Psychoanalysis* issue of 1952 and was later revised and expanded into *New Directions in Psychoanalysis*, 1955.

13 June 1949

Dear Money-Kyrle,

I am very grateful indeed to be asked to co-operate in the preparation of a book to commemorate Mrs. Klein's 70th birthday. It is very difficult to know what to offer. I would like at this stage, however, to say that I feel very inclined to tackle a subject which is not on your list, namely, the Classification of Environmental Factors. I feel that it is important that this should be done because it is so often thought that Mrs. Klein ignores environmental factors, which of course is absurd. At first she had to fight for the importance of the internal factors because the extreme child guidance view of twenty years ago was finding support from the Viennese child analysis group.

At any rate I would like you to consider putting this somewhere in the programme and to consider asking me to tackle this. I can already begin to show you the method which I should adopt. Obviously the classification has to be based on the classification of individual needs.

Yours sincerely,
D. W. Winnicott

11

Notes on the Discussion Held on Dr Winnicott's Paper 'The Birth Trauma'

'Birth Memories, Birth Trauma, and Anxiety' [CW 3:4:8] was given to the British Psychoanalytical Society on 18 May 1949, and the discussion continued at the subsequent Scientific Meeting, 15 June. These typed notes include several pages of Winnicott's own remarks, before moving on to a report of the general discussion.

16 June 1949

Dr Gillespie said that he wondered whether anything could be done in the way of observation from outside comparable with the correlations between the breast feeding and subsequent behaviour made by G . . . He asked whether there was any clinical picture which one could expect to be correlated with birth trauma.

Answer That Might Have Been Made

I feel that I am not yet in a position to answer this question although it interests me very much. It seems to me that if in one group of such cases an apparently successful and acceptable person begins to seek treatment one can see that there is something disturbing the individual and one can get the flavour of paranoia although recognising the value and in many ways health of the individual. On analysis, however, if the person comes to analysis, one finds that there is a very powerful paranoid organisation which has been latent. In such an analysis one is astonished by the intensity of the illness when one meets it, which is in such contrast with the opinion that is held of the same individual in ordinary life. At the other extreme there seem to me to be certain cases of fairly frank paranoia in which, however, the person manages to be sane but is compelled to seek and meet a succession of actual persecutions or alternatively he (or she) complains continuously of headaches and breathing disorders and so on. In other words, this individual is ill and one can see the paranoid organisation that underlies the illness, but still the case is not a frank paranoid insanity.

I imagine that in all these cases a more detailed early infancy history would support the diagnosis of a disturbance at an early level. It is this point that interests me so very much because in taking histories of timid and more frankly paranoid child cases in a certain proportion one finds that the troubles go right back to the first few days of life, if not to the very beginning. In such cases one would have to postulate a very powerful inherited factor were it not for the possibility that there is this very important early environmental disturbance which has made me use the word congenital (but not inherited) paranoia. I really feel extremely diffident about all these suggestions that I made in my paper, and in any case I am only too well aware that I did not properly bring my views into relationship with the accepted views. To do this requires a good deal of work and I am not prepared at present to devote more than a certain amount of time to one limited subject in this huge field of ours. In any case I feel that Greenacre has made a very wide survey.

Dr Heimann referred to the normal birth, if it exists, and the way in which it might follow on a preparation for impingement and reaction to impingement, the preparation having been started in intrauterine life. In other words, she was exploring the possibilities mentioned in the paper that the birth process, if fairly normal, and within range of the phases of disturbances already expected, might be actually a valuable experience, for the infant. She also referred to the way in which refugees coming in distress from Germany found themselves reborn and for a time being were notoriously in a paranoid condition. She felt that this transfer from one life to another might have seemed to them like a compulsory reliving of the birth situation followed by a sensitivity to persecution comparable to that of the baby born with more or less trauma.

Dr Winnicott took up this matter of the temporary paranoid phases of refugees and linked it with other phenomena equally well known, such as the need for soldiers returning from prison camps to be given special conditions for a time being in which they could recover, they too being liable to experiences of temporary paranoid phases. Children who have been in a pathological introverted state regularly, on recovery from this, which is a kind of self-imprisonment, show paranoid reactions which require special management if the passage is to be made through to extraversion and to the ordinary state in which neither introversion nor extraversion is obligatory. He pointed out that in the analysis of such cases there would be found to be much complex psychology belonging to later stages of emotional development, but he felt that in some cases a full understanding would not come without the inclusion of the original apparently paranoid phase following traumatic birth. He referred here to the need which is very great when an infant has been born with difficulty for an initial period of very quiet handling. This is not always recognised. It was illustrated by the dream referred to in the paper in which the patient's skin was burned all over and she was covered with gravel. Removal of the gravel would be intolerable and she expected it. Nevertheless oil was poured over the gravel and she was left alone for three weeks, after which everything could be taken away without trouble because the skin had healed. This dream represented the new hope that this patient had because of analysis, because she felt that the analyst would respect the terrible sensitivity that followed the birth process in her case.

Dr Winnicott referred to the writing of Lady Pennington in 'Advice to her daughters in 1824'. Here was a most astonishing understanding of infant needs derived not from the study of psychology but from an innate ability on the part of a mother to feel herself into her infant's position. One of the things she recommended her daughter was that after the birth of a baby someone should hold the baby absolutely quiet for half an hour.

Dr Scott quoted from Greenacre's article and referred especially to her description of pre-natal narcissism as a libidinal component of growth. He referred to the continuity which he had also described as a going-alongness which referred to both time and space. He added to the idea of awareness of phases and of pressure an awareness of movements, of muscle erotism, of posture and shape.

Dr Winnicott suggested that it might be better to refer to a libidinal component of existing rather than of growth because of the uncertainty that there is in awareness of growth itself.

Dr Scott gave psycho-analytic Illustrations of the very close feeling that the pregnant mother can have towards the end of her time for the infant so that she is as much aware of the infant's body and posture and position and movements as if she were the infant and in her dreams she can show that she can be as much the infant as the mother.

Later Dr Wilson gave a case illustrating the way in which the father can be involved in the same way even when living at a distance.

Dr Winnicott took up this point and said that he felt it was important because it was one of the ways of saying that the proper person to look after a new-born infant is the mother. Only she can get into the state of knowing exactly what is the infant's position and what are the infant's needs to be able to make the 100% adaptation which is required. Only the mother of the infant can know things like the infant's great need to be held quietly for a period of time after birth, for instance. On routine questioning of ordinary mothers attending Paddington Green Children's Hospital he finds that mothers insist that they prefer to be conscious at the time of the infant's birth. Sometimes in the description of an infant's needs by psycho-analysts there creeps in the idea that at the beginning anyone is good enough who does the job well. The point is, however, that no-one can do the job well enough except the mother because no-one other than the mother can have the degree of sensitivity to the infant's needs which is required at the beginning.

Dr Rosenberg referred to her recent paper and to the value of sorting out primary from secondary anxiety. She felt that it would not be useful to follow Dr Winnicott's line and to think of anxiety at a later stage as something qualitatively different from psychotic anxiety or the anxieties belonging to disintegration and comparable phenomena. The concept of primary and secondary anxiety contained the relationship between the two. In secondary anxiety, however, there is the defensive quality referred to by Freud, who points out that anxiety is a useful function enabling the individual to avoid what Dr Rosenberg has described as primary anxiety.

Letter to Roger Money-Kyrle

Roger Money-Kyrle (1898–1980) was a British psychoanalyst and follower of Melanie Klein.

22 June 1949

Dear Money-Kyrle,

Thank you for you further letter about the Birthday book.[i] I would like to co-operate in whatever way you and Paula Heimann feel would be best, and I am so keen that the book should be a really good one that I should be perfectly willing to submit one or two trial papers for you to consider in relation to the rest of the book. It would be important to know just how urgent the matter is. Probably you would like to know where you are by the end of the summer?

You will understand that if someone else felt like doing the Environmental thing I would only be too glad. Also when I come to write about psychosis I am terribly aware that Scott is miles ahead of anything I can do on this subject. I think the only thing to do is for me to go ahead along the lines you suggest, and then let the matter of decision as to whether it is suitable for the book or not rest with the Editors.

With good wishes,
Yours,
D. W. Winnicott

---

[i] See also letters [CW 3:4:10; CW 3:4:13; CW 3:5:9; CW 3:5:11; CW 3:5:13].

13

Letter to Roger Money-Kyrle

Roger Money-Kyrle (1898–1980) was a British psychoanalyst and follower of Melanie Klein.

24 June 1949

Dear Money-Kyrle,

Thank you for your further letter, which does not need to be answered except in regard to the last detail. I cannot see how tension in the Society could be increased in any way that one ought to avoid increasing it by the publication of this book. It seems to me usual for a 70th Birthday book[i] to be got together by colleagues. I should think that an official book at the present time would have to be spoilt by the need for the official policy to avoid treading on people's corns. I suppose the whole thing is open to argument, but you might like to have my view.

Yours,
D. W. Winnicott

---

[i] See also letters [CW 3:4:10; CW 3:4:12; CW 3:5:9; CW 3:5:11; CW 3:5:13].

14

Letter to Joan Riviere

[Excerpts] Originally published in Rodman, F. R. *Winnicott: Life and work* (pp. 155–156) Cambridge, MA: Perseus, 2003.

Joan Riviere (1883–1962) was a psychoanalyst, supporter, and follower of Melanie Klein, and Winnicott's second analyst. Riviere was also a cofounder of the British Society and an early translator of the works of Freud.

24 June 1949

... M's relation to you was undoubtedly very disturbed and one could say that M is only just coming round into being able to be a human being in your presence.[i] You might of course have got round this by taking what M had to say and seeing what there was that was good or bad in it and pointing out M's deficiencies. Probably the method that you adopted was the better one, by which I think you told M what to do and rather expected M to put it into practice. This method, however, had to generate difficulties because of the particular quality of M's mother's attitude towards M in which M was dominated and had no other method but to be dominated from early infancy, the mother being a teacher and not being able to stop teaching or to do anything much else ...

There was no question of your being asked to do this supervision in order that I should avoid the negative mother transference. You have suggested this in conversation with me, and I want to make it quite clear that this suggestion is not founded on fact. It is important for me that you should understand that this is so because I do not like to be misunderstood, especially by yourself. Dr Heimann has also expressed a view that I try to avoid the negative transference, especially the transference in which I am the bad mother ...

---

[i] M was a candidate for membership at the British Psychoanalytical Society who was in analysis with Winnicott and had consulted Riviere for supervision.

I think the misunderstanding . . . comes from my pointing out that in the treatment of a severely regressed patient the analyst needs to adapt to the regression of the patient. It is easy to feel that I am saying that the analyst has to be a good mother if the patient is a small infant. What I really do say, however, is not that, but it is that in the transference situation when the patient is in the very early stages of infancy the analyst is in the role of the devoted mother. This is quite different from good mother. In fact it antedates a splitting of the good and bad mother. It pays tribute to the fact that at the beginning the infant is absolutely dependent on the devotion of a mother figure, without which the very early stages of emotional development cannot be made.[ii]

> . . . With good wishes

[ii] F. R. Rodman (2003) reported that Winnicott went on to argue in this letter that supervisors should be more concerned with the teaching of the candidate than the progress of the case itself. Winnicott stated his difference of opinion with Riviere regarding the candidate's ability and went on to insist that he had the authority to judge when the candidate was ready to undertake the case in question at the right moment and not too early.

15

Review: *Handbook of Child Guidance*

EDITED BY ERNEST HARMS (NEW YORK: CHILD CARE PUBLICATIONS, 1947)

Review originally published in *British Medical Journal*, 6 August 1949, 2(4622), 321.

Dr Ernest Harms has gathered together many workers in child guidance; each has written on some aspect of theory or practice; and the result is a book of 751 pages of beautiful paper.

Every feature is covered: one wonders whether any more need ever be written on the subject. It may be that from now on the matter of child guidance must be considered closed. Every library should have this volume on its shelves, and there are probably people who, unlike this reviewer, love to read books of 751 pages which cover everything.

I have looked through the pages for annoying features and obvious errors, and I cannot find any. The English is clear and good. There is even an attempt to present Freud's and Jung's theories which must be described as serious. Frances G. Wickes's chapter on Jung's theories is one of the best. Beside this there are references to Anna Freud's work, and there are attempts to state or evaluate a few of Melanie Klein's concepts.

I have also looked for an original idea, and the fact that I have not found one must not be taken as meaning anything. Such volumes can easily be burial grounds for new ideas. In any case the book remains a monument to the personal drive of Dr Harms.

16

Letter to *The Times*

PUNISHMENT AND CRIME: A PSYCHOLOGIST'S VIEW

Originally published in *The Times*, issue 51467 (p. 6); also published in Rodman, F. R. (Ed.), *The spontaneous gesture. Selected letters of D. W. Winnicott* (Letter 12, pp. 15–16). Cambridge, MA: Harvard University Press, 1987.

10 August 1949

Sir: In your faithful reporting of public affairs you have published several reports, comments and letters in this past week on juvenile delinquency and on the management of Holloway Gaol and on the knotty problem of crime and insanity. It is very seldom that the comments of a psycho-analyst are asked for or printed; instead it is assumed that the psychologist has an attitude, probably a sentimental one. The idea that psycho-analysis has no attitude, but that it can enlighten, seldom percolates.

There is a great danger in the present trend, which some of us predicted. A sentimental swing toward the antisocial child or adult must sooner or later be followed by a reaction. Indeed the sentimentalist in regard to crime is using the criminal for the expression of his own hidden criminality, and is in the same position (but less openly so) as the ordinary man or woman who enjoys crime in the Sunday papers or who reads detective stories. The practice of the Courts must be founded on something more sure than sentimentalism, either on the deep feelings of unsentimental people who can reach to the criminal in themselves, or else on the thinking-out of those who can take into account the unconscious.

There is a very real contribution which psycho-analysis could make, even now, if it were asked to do so. One example could be given right away, and perhaps usefully given. It is this:

Whatever the state of the criminal, old or young, sane or insane, male or female, there is another half of every antisocial act to be considered—society's revenge feelings.

Now public revenge is not necessarily felt in respect of each individual antisocial act, but unpunished misdemeanour or crime swells the reservoir of unconscious public revenge, and unless this revenge is expressed periodically it will come out in some ugly form. The main function of legal procedure is the prevention of lynch-law, which always hangs round the corner even in this country where (because of the success of legal procedure) it is never seen. I have found this view is an extremely unpopular one especially among the sentimentalists in the penal reform movement. The public must be avenged.

What about public education? Cannot the public be educated to see the criminal as an ill person? The answer is that in so far as men and women are conscious of their feelings they can be educated to whatever is truly discovered about the psychology of crime. But people are not like that, and groups of people have always a large central core that is unconscious, and to a large extent unavailable to consciousness even with the help which poets, artists, and philosophers can give those who allow time for that help to operate.

In other words there is a limit to the capacity for each one of us to become fully educated even to what we know to be true. There must therefore always be two points of view. The doctor (psychoanalyst) will surely be more and more liable as time goes on to say: this antisocial child or adult is antisocial because ill. And then the law must follow on by considering how far public (unconscious) feeling needs punishment to be given, regardless of the psychiatric diagnosis.

Only if this simple separation of the two points of view can be made and maintained can the physician of the psyche hope to retain the opportunity to study the antisocial individual as an ill person and to present that point of view when asked!

I am,
Yours etc.
D. W. Winnicott, F.R.C.P.

17

Letter to R. S. Hazlehurst

Originally published in Rodman, F. R. (Ed.), *The spontaneous gesture. Selected letters of D. W. Winnicott* (Letter 13, p. 17). Cambridge, MA: Harvard University Press, 1987.

R. S. Hazlehurst was a British minister who responded to Winnicott's letter to the *Times*, 10 August 1949, 'Punishment and Crime, a Psychologist's View' [CW 3:4:16].

1 September 1949

Dear Mr Hazlehurst:

Thank you for your letter about mine to the Times. I like your classification into two essentials and two accidentals.

It would interest you, I am sure, how in psycho-analytic and also ordinary psycho-therapeutic work, especially with children, the anti-social compulsions come out as symptoms of illness. Especially at their earliest stages it is often quite clear that stealing is an unwelcome thing turning up in the life of the child and bewildering him (or her). Soon, as the child does not understand why he must steal, there comes about a hardening and a whole host of secondary motives, and by that time there is almost no hope of effecting a cure. In the early stages we do seem to bring about a cure in many cases.

Stealing has practically no more relation to poverty and want than civil murder has to persecution.

Yours truly,
D. W. Winnicott

18

Letter to S. H. Hodge

Originally published in Rodman, F. R. (Ed.), *The spontaneous gesture. Selected letters of D. W. Winnicott* (Letter 14, pp. 17–19), Cambridge, MA: Harvard University Press, 1987.

S. H. Hodge was a British minister who responded to Winnicott's letter to the *Times*, 10 August 1949, 'Punishment and Crime, a Psychologist's View' [CW 3:4:16].

1 September 1949

Dear Mr Hodge:

Thank you for writing to me about my letter printed in the Times. I am interested in what you say.

You will easily understand that in my view the punishment of crime has nothing to do with doing the criminal good. He should really be treated as ill, if the community could allow it, which it can only do to some extent. It could allow it more if there were knowledge and facilities available for *successful* treatments, but it does not interest the public unconscious that criminal symptoms could be treated, i.e. theoretically could be treated.

Your point about the value to the criminal of expiation and propitiation is an immensely interesting one. To some extent the criminal comes in (as a member of society) in his relief at punishment for (even his own) crime. Nevertheless psychology must diverge from the theological view here because the latter have not yet (I feel) been adjusted to the new findings in respect of the unconscious.

We regularly find that at the start of anti-social tendencies in a human being (always in childhood) there is an ordinary strong sense of guilt which (as part of the illness) does not become attached to stealing (or whatever the symptom is) because the individual becomes split. Help given at this point enables the patient to become conscious of a great deal of the conflict and so to reintegrate and to become able to feel guilty about the stealing.

As an example, a child may start stealing because of a feeling of loss of being loved, without knowing at all what is happening. When asked why do you steal, he at first says, truthfully, that he does not know. If the question is repeated he invents reasons rather than feel an ass, or mad, and then (lest the question be asked again) he steals for definite reasons, which he knows. But this third stage is part of a process of hardening. There is no guilt feeling available because the whole thing has become a defensive construction. To reach the guilt one has to get to the individual's original conflict which was there before the stealing started and before he felt a loss of being loved, in fact to that which is common to all human beings: the destructive ideas in the original love impulses. At any stage later than this the individual feels no guilt and in any case his symptom is a reaction to environmental failure—a weakness in the framework life should provide for the developing individual.

I think that in your work you have to take people as they are, apart from their developmental history; also you have to leave out consideration of the repressed unconscious. These two things hamper your work a great deal as in a way you can only deal with the healthy (psychiatrically) personality; yet it is so often the rather unhealthy person who needs help. And it will be many decades before there are enough psycho-therapists competent to help people by freeing their unconscious and with it (in many cases) their guilt feelings and in a more positive sense their sense of concern.

I do hope what I have said may help a little in your understanding of my point of view.

Yours truly,
D. W. Winnicott

Letter to the *British Medical Journal*

PADDINGTON GREEN CHILDREN'S HOSPITAL

Originally published in *British Medical Journal*, 2 (4629), 711.

24 September 1949

Sir: The Paddington Green Children's Hospital is to be closed down. I think that this news should be widely spread, and I ask you to allow me to give my personal view of this, which I consider to be a tragedy.

The following general facts should be advertised, if only that they can be corrected if wrongly stated. After the war the idea was spread around that the small hospitals would not survive unless they got under the wing of larger institutions. Reluctantly, Paddington Green allowed itself to be taken over by St Mary's, with which teaching hospital it had always been on the friendliest terms. Since it was taken over there has been a happy experience of co-operation between the parent and the adopted child. Subsequently St Mary's took over other hospitals, including the Princess Louise Hospital for Children.

Suddenly the St Mary's Hospital Board announced its intention of destroying Paddington Green and of using its walls as the basis for a new wing for the care of adult skin and throat cases. In the printed statement (marked 'confidential' for some reason not given) it is made clear that regional needs are not under consideration, but only the needs of St Mary's as an undergraduate teaching hospital. Apparently someone at St Mary's has blundered, and more children's beds have been taken over than are specified as minimum requirements in the Goodenough Report.[i] The board's way out is to destroy one of the

---

[i] A report of the Interdepartmental Committee on Medical Schools, under the chairmanship of Sir William Goodenough, published by the Ministry of Health in 1944.

two children's hospitals adopted and so make the numbers of skin and throat beds add up nicely. No mention is made of out-patient and casualty needs.

This state of affairs must surely interest the profession and also the general public. The teaching of medical students is apparently a matter of compliance with the Goodenough recommendations, and it is not a matter of letting students feel that the direct needs of the public are also important.

It is not for us to praise our own hospital, but who will defend it if we do not do so? I personally think that mothers and children get excellent service at Paddington Green, and 39,000 mothers bring their children to the hospital every year. No alternative provision whatever is to be made for these mothers. Certainly these 78,000 persons (mothers and children) cannot be wanted in the terribly overcrowded out-patient department at St Mary's.

As my specialty is towards the psychological side, I can perhaps say that the physical paediatrics practised by my colleagues is as good as any. Moreover, the parents and children are treated as human beings. Any children's hospital is a very specialized affair. The matron, the nurses, the dispenser, the almoner, the telephone girl are all there because mothers and children interest them. The special departments are adapted to the handling of parents and children. Such an institution cannot be created suddenly. Paddington Green has been 80 years in the making. Many of the parents came to the hospital when they were children themselves. Locally, a children's hospital has a value even when it is not used, as a place that is known and that can be used in case of doubt or emergency.

It seems to me that it is a disgrace and a very irresponsible thing that a teaching hospital board should come to a decision like this without reference to local out-patient needs. I feel that if the scheme is carried through the reputation of St Mary's will suffer for a long time, both locally and generally in the profession.

I am near enough to the end of my service to Paddington Green to be able to publish my personal view without its being thought that I am just annoyed about my personal loss. As a matter of fact I do feel annoyed and insulted—in fact, we have all been stunned. This was one of those things that could not happen, the destruction of a good thing and for a paltry reason.

There seems to be no way of getting this matter brought into the open except in your invaluable correspondence columns.—I am, etc.,

London, W.1.   D. W. WINNICOTT

20

Mind and Its Relation to the Psyche-Soma

Originally published in *British Journal of Medical Psychology*, 1954, 27(4), 201–209. Also published in *Collected papers: Through paediatrics to psycho-analysis* (pp. 243–254). London: Tavistock, 1958.

Read before the Medical Section of the British Psychological Society on 14 December 1949 and revised October 1953.

To ascertain what exactly comprises the irreducible mental elements, particularly those of a dynamic nature, constitutes in my opinion one of our most fascinating final aims. These elements would necessarily have a somatic and probably a neurological equivalent, and in that way we should by scientific method have closely narrowed the age-old gap between mind and body. I venture to predict that then the antithesis which has baffled all the philosophers will be found to be based on an illusion. In other words, *I do not think that the mind really exists as an entity*—possibly a startling thing for a psychologist to say [my italics]. When we talk of the mind influencing the body or the body influencing the mind we are merely using a convenient shorthand for a more cumbrous phrase . . . (Jones, 1946)

This quotation by Scott (1949) stimulated me to try to sort out my own ideas on this vast and difficult subject. The body scheme with its temporal and spatial aspects provides a valuable statement of the individual's diagram of himself, and in it I believe there is no obvious place for the mind. Yet in clinical practice we do meet with the mind as an entity localized somewhere by the patient; a further study of the paradox that 'mind does not really exist as an entity' is therefore necessary.

Mind as a Function of Psyche-Soma

To study the concept of mind one must always be studying an individual, a total individual, and including the development of that individual from the very beginning of psychosomatic existence. If one accepts this discipline then one can study the mind of an individual as it specializes out from the psyche part of the psyche-soma.

The mind does not exist as an entity in the individual's scheme of things provided the individual psyche-soma or body scheme has come satisfactorily through the very early developmental stages; mind is then no more than a special case of the functioning of the psyche-soma.

In the study of a developing individual the mind will often be found to be developing a *false entity,* and a *false localization*. A study of these abnormal tendencies must precede the more direct examination of the mind-specialization of the healthy or normal psyche.

We are quite used to seeing the two words mental and physical opposed and would not quarrel with their being opposed in daily conversation. It is quite another matter, however, if the concepts are opposed in scientific discussion.

The use of these two words physical and mental in describing disease leads us into trouble immediately. The psychosomatic disorders, half-way between the mental and the physical, are in a rather precarious position. Research into psychosomatics is being held up, to some extent, by the muddle to which I am referring (MacAlpine, 1952). Also, neuro-surgeons are doing things to the normal or healthy brain in an attempt to alter or even improve mental states. These 'physical' therapists are completely at sea in their theory; curiously enough they seem to be leaving out the importance of the physical body, of which the brain is an integral part.

Let us attempt, therefore, to think of the developing individual, starting at the beginning. Here is a body, and the psyche and the soma are not to be distinguished except according to the direction from which one is looking. One can look at the developing body or at the developing psyche. I suppose the word psyche here means the *imaginative elaboration of somatic parts, feelings, and functions,* that is, of physical aliveness. We know that this imaginative elaboration is dependent on the existence and the healthy functioning of the brain, especially certain parts of it. The psyche is not, however, felt by the individual to be localized in the brain, or indeed to be localized anywhere.

Gradually the psyche and the soma aspects of the growing person become involved in a process of mutual interrelation. This interrelating of the psyche with the soma constitutes an early phase of individual development (see Primitive Emotional Development [CW 2:7:8]). At a later stage the live body, with its limits, and with an inside and an outside, is *felt by the individual* to form the core for the imaginative self. The development to this stage is extremely complex, and although this development may possibly be fairly complete by the time a baby has been born a few days, there is a vast opportunity for distortion of the natural course of development in these respects. Moreover, whatever applies to very early stages also applies to some extent to all stages, even to the stage that we call adult maturity.

Theory of Mind

On the basis of these preliminary considerations I find myself putting forward a theory of mind. This theory is based on work with analytic patients who have needed to regress to an extremely early level of development in the transference. In this paper I shall only give one piece of illustrative clinical material, but the theory can, I believe, be found to be valuable in our daily analytic work.

Let us assume that health in the early development of the individual entails *continuity of being*. The early psyche-soma proceeds along a certain line of development provided its *continuity of being is not disturbed*; in other words, for the healthy development of the early psyche-soma there is a need for a *perfect* environment. At first the need is absolute.

The perfect environment is one which *actively adapts* to the needs of the newly formed psyche-soma, that which we as observers know to be the infant at the start. A bad environment is bad because by failure to adapt it becomes an *impingement* to which the psyche-soma (i.e. the infant) must *react*. This reacting disturbs the continuity of the going-on-being of the new individual. In its beginnings the good (psychological) environment is a physical one, with the child in the womb or being held and generally tended; only in the course of time does the environment develop a new characteristic which necessitates a new descriptive term, such as emotional or psychological or social. Out of this emerges the ordinary good mother with her ability to make active adaptation to her infant's needs arising out of her devotion, made possible by her narcissism, her imagination, and her memories, which enable her to know through identification what are her baby's needs.

The need for a good environment, which is absolute at first, rapidly becomes relative. *The ordinary good mother is good enough*. If she is *good enough* the infant becomes able to allow for her deficiencies by mental activity. This applies to meeting not only instinctual impulses but also all the most primitive types of ego need, even including the need for negative care or an alive neglect. The mental activity of the infant turns a *good-enough* environment into a perfect environment, that is to say, turns relative failure of adaptation into adaptive success. What releases the mother from her need to be near-perfect is the infant's understanding. In the ordinary course of events the mother tries not to introduce complications beyond those which the infant can understand and allow for; in particular she tries to insulate her baby from coincidences and from other phenomena that must be beyond the infant's ability to comprehend. In a general way she keeps the world of the infant as simple as possible.

The mind, then, has as one of its roots a variable functioning of the psyche-soma, one concerned with the threat to continuity of being that follows any failure of (active) environmental adaptation. It follows that mind-development is very much influenced by factors not specifically personal to the individual, including chance events.

In infant care it is vitally important that mothers, at first physically, and soon also imaginatively, can start off by supplying this active adaptation, but also it is a characteristic maternal function to provide *graduated failure of adaptation,* according to the growing ability of the individual infant to allow for relative failure by mental activity, or by understanding. Thus there appears in the infant a tolerance in respect of both ego need and instinctual tension.

It could perhaps be shown that mothers are released slowly by infants who eventually are found to have a low I.Q. On the other hand, an infant with an exceptionally good brain, eventually giving a high I.Q., releases the mother earlier.

According to this theory then, in the development of every individual, the mind has a root, perhaps its most important root, in the need of the individual, at the core of the self, for a perfect environment. In this connection, I might refer to my view of psychosis as an environmental deficiency disease (see Psychoses and Child Care [CW 4:1:5]). There are certain developments of this theory which seem to me to be important. Certain kinds of failure on the part of the mother, especially erratic behaviour, produce over-activity of the mental functioning. Here, in the overgrowth of the mental function reactive to erratic mothering, we see that there can develop an opposition between the mind and the psyche-soma, since in reaction to this abnormal environmental state the thinking of the individual begins to take over and organize the caring for the psyche-soma, whereas in health it is the function of the environment to do this. In health the mind does not usurp the environment's function, but makes possible an understanding and eventually a making use of its relative failure.

The gradual process whereby the individual becomes able to care for the self belongs to later stages in individual emotional development, stages that must be reached in due course, at the pace that is set by natural developmental forces.

To go a stage further, one might ask what happens if the strain that is put on mental functioning organized in defence against a tantalizing early environment is greater and greater? One would expect confusional states, and (in the extreme) mental defect of the kind that is not dependent on brain-tissue deficiency. As a more common result of the lesser degrees of tantalizing infant care in the earliest stages we find *mental functioning becoming a thing in itself,* practically replacing the good mother and making her unnecessary. Clinically, this can go along with dependence on the actual mother and a false personal growth on a compliance basis. This is a most uncomfortable state of affairs, especially because the psyche of the individual gets 'seduced' away into this mind from the intimate relationship which the psyche originally had with the soma. The result is a mind-psyche, which is pathological.

A person who is developing in this way displays a distorted pattern affecting all later stages of development. For instance, one can observe a tendency for easy identification with the environmental aspect of all relationships that involve dependence, and a difficulty in identification with the dependent individual. Clinically one may see such a person develop into one who is a *marvellously good mother to others* for a limited period; in fact a person who has developed along these lines may have almost magical *healing properties* because of an extreme capacity to make active adaptation to primitive needs. The falsity of these patterns for expression of the personality, however, becomes evident in practice. Breakdown threatens or occurs, because what the individual is all the time needing is *to find someone else* who will make real this 'good environment' concept, so that the individual may return to the dependent psyche-soma which forms the only place to live from. In this case, 'without mind' becomes a desired state.

There cannot of course be a direct partnership between the mind-psyche and the body of the individual. But the *mind-psyche* is localized by the individual, and is placed either inside the head or outside it in some special relation to the head, and this provides an important source for headache as a symptom.

The question has to be asked why the head should be the place inside which the mind tends to become localized by the individual, and I do not know the answer. I feel that an important point is the individual's need to localize the mind because it is an enemy, that is to say, for control of it. A schizoid patient tells me that the head is the place to put the mind because, *as the head cannot be seen by oneself,* it does not obviously exist as part of oneself. Another point is that the head has special experiences during the birth process, but in order to make full use of this latter fact I must go on to consider another type of mental functioning which can be specially activated during the birth process. This is associated with the word 'memorizing'.

As I have said, the continuity of being of the developing psyche-soma (internal and external relationships) is disturbed by reactions to environmental impingements, in other words by the results of failures of the environment to make active adaptation. By my theory a rapidly increasing amount of reaction to impingement disturbing continuity of psyche-soma becomes expected and allowed for according to mental capacity. Impingements demanding *excessive* reactions (according to the next part of my theory) cannot be allowed for. All that can happen apart from confusion is that the reactions can be *catalogued.*[1]

Typically at birth there is apt to be an excessive disturbance of continuity because of reactions to impingements, and the mental activity which I am describing at the moment is that which is concerned with exact memorizing during the birth process. In my psycho-analytic work I sometimes meet with regressions fully under control and yet going back to prenatal life. Patients regressed in an ordered way go over the birth process again and again, and I have been astonished by the convincing proof that I have had that an infant during the birth process not only memorizes every reaction disturbing the continuity of being, but also appears to memorize these in the correct order. I have not used hypnosis, but I am aware of the comparable discoveries, less convincing to me, that are achieved through use of hypnosis. Mental functioning of the type that I am describing, which might be called memorizing or cataloguing, can be extremely active and accurate at the time of a baby's birth. I shall illustrate this by details from a case, but first I want to make clear my point that *this type of mental functioning is an encumbrance to the psyche-soma*, or to the individual human being's continuity of being which constitutes the self. The individual may be able to make use of it to relive the birth process in play or in a carefully controlled analysis. But this cataloguing type of mental functioning acts like a foreign body if it is associated with environmental adaptive failure that is beyond understanding or prediction.

No doubt in health it may happen that the environmental factors are held fixed by this method until the individual is able to make them his own after having experienced libidinous and especially aggressive drives, which can be projected. In this way, and it is essentially a false way, the individual gets to feel responsible for the bad environment for which in fact he was not responsible and which he could (if he knew) justly blame on the world because it disturbed the continuity of his innate developmental processes before the psyche-soma had become sufficiently well organized to hate or to love. Instead of hating these environmental failures the individual became disorganized by them because the process existed prior to hating.

Clinical Illustration

The following fragment of a case history is given to illustrate my thesis. Out of several years' intensive work it is notoriously difficult to choose a detail; nevertheless, I include this fragment in order to show that what I am putting forward is very much a part of daily practice with patients.

> A woman[2] who is now 47 years old had made what seemed to others but not to herself to be a good relationship to the world and had always been able to earn her own living. She had achieved a good education and was generally liked; in fact I think she was never actively disliked. She herself,

however, felt completely dissatisfied, as if always aiming to find herself and never succeeding. Suicidal ideas were certainly not absent but they were kept at bay by her belief which dated from childhood that she would ultimately solve her problem and find herself. She had had a so-called 'classical' analysis for several years but somehow the core of her illness had been unchanged. With me it soon became apparent that this patient must make a very severe regression or else give up the struggle. I therefore followed the regressive tendency, letting it take the patient wherever it led; eventually the regression reached the limit of the patient's need, and since then there has been a natural progression with the true self instead of a false self in action.

For the purpose of this paper I choose for description one thing out of an enormous amount of material. In the patient's previous analysis there had been incidents in which the patient had thrown herself off the couch in an hysterical way. These episodes had been interpreted along ordinary lines for hysterical phenomena of this kind. In the deeper regression of this new analysis light was thrown on the meaning of these falls. In the course of the two years of analysis with me the patient has repeatedly regressed to an early stage which was certainly prenatal. The birth process had to be relived, and eventually I recognized how this patient's unconscious need to relive the birth process underlay what had previously been an hysterical falling off the couch.

A great deal could be said about all this, but the important thing from my point of view here is that evidently every detail of the birth experience had been retained, and not only that, but the details had been retained in the exact sequence of the original experience. A dozen or more times the birth process was relived and each time the reaction to one of the major external features of the original birth process was singled out for re-experiencing.

Incidentally, these relivings illustrated one of the main functions of acting out; by acting out the patient informed herself of the bit of psychic reality which was difficult to get at at the moment, but of which the patient so acutely needed to become aware. I will enumerate some of the acting-out patterns, but unfortunately I cannot give the sequence which nevertheless I am quite sure was significant.

> The breathing changes to be gone over in most elaborate detail.
> The constrictions passing down the body to be relived and so remembered.
> The birth from the fantasy inside of the belly of the mother, who was a depressive, unrelaxed person.
> The changeover from not feeding to feeding from the breast, and then from the bottle.
> The same with the addition that the patient had sucked her thumb in the womb and on coming out had to have the fist in relation to the

breast or bottle, thus making continuity between object relationships within and without.
- The severe experience of pressure on the head, and also the extreme of awfulness of the release of pressure on the head; during which phase, unless her head were held, she could not have endured the re-enactment.
- There is much which is not yet understood in this analysis about the bladder functions affected by the birth process.
- The changeover from pressure all round (which belongs to the intra-uterine state) to pressure from underneath (which belongs to the extra-uterine state). Pressure if not excessive means love. After birth therefore she was loved on the under side only, and unless turned round periodically became confused.

Here I must leave out perhaps a dozen other factors of comparable significance.

> Gradually the re-enactment reached the worst part. When we were nearly there, there was the anxiety of having the head crushed. This was first got under control by the patient's identification with the crushing mechanism. This was a dangerous phase because if acted out outside the transference situation it meant suicide. In this acting-out phase the patient existed in the crushing boulders or whatever might present, and the gratification came to her then from *destruction* of the head (including mind and false psyche) which had lost significance for the patient as part of the self.
>
> Ultimately the patient had to accept annihilation. We had already had many indications of a period of blackout or unconsciousness, and convulsive movements made it likely that there was at some time in infancy a minor fit. It appears that in the actual experience there was a loss of consciousness which could not be assimilated to the patient's self until accepted as a death. When this had become real the word death became wrong and the patient began to substitute 'a giving-in', and eventually the appropriate word was 'a not-knowing'.

In a full description of the case I should want to continue along these lines for some time, but development of this and other themes must be made in future publications. Acceptance of not-knowing produced tremendous relief. 'Knowing' became transformed into 'the analyst knows', that is to say, 'behaves reliably in active adaptation to the patient's needs'. The patient's whole life had been built up around mental functioning which had become falsely the place (in the head) from which she lived, and her life which had rightly seemed to her false had been developed out of this mental functioning.

Perhaps this clinical example illustrates what I mean when I say that I got from this analysis a feeling that the cataloguing of reactions to environmental impingements belonging to the time around about birth had been exact and complete; in fact I felt that the only alternative to the success of this cataloguing was absolute failure, hopeless confusion and mental defect.

But the case illustrates my theme in detail as well as generally.

I quote again from Scott (1949):

> Similarly when a patient in analysis loses his mind in the sense that he loses the illusion of needing a psychic apparatus which is separate from all that which he has called his body, his world, etc., etc., this loss is equivalent to the gain of all that conscious access to and control of the connections between the superficies and the depths, the boundaries and solidity of his Body Scheme—its memories, its perceptions, its images, etc., etc., which he had given up at an earlier period in his life when the duality soma-psyche began.
>
> Not infrequently in a patient whose first complaint is of fear of 'losing his mind'—the desire to lose such a belief and obtain a better one soon becomes apparent.

At this point of not-knowing in this analysis there appeared the memory of a bird that was seen as 'quite still except for the movements of the belly which indicated breathing'. In other words, the patient had reached, at 47 years, the state in which physiological functioning in general constitutes living. The psychical elaboration of this could follow. This psychical elaboration of physiological functioning is quite different from the intellectual work which so easily becomes artificially a thing in itself and falsely a place where the psyche can lodge.

Naturally only a glimpse of this patient can be given, and even if one chooses a small part, only a bit of this part can be described. I would like, however, to pursue a little the matter of the gap in consciousness. I need not describe the gap as it appeared in more 'forward' terms, the bottom of a pit, for instance, in which in the dark were all sorts of dead and dying bodies. Just now I am concerned only with the most primitive of the ways in which the gap was found, by the patient, by the reliving processes belonging to the transference situation. The gap in continuity, which throughout the patient's life had been actively denied, now became something urgently sought. We found a need to have the head broken into, and violent head-banging appeared as part of an attempt to produce a blackout. At times there was an urgent need for the destruction of the mental processes located by the patient in the head. A series of defences against full recognition of the desire to reach the gap in continuity of consciousness had to be dealt with before there could be acceptance of the not-knowing state. It happened that on the day on which this work reached its climax the patient stopped writing her diary.[3] This diary had been kept throughout the analysis, and it would be possible to reconstruct the whole of her analysis up to this time from it. There is little that the patient could perceive that has not been at least indicated in this diary. The meaning of the diary now became clear—it was a projection of her mental apparatus, and not a picture of the true self, which, in fact, had never lived till, at the bottom of the regression, there came a new chance for the true self to start.

The results of this bit of work led to a temporary phase in which there was no mind and no mental functioning. There had to be a temporary phase in which the breathing of her body was all. In this way the patient became able to accept the not-knowing condition because I was holding her and keeping a continuity by my own breathing, while she let go, gave in, knew nothing; it could not be any good, however, if I held her and maintained my own continuity of life if she were dead. What made my part operative was that I could see and hear her belly moving as she breathed (like the bird) and therefore I knew that she was alive.

Now for the first time she was able to have a psyche, an entity of her own, a body that breathes and in addition the beginning of fantasy belonging to the breathing and other physiological functions.

We as observers know, of course, that the mental functioning which enables the psyche to be there enriching the soma is dependent on the intact brain. But we do not place the psyche anywhere, not even in the brain on which it depends. For this patient, regressed in this way, these things were at last not important. I suppose she would now be prepared to locate the psyche wherever the soma is alive.

This patient has made considerable progress since this paper was read. Now in 1953 we are able to look back on the period of the stage I have chosen for description, and to see it in perspective. I do not need to modify what I have written. Except for the violent complication of the birth process body-memories, there has been no major disturbance of the patient's regression to a certain very early stage and subsequent forward movement towards a new existence as a real individual who feels real.

Mind Localized in the Head

I now leave my illustration and return to the subject of the localizing of the mind in the head. I have said that the imaginative elaboration of body parts and functions is not localized. There may, however, be localizations which are quite logical in the sense that they belong to the way in which the body functions. For instance, the body takes in and gives out substances. An inner world of personal imaginative experience therefore comes into the scheme of things, and shared reality is on the whole thought of as outside the personality. Although babies cannot draw pictures, I think that they are capable (except through lack of skill) of depicting themselves by a circle at certain moments in their first months. Perhaps if all is going well, they can achieve this soon after birth; at any rate we have good evidence that at six months a baby is at times using the circle or sphere as a diagram of the self. It is at this point that Scott's body scheme is so illuminating and especially his reminder that we are referring to time as well as to space. In the body scheme as I understand it there seems to me to be no place for the mind, and this is not a criticism of the body scheme as a diagram; it is a comment on the falsity of the concept of the mind as a localized phenomenon.

In trying to think out why the head is the place where either the mind is localized, or else outside which it is localized, I cannot help thinking of the way in which the head of the human baby is affected during birth, the time at which the mind is furiously active cataloguing reactions to a specific environmental persecution.

Cerebral functioning tends to be localized by people in the head in popular thought, and one of the consequences of this deserves special study. Until quite recently surgeons could be persuaded to open the skulls of mentally defective infants to make possible further development of their brains which were supposed to be constricted by the bones of the skull. I suppose the early trephining of the skull was for relief of *mind* disorders, i.e. for cure of persons whose mental functioning was their enemy and who had falsely localized their mental functioning in their heads. At the present time the curious thing is that once again in medical scientific thought the brain has got equated with the mind, which is felt by a certain kind of ill person to be an enemy, and a thing in the skull. The surgeon who does a leucotomy would *at first* seem to be doing what the patient asks for, that is, to be relieving the patient of mind activity, the mind having become the enemy of the psyche-soma. Nevertheless, we can see that the surgeon is caught up in the mental patient's false localization of the mind in the head, with its sequel, the equating of mind and brain. When he has done his work he has failed in the second half of his job. The patient wants to be relieved of the *mind activity* which has become a threat to the psyche-soma, but the patient next needs the full-functioning brain tissue *in order to be able to have psyche-soma existence*. By the operation of leucotomy with its irreversible brain changes the surgeon has made this impossible. The procedure has been of no use except through what the operation means to the patient. But the imaginative elaboration of somatic experience, the psyche, and for those who use the term, the soul, depend on the intact brain, as we know. We do not expect the *unconscious* of anyone to know such things, but we feel the neuro-surgeon ought to be *to some extent* affected by intellectual considerations.

In these terms we can see that one of the aims of *psychosomatic illness* is to draw the psyche from the mind back to the original intimate association with the soma. It is not sufficient to analyse the hypochondria of the psychosomatic patient, although this is an essential part of the treatment. One has also to be able to see the *positive value of the somatic disturbance* in its work of counteracting a 'seduction' of the psyche into the mind. Similarly, the aim of physiotherapists and the relaxationists can be understood in these terms. They do not have to know what they are doing to be successful psychotherapists. In one example of the application of these principles, if one tries to teach a pregnant woman how to do all the right things one not only makes her anxious, but one feeds the tendency of the psyche to lodge in the mental processes. *Per contra,* the relaxation methods at their best enable the mother to become body-conscious, and (if she is not a mental case) these methods help her to a continuity of being, and enable her to live as a psyche-soma. This is essential if she is to experience child-birth and the first stages of mothering in a natural way.

Summary

1. The true self, a continuity of being, is in health based on psyche-soma growth.
2. Mental activity is a special case of the functioning of the psyche-soma.
3. Intact brain functioning is the basis for psyche-being as well as for mental activity.
4. There is no localization of a mind self, and there is no thing that can be called mind.
5. Two distinct bases for normal mental functioning can already be given, viz.: (*a*) conversion of good enough environment into perfect (adapted) environment, enabling minimum of reaction to impingement, and maximum of natural (continuous) self-development; and (*b*) cataloguing of impingements (birth trauma, etc.) for assimilation at later stages of development.
6. It is to be noted that psyche-soma growth is universal and its complexities are inherent, whereas mental development is somewhat dependent on variable factors such as the quality of early environmental factors, the chance phenomena of birth and of management immediately after birth, etc.
7. It is logical to oppose psyche and soma and therefore to oppose the emotional development and the bodily development of an individual. It is not logical, however, to oppose the mental and the physical as these are not of the same stuff. Mental phenomena are complications of variable importance in psyche-soma continuity of being, in that which adds up to the individual's 'self'.

Notes

1. Cf. Freud's theory of obsessional neurosis (1909).
2. Case referred to again in 'Metapsychological and Clinical Aspects of Regression Within the Psycho-Analytical Set-Up' [CW 4:3:6].
3. The diary was resumed at a later date, for a time, with a looser function, and a more positive aim including the idea of one day using her experiences profitably.

21

Leucotomy

Originally published in *British Medical Student's Journal*, 1949, 3. Also published in C. Winnicott, R. Shepherd, & M. Davis (Eds.), *Psycho-analytic explorations* (pp. 543–547, part of the chapter 'Physical therapy of mental disorder: Leucotomy'). Cambridge, MA: Harvard University Press, 1989.

In many respects the medical student is out to learn, postponing till after qualification the attitude of inquiry which belongs to maturity and health. Perhaps leucotomy, the treatment of mental disorder by a surgical procedure that is destructive of brain tissue, provides a good example of a therapy that is open to question, and that need not be accepted even for the purpose of satisfying the examiners.

In the medical press I have expressed my personal criticism of leucotomy in the strongest possible terms, because I believe it to represent the worst possible trend in medical practice; but this criticism has always been made in respect of the opinions held by those who use the method, and never in respect of the medical men themselves, who are known to me as ordinary people doing the best they know for their patients, and experimenting only when they genuinely believe they see justification for experiment.

It should be remembered that there exist in large numbers insane people in asylums in the British Isles, and this represents a tremendous drain on medical and nursing man-hours. No one could be criticised for trying to lessen the burden on the community provided by the hopelessly insane. Leucotomy does make some very difficult patients less difficult, and relieves some acute sufferers from prolonged suffering. No wonder the neurosurgeons turn from the very highly skilled technique which enables them to remove rare brain tumours to the far less skilled cutting of nervous tissue in respect of a common condition. In any case, it could be argued, the brains of the worst mental cases are already diseased—syphilitic, arteriosclerotic, scarred after inflammatory processes.

What, then, are the reasons which make it seem to me that the operation should be abandoned?

First, I would say that if it is intended to relieve the community of the burden of the hopelessly insane, why not a more complete cut, say of the brain stem, or a deliberate policy of euthanasia? The answer is that this puts a responsibility on the medical man that he should not have—the responsibility for deciding as to life or death in respect of a fellow human being. This is a different matter from the decisions doctors make every day in respect of their opinions as to diagnosis and treatment to cure from disease.

The simple argument, that anything is justified that relieves the community or relieves personal suffering, is not good enough. Argument in favour of leucotomy can start with the claim that it is a good treatment for a patient who is mentally ill, that is to say, on the likelihood of its effecting a cure, but it must go further and show that it is not harmful to people in general.

It should be remembered, here, that it is one thing to cure a patient of cancer of the breast by removing a breast, and quite another thing to 'cure' a patient of mental disorder by removal of a part of the brain function. In the first case the person is left intact, and in the second it is the person that is maimed.

The theory of today is that it is the brain tissue that is needed before the mind can even start to be, and any other theory must first displace this one if it is to be accepted. Those who practise leucotomy have not tried to give a new theory, but have let it be assumed that the brain is the physical organ which is needed for the functioning of mind and consequently the organisation of personality.

At this point in the argument we must consider the fact that certain very ill patients have been considerably helped by leucotomy, have even left hospital and returned to work and to family life. If the treatment has only been given to very ill patients, then no harm has been done, and to some there has been benefit.

Unfortunately, a treatment cannot exist in a circumscribed way like this. It soon becomes applied to less severe cases. Theories arise and (in the case of leucotomy) the possibility of treatment gives power and direction in the mental hospital to the neurosurgeon, whose skill is in surgery of the brain and who is not trained to be a student of human nature.

First, in regard to the wider application of the treatment, it is natural that each unit should wish to do its thousand cases in order to have a round number for a report, and some of the thousand will be diagnostically at the less ill end, and in fact it will be seen in the reports that patients have already been leucotomised who have been diagnosed as suffering from depression, obsessional neurosis, etc.—certainly the cases are not confined to the brain-diseased.

This raises the vast question of the psycho-genesis of insanity. It can be said that it is impossible to be a brain-surgeon and also to be well informed psychologically. The two disciplines are too exacting for one doctor to grasp both fully, at one and the same time. And it would be easier for a really first-rate psychologist to learn to be a neurosurgeon than for the latter to learn to be a psychologist, simply because psychology can only be learned over a period of time in which the learner has to grow to meet the emotional demands that psychology puts on himself. No medical student, however brilliant, can just *learn* psychology; he has to spend years maturing and developing his own personality, while gradually coming to grips with the subject. In fact, experience shows that psychology taught to medical students can easily upset even what appeared to be stable personalities. The psycho-analysts' rule is undoubtedly sound: that the psychology of the unconscious can only be taught to people if they are themselves being analysed or if they have had previous successful analysis.

Reports on the psychology of patients before and after leucotomy and given in good faith by neurosurgeons are apt to look naive in the extreme to the psycho-analyst, who is perforce used to the extreme complexity of human material, and who is more aware than most people of the areas of ignorance in the understanding of persons.

There is a vast amount of evidence available to those who care to study the deeper aspects of psychology that the ordinary insanities—schizophrenia, the depressions, paranoia, as well as obsessional neurosis and delinquency—are disorders of emotional development, *not disorders dependent on brain-tissue changes*. Obviously, brain-tissue changes produce personality and behaviour changes, but people who are ill mentally on the whole are ill in spite of having healthy brain tissue. Mental illness that is not just a confusional state is an organised pattern, an organisation of defences, and of resistances, and of postponements of forward emotional development. This pattern would appear logical to the investigator if the whole truth were known. If an insane person is studied in sufficient detail the course of the illness becomes intelligible as an expression of the difficulties inherent in life, difficulties in personal development, in environmental influence, and in the interaction of the two. It cannot be argued that because brain syphilis produces ideas of grandeur and because arteriosclerosis produces perseverance of ideas or narrowing of intellect, therefore emotional disturbance spells underlying brain-tissue changes. In fact, the whole evidence points the other way.

The neurosurgeon, however, who starts off with a readiness to see insanity as a collection of separate illnesses, with brain-tissue changes, is not easily persuaded that his patients are still human beings. Even when they are withdrawn, degenerate and incontinent, they are still struggling with the problems of life which for the more fortunate of us have merely been a little easier to solve. When those who are not psychologists see symptoms and resistances disappear after leucotomy they feel supported in their theories, and have no idea that the removal of resistances can mean the final loss of the individuality of the person concerned.

It is really only the psycho-analysts who respect resistances, and see in them the unconscious struggle of the person to find himself. The whole tendency of modern (non-psycho-analytic) therapy is to bypass resistance.

Perhaps the best example that there will ever be of the bypassing of resistance is the operation of leucotomy. In fact, every person who feels he is going ill in a mental way in these days cannot be sure that he or she will not be insulted by physical interference with the brain tissue. This is not exactly the best way to get people to apply to be voluntary boarders in the early stages of psychiatric disorder. Many who would recover spontaneously with a few months of being tolerated, and if possible cherished somewhere and kept from suicide while in a depressed state, do in fact struggle on in their ordinary life through fear (well founded) that they will not recover without having at least been given a series of fits, and perhaps having had the brain irreversibly altered. After interference with the physical brain no man or woman can be sure of his identity: he is not there to be sure, because the person built up over the whole time since birth is not there.

If I behave today in an acceptable way this is a build-up of all my life, and a positive social contribution, an infinitely complex and actively meaningful example of the relation between all of me since my birth to all my environment. If I behave still better because I have had a leucotomy I am not making a better contribution, because it is not me behaving.

Human beings are entitled to all manner of dreams, including the most sadistic, and our job as medical practitioners with a scientific training is to provide the public with a reality against which they can match their dreams. Patients dream that their doctors are in love with them, but the doctors' oath forestalls this, and it very seldom happens that a doctor abuses his opportunities for intimacy. Dreams can be matched against reality.

In the same way patients dream of bad doctors doing fantastic and mutilating operations. On the whole doctors do not operate except under very highly controlled conditions, employing scientific principles in complete justification of their actions. Leucotomy seems, to me personally, to be on the borderline between science and superstition. I think people should not have to undergo this ordeal of which they are frightened even to dream. Those who practise leucotomy are frightening patients very much more than relieving the suffering of a few individuals under their care, they are producing a fear of doctors and increasing the fear of madness. This has far-reaching effects. Fear of madness leads to a flight to an extreme of sanity which is a false step in civilisation; it means a flight to the logical and the conscious and the easily planned, and a loss of contact with individual integrity, and the hidden depths of the personality of each person.

In my opinion the responsibility taken by those who blindly cut about the brains of persons just because they are insane is tremendous, and it is for them to take much more trouble than they have taken hitherto to show that they recognise the wider implications of their practice.

22

Review: *Art Versus Illness*
BY ADRIAN HILL (LONDON: GEORGE ALLEN AND UNWIN LTD., 1948, 2ND EDITION)

Review originally published in *British Journal of Medical Psychology*, 1949, 22. Also published in C. Winnicott, R. Shepherd, & M. Davis (Eds.), *Psycho-analytic explorations* (pp. 555–557, part of the chapter 'Occupational therapy'). Cambridge, MA: Harvard University Press, 1989.

I think this book is good. Adrian Hill, himself an artist and art teacher, had a period of enforced idleness as a phthisical subject in a sanatorium, and he discovered a new reason for drawing and painting. It made him feel better, and perhaps indirectly affected the physical healing process. What could be more natural than for him to become, on discharge from the sanatorium, a militant protagonist of Art versus Illness?

The book tells the story of his adventures. In order to sell the idea that burned holes in him when he had to hang round for various kinds of permission, he needed much self-control and patient understanding of the mentality of doctors and nurses and committees of management.

The main idea is that when ill people are not too ill they absolutely need help in the management of their souls, or inner worlds, or whatever you call it. The time of enforced idleness is either a time wasted or else time for inner growth and development. It is well known that children as well as adults can develop depth and poise during an illness with rheumatic heart disease, or when immobilized by tuberculosis or a fractured femur; but it is touch and go, whether the strain of simple contemplation may not prove too great, and the result be disruptive rather than productive.

Adrian Hill clearly sees that a good teacher can make all the difference between disruption and integration, by personally sponsoring art interest and activity. In some cases he does no more than provide a frame on the wall opposite the bed into which a series of interesting prints can be inserted, whereas in other cases he organizes actual drawing and painting, but he always aims at finding the true personal contribution that the individual patient has the capacity to make.

One wants to know, can the author see that his idea, though original in one sense, is not new, that many, indeed, have had the same idea and have put it into practice, although not perhaps on a wide scale? If he can, then we can be glad of his personal enthusiasm and wish him well in his crusade.

What is the relation of all this to Occupation Therapy? This question may have been answered somewhere, and the answer is not in this book. I would say that at its worst, occupation therapy is an organized attempt to keep people from themselves, and that this is opposite to the aim that Adrian Hill sponsors. Some think that the official occupation therapy teaching is dangerously veering towards a training in skills, an immense number of skills, the training being enough to put off the true artists, potters, musicians. Yet, of course, there has to be an official course and qualification, and there would be chaos if occupation therapy were to be handed over to artists.

In the war my wife, herself an artist, potter and modeller (working in the occupation therapy department at the Maudsley Hospital, then at Mill Hill), found that constructive clay work could be used in this same self-revealing way with men and women who had various kinds of psychiatric disorders, in psychiatric work there is a need for close co-operation between the artist (potter, etc.) and the medically responsible psychiatrist, and this is not always forthcoming. It is more likely to develop if the artist is a qualified occupation therapist.

At its best occupation therapy is in fact just what Adrian Hill is describing. An artist, potter, musician, sculptor, modeller, who lives in his own chosen medium, takes the trouble to reach a group of bedridden or immobilized patients, and by personal contact enables each patient, in his or her own way, to create a bridge between the unconscious and ordinary conscious living, a bridge with two-way traffic. Much happens, but the main thing is that the patient, by gradually discovering his or her creative urges and positive integrative forces, is enabled to look at what is inside the self to see whatever is there, the chaos, the tensions, the death, as well as the beauty and the innate liveliness.

As an example of the use of music I remember a long-term convalescent home for rheumatic children in Warwickshire at which all the children were making pipes, playing them, writing original themes, conducting, or in some other way contributing to the musical pool. A musician (not an occupation therapist) was on the staff. This was an immensely enriching experience for the children, and it is of no significance if none of them later became musicians. It would, of course, be a nuisance to be forced to become musical if one happened to be ill in a music-mad institution.

The wireless can be a tremendous help to the ill person, provided the knobs and the *Radio Times* are within easy reach. One can use the various programmes for personal growth. On the other hand, to be subjected, when ill, to a programme chosen by the engineer in the hospital basement is to be 'occupied', and prevented from finding oneself or from growing.

This book can be used, then, as a corrective to the bad tendencies (if they exist) in the official occupation therapy outlook, and as a support to the good tendencies. It is unfortunate that the words 'occupation therapy' seem to divert attention away from the enriching experience to the manufacture of an article that can be shown on view day.

23

A Man Looks at Motherhood

> Originally published as the Introduction to *The ordinary devoted mother and her baby* (pp. 3–6). London: C. A. Brock, 1949. Also published in *The child and the family: First relationships* (pp. 3–6). London: Tavistock, 1957; and *The child, the family, and the outside world* (pp. 15–18). Harmondsworth, UK: Penguin Books, 1964. Broadcast 5 October 1949, as 'Caring for Children and How Babies Develop Their Personalities'. Benzie, I. (Producer), the first in the series *How's the baby?* Home Service. London: British Broadcasting Corporation (see the broadcast list [CW 12:3:2]). Recorded as part of 'The Ordinary Devoted Mother and Her Baby' [CW 12:3:3].

To begin with, you will be relieved to know that I am not going to be telling you what to do. I am a man, and so I can never really know what it is like to see wrapped up over there in the cot a bit of my own self, a bit of me living an independent life, yet at the same time dependent and gradually becoming a person. Only a woman can experience this, and perhaps only a woman can imaginatively experience it, as she has to do when by bad luck of one kind or another the actual experience is lacking.

What is there for me to do, then, if I am not going to give instructions? I'm used to having mothers bring their children to me, and when this happens we see what we want to talk about right before our eyes. The baby is jumping about on the mother's knee, reaching out for things on my desk, climbing down on to the floor and crawling round; clambering up on the chairs, or pulling books out of the book-cases; or perhaps clinging to mother in dread of the white-coated doctor who will surely be a monster who eats children if they are nice, and who does worse things if they are nasty. Or an older child is at a separate table drawing pictures while mother and I are trying to piece together the history of his development, and trying to see where things started to go wrong. The child is listening out of one ear to make sure we are up to no mischief, and at the same time is communicating with me without speaking, by the drawings which I go over to see from time to time.

How easy is all this, and how different is my task now, when I have to build baby and small child out of my imagination and experience!

You have had the same difficulty. If I cannot communicate with you, what did you feel like having a baby a few weeks old, not knowing what was or was not there to communicate with? If you are thinking this out, try to remember at what age your baby or babies seemed to notice you as a person, and what made you feel fairly sure at that exciting moment that you were two people communicating with each other. You did not have to do everything from different sides of the room, by talking. What language would you have used? No, you found yourself concerned with management of the baby's body, and you liked it to be so. You knew just how to pick the baby up, how to put the baby down, and how to leave well alone, letting the cot act for you; and you had learnt how to arrange the clothes for comfort and for preserving the baby's natural warmth. Indeed, you knew all this when you were a little girl and played with dolls. And then there were special times when you did definite things, feeding, bathing, changing napkins, and cuddling. Sometimes the urine trickled down your apron or went right through and soaked you as if you yourself had let slip, and you didn't mind. In fact by these things you could have known that you were a woman, and an ordinary devoted mother.

I am saying all this because I want you to know that this man, nicely detached from real life, free from the noise and smell and responsibility of child care, does know that the mother of a baby is tasting real things, and that she would not miss the experience for worlds. If we understand each other thus far, you will perhaps let me talk about being an ordinary devoted mother and managing the earliest stages of the life of a new human being. I cannot tell you exactly what to do, but I can talk about what it all means.

In the ordinary things you do you are quite naturally doing very important things, and the beauty of it is that you do not have to be clever, and you do not even have to think if you do not want to. You may have been hopeless at arithmetic at school, or perhaps all your friends got scholarships, but you didn't like the sight of a history book, and so failed and left school early; or perhaps you would have done well if you hadn't had measles just before the exam. Or you may be really clever. But all this does not matter, and it hasn't anything to do with whether you are a good mother or not. If a child can play with a doll, you can be an ordinary devoted mother, and I believe you are just this most of the time. Isn't it strange that such a tremendously important thing should depend so little on exceptional intelligence!

If human babies are to develop eventually into healthy, independent, and society-minded adult individuals, they absolutely depend on being given a good start, and this good start is assured in nature by the existence of the bond between the baby's mother and the baby, the thing called love. So if you love your baby he or she is getting a good start.

Let me quickly say that I am not talking about sentimentality. You all know the kind of person who goes about saying, 'I simply *adore* babies'. But you wonder, do they love them? A mother's love is a pretty crude affair. There's possessiveness in it, appetite, even a 'drat the kid' element; there's generosity in it, and power, as well as humility. But sentimentality is outside it altogether, and is repugnant to mothers.

Now, it may be that you are an ordinary devoted mother, and you like being one without thinking about it. Artists are often the very people who hate thinking about art, and about the purpose of art. You, as a mother, may prefer to avoid thinking things out, so I want to warn you that in this book we are going to talk about the things a devoted mother does by just being herself. But a few will like to consider what they are doing. Probably some of you have finished with actual mothering, and your children have grown up and gone to school; you may then like to look back on the good things you did, and think about the way in which you laid the foundation for your children's development. If you did it all intuitively, probably that was the best way.

It is vitally important that we should get to understand the part played by those who care for the infant, so that we can protect the young mother from whatever tends to get between herself and her child. If she is without understanding of the thing she does so well she is without means to defend her position, and only too easily she spoils her job by trying to do what she is told, or what her own mother did, or what the books say.

Fathers come into this, not only by the fact that they can be good mothers for limited periods of time, but also because they can help to protect the mother and baby from whatever tends to interfere with the bond between them, which is the essence and very nature of child care.

In the following pages I shall be deliberately trying to put into words what a mother does when she is ordinarily and quite simply devoted to her baby.

We still have much to learn about infants at the beginning, and perhaps only mothers can tell us what we want to know.

24

The Baby as a Going Concern

> Originally published in *The ordinary devoted mother and her baby* (pp. 7–11). London: C. A. Brock, 1949. Also published in *The child and the family: First relationships* (pp. 13–17). London: Tavistock, 1957; and *The child, the family, and the outside world* (pp. 25–29). Harmondsworth, UK: Penguin, 1964. Broadcast 12 October 1949, as 'The Mind of a Child'. I. Benzie (Producer), the second in the series *How's the baby?* Home Service. London: British Broadcasting Corporation (see the broadcast list [CW 12:3:2]). Recorded as part of 'The Ordinary Devoted Mother and Her Baby' [CW 12:3:3].

I have been writing generally about mothers and their own babies. I was not specially out to tell mothers what to do, because they can get advice over details quite easily from Welfare Centres. In fact advice over details comes to them almost too easily, sometimes causing a feeling of muddle. I have chosen instead to write for those mothers who are ordinarily good at looking after their own babies, intending to help them to know what babies are like, and to show them a little of what is going on. The idea is that the more they know, the more they will be able to afford to trust their own judgement. It is when a mother trusts her own judgement that she is at her best.

It is surely tremendously important for a mother to have the experience of doing what she feels like doing, which enables her to discover the fullness of the motherliness in herself; for just as a writer is surprised by the wealth of ideas that turn up when he puts his pen to paper, so the mother is constantly surprised by what she finds in the richness of her minute-to-minute contact with her own baby.

In fact, one might ask how can a mother learn about being a mother in any other way than by taking full responsibility? If she just does what she is told, she has to go on doing what she is told, and to improve she can only choose somebody better to tell her what to do. But if she is feeling free to act in the way that comes naturally to her, she grows in the job.

This is where the father can help. He can help provide a space in which the mother has elbow-room. Properly protected by her man, the mother is saved from having to turn outwards to deal with her surroundings at the time when she is wanting so much to turn inwards, when she is longing to be concerned with the inside of the circle which she can make with her arms, in the centre of which is the baby. This period of time in which the mother is naturally preoccupied with the one infant does not last long. The mother's bond with the baby is very powerful at the beginning, and we must do all we can to enable her to be preoccupied with her baby at this, the natural time.

Now it so happens that it is not only the mother that this experience is good for; the baby undoubtedly needs exactly this kind of thing too. We are only just beginning to realize how absolutely the new-born infant needs love of the mother. The health of the grown-up person is being founded throughout childhood, but the foundation of the health of the human being is laid by you in the baby's first weeks and months. Perhaps this thought can help a little when you feel strange at the temporary loss of your interest in world affairs. You are founding the health of a person who will be a member of our society. This is worth doing. The odd thing is that it is generally thought that the care of children is more difficult the greater the number being cared for. Actually I am sure that the fewer the children, the greater the emotional strain. Devotion to one child is the greatest strain of all, and it is a good job it only lasts for a while.

So here you are with all your eggs in one basket. What are you going to do about it? Well, enjoy yourself! Enjoy being thought important. Enjoy letting other people look after the world while you are producing a new one of its members. Enjoy being turned-in and almost in love with yourself, the baby is so nearly part of you. Enjoy the way in which your man feels responsible for the welfare of you and your baby. Enjoy finding out new things about yourself. Enjoy having more right than you have ever had before to do just what you feel is good. Enjoy being annoyed with the baby when cries and yells prevent acceptance of the milk that you long to be generous with. Enjoy all sorts of womanly feelings that you cannot even start to explain to a man. Particularly, I know you will enjoy the signs that gradually appear that the baby is a person, and that you are recognized as a person by the baby.

Enjoy all this for your own sake, but the pleasure which you can get out of the messy business of infant care happens to be vitally important from the baby's point of view. The baby does not want to be given the correct feed at the correct time, so much as to be fed by someone who loves feeding her own baby. The baby takes for granted all things like the softness of the clothes and having the bath water at the right temperature. What cannot be taken for granted is the mother's pleasure that goes with the clothing and bathing of her own baby. If you are there enjoying it all, it is like the sun coming out, for the baby. The mother's pleasure has to be there or else the whole procedure is dead, useless, and mechanical.

This enjoyment, which comes naturally in the ordinary way, can of course be interfered with by your worries, and worry depends a great deal on ignorance. It is rather like the relaxation methods in childbirth, about which you may perhaps have read. The people who write these books do all they can to explain just what happens during pregnancy and childbirth, so that mothers can relax, which means stop worrying about the unknown, and, as it were, lie back on natural processes. So much of the pain of childbirth does not belong to childbirth itself but to the tightness that comes from fear, chiefly from fear of the unknown. That is all explained to you, and if you have a good doctor and nurse available you can bear the pain which cannot be avoided.

In the same way, after the child is born, the pleasure that you get looking after the baby depends on your not being tense and worried because of ignorance and fear.

In these pages I want to give mothers information, so that they will know more than they did about what is going on in the baby, and so that they will see how the baby needs just exactly what a mother does well if she is easy, natural, and lost in the job.

I shall talk about the baby's body and what goes on inside; and I shall talk about the baby's developing person, and I shall talk about the way you introduce the world in small doses, so that the baby is not confused.

Now I want to make just one thing clear. It is this. Your baby does not depend on you for growth and development. Each baby is a *going concern.* In each baby is a vital spark, and this urge towards life and growth and development is a part of the baby, something the child is born with and which is carried forward in a way that we do not have to understand. For instance, if you have just put a bulb in the window-box you know perfectly well that you do not have to make the bulb grow into a daffodil. You supply the right kind of earth or fibre and you keep the bulb watered just the right amount, and the rest comes naturally, because the bulb has life in it. Now, the care of infants is very much more complicated than the care of a daffodil bulb, but the illustration serves my purpose because, both with the bulb and with the infant, there is something going on which is not your responsibility. The baby was conceived in you and from that moment became a lodger in your body. After birth the baby became a lodger in your arms. This is a temporary affair. It will not last for ever, in fact it will not last for long. The baby will only too soon be at school. Just at the moment this lodger is tiny and weak in body, and needing the special care that comes from your love. This does not alter the fact that the tendency towards life and growth is something inherent in the baby.

I wonder whether you feel at all relieved to hear somebody say this? I have known mothers whose enjoyment of their motherhood was spoiled by the fact that they felt somehow responsible for the aliveness of the baby. If the baby slept they would go over to the cot rather hoping that he or she would wake and so show signs of liveliness. If the baby were sullen they would play about, and poke his face, trying to produce a smile, which of course meant nothing to the infant. It was just a reaction. Such people are always jogging babies up and down on their knees trying to produce a giggle, or anything that reassures them themselves by indicating that the life process in the infant continues.

Some children are never allowed even in earliest infancy just to lie back and float. They lose a great deal and may altogether miss the feeling that they themselves want to live. It seems to me that if I can convey to you that there really is this living process in the baby (which, as a matter of fact, it is quite difficult to extinguish) you may be better able to enjoy the care of your baby. Ultimately, life depends less on the will to live than on the fact of breathing.

Some of you have created works of art. You have done drawings and paintings, or you have moulded out of clay, or you have knitted jumpers or made dresses. When you did these things, what turned up was made by you. Babies are different. The baby grows, and you are the mother providing a suitable environment.

Some people seem to think of a child as clay in the hands of a potter. They start moulding the infant, and feeling responsible for the result. This is quite wrong. If this is what you feel, then you will be weighed down with responsibility which you need not take at all. If you can accept this idea of a baby as a going concern you are then free to get a lot of interest out of looking to see what happens in the development of the baby while you are enjoying responding to his or her needs.

25

Where the Food Goes

> Originally published in *The ordinary devoted mother and her baby* (pp. 12–16). London: C. A. Brock, 1949. Also published in *The child and the family: First relationships* (pp. 23–27). London: Tavistock, 1957; and *The child, the family, and the outside world* (pp. 35–39). Harmondsworth, UK: Penguin, 1964. Broadcast 19 October 1949, as 'The Baby and its Food'. I. Benzie (Producer), the third in the series *How's the baby?* Home Service. London: British Broadcasting Corporation (see the broadcast list [CW 12:3:2]). Recorded as part of 'The Ordinary Devoted Mother and Her Baby' [CW 12:3:3].

When babies begin to feel hungry something is beginning to come alive in them which is ready to take possession of them. You yourself begin to make certain noises to do with the preparation of the feed which the baby knows as a sign that the time is coming when it will be safe to let eagerness for food ripen into a terrific urge. You can see saliva flowing out, because small babies don't swallow their saliva—they show the world by dribbling that they have an interest in things they can get hold of with their mouths. Well, this is only saying that the baby is getting excited, and particularly excited in the mouth. The hands also play their part in the search for satisfaction. So when you give the baby food, you are fitting in with a tremendous desire for food. The mouth is prepared. The pads on the lips are very sensitive at this time and they help to provide a high degree of pleasurable mouth sensation which the baby will never have again in later life.

A mother actively adapts to her baby's needs. She likes to. Because of her love she is expert at making delicate adjustments in her management which other people wouldn't think worth while, and wouldn't be able to know about. Whether you are feeding at the breast or the bottle, the baby's mouth becomes very active and milk goes from you or the bottle into the mouth.

There is generally thought to be a difference here between the breast- and bottle-fed baby. The breast-fed baby gets behind the root of the nipple and chews with the gums. This can be quite painful for the mother, but the pressure there pushes the milk that is in the nipple into the mouth. The milk is then swallowed. The bottle-fed baby, however, has to employ a different technique. In this case the accent is on the sucking, which can be a relatively minor matter in the breast experience.

Some babies on the bottle need a fairly large hole in the teat because they want to get the milk without sucking until they have learned to suck. Others suck right away and get swamped if the hole is too big.

If you are using a bottle, you will have to be prepared to make changes in what you are doing in a more conscious way than you would be if you were feeding at the breast. The breast-feeding mother relaxes, she feels the blood going to her breasts, and the milk just comes. When she is bottle-feeding she has to keep her wits about her. She keeps on taking the bottle out of the baby's mouth and letting some air into it, because otherwise the vacuum in the bottle becomes so great that the baby can't get any milk out. She lets the milk cool to almost the right temperature, and tests it by putting the bottle against her arm; and she has a can of hot water by her to stand the bottle in, in case the baby is slow and the milk cools down too much.

Well, now we are concerned with what happens to the milk. We could say that the baby knows a lot about the milk up to the moment when it is swallowed. There it is going into the mouth, and giving a definite sensation to the mouth, and having a definite taste. This is undoubtedly very satisfactory. And then it is swallowed. This means it is almost lost from the baby's point of view. Fists and fingers are better in this respect, for they stay put, and remain available. Swallowed food is not completely lost, however, not while it is in the stomach. From this the food can still be returned. Babies seem to be able to know of the state of their stomachs.

You probably know that the stomach is a small organ shaped rather like a baby's bottle swung across from left to right under the ribs, and it is a muscle, rather a complicated one, with a wonderful capacity for doing just what mothers do to their babies; that is, it adapts to new conditions. It does this automatically unless disturbed by excitement, fear, or anxiety, just as mothers are naturally good mothers unless they are tense and anxious. It is rather like a miniature good mother inside. When a baby feels at ease (or what we call relaxed when we are talking about grown-up people) this muscular container, which we call the stomach, behaves itself well. That means that it keeps up a certain tension within itself and yet maintains its shape and its position.

So the milk is in the stomach, and is held there. And now starts a series of processes which we call digestion. There is always fluid in the stomach, digestive juices, and at the top end there is always air. This air has a special interest for mothers and babies. When the baby swallows the milk there is an increase in the amount of fluid in the stomach. If you and the baby are fairly calm the pressure in the stomach-wall adapts itself and loosens up a bit; the stomach gets bigger. The baby is usually a bit excited, however, and the stomach therefore takes a little while to adapt. The temporarily increased pressure in the stomach is uncomfortable, and a quick way out of the trouble is for the baby to belch a little wind. For this reason, after you have fed your baby, or even in the middle of a feed, you may find it a good idea to expect a little wind, and if the baby is upright when belching you are much more likely to get wind by itself, instead of a return of some of the milk along with it. That is why you can see mothers putting their babies up on their shoulders and just patting the back a little, because the patting stimulates the stomach muscle and makes the baby more liable to belch.

Of course it very often happens that the baby's stomach adapts so quickly to the feed, and accepts the milk so easily, that there is no need for any belching at all. But if the mother of the baby is in a tense state herself (as she may well be sometimes) then the baby gets into a tense state too, and in that case the stomach will take longer to adapt to the increase in the amount of food in it. If you understand what is going on, you will be able to manage this wind business quite easily, and you will not be puzzled when one feed is quite different from another, or when one baby is different from another baby in this matter of wind.

If you do not understand what is going on, you are bound to be flummoxed. A neighbour says to you, 'Be sure you get some wind up after the baby's feed!' Not knowing the facts you can't argue so you plant the baby on your shoulder and vigorously pat the back, trying to get up this wind which you feel *has* to be produced. It can become a kind of religion. In that way you are imposing your own (or your neighbour's) ideas on the baby, and interfering with the natural way, which is after all the only good kind of way.

Well, this little muscular container keeps the milk for a certain length of time, until the first stage in digestion has occurred. One of the first things that happens to the milk is that it becomes curdled. That is the first stage in the natural process of digestion. In fact in making a junket you imitate what happens in the stomach. Don't be alarmed, therefore, if your baby brings up some curdled milk. It ought to be so. Also babies are very easily a little bit sick.

In this period, in which things are going on in the stomach itself, it is a very good idea if the baby is able to be quiet. Whether you manage this best by putting the baby in a cot after the feed, or by gently carrying him round for a little while, I must leave to you, because no two mothers and no two babies are alike. In the easiest circumstances the baby just lies back and seems to be contemplating the inside. There can be a good feeling inside at this time, because the blood goes to the active part, and this gives a nice warm sensation in the baby's belly. Disturbances, distractions, and excitements during this early part of the digestive processes can easily cause discontented crying, or can lead either to vomiting, or else to a too early passing on of the food before it has really undergone all the changes which it should undergo in the stomach itself. I think you know how important it is to keep neighbours out when you are feeding your child. This does not apply simply to the time when you are giving the feed. The feeding time continues right on to the time when the food leaves the stomach, and it is rather like the important part of a solemn occasion which seems to be spoiled if an aeroplane passes overhead. This solemn period extends to include the period after feeding, when the food is not yet fully accepted.

If all goes well, there comes an end to the particular sensitive time, and you begin to hear gurglings and rumblings. This means that the part of the digestion of the milk which goes on in the stomach is becoming completed, and quite automatically the stomach now tends to squirt more and more of the partially digested milk through a valve into what we might call the guts.

Now, you do not have to know much about what happens in the guts. The continuation of the digestion of the milk is a very complex process, but gradually the digested milk starts to get absorbed into the blood and to be carried to every part of the body. It is interesting to know that soon after the milk leaves the stomach bile is added. This comes down from the liver at the appropriate moment, and it is because of bile that the contents of the guts have their particular colour. You may have had catarrhal jaundice yourself and so you know how horrid it feels when the bile cannot go from the liver into the guts, in that case because of inflammatory swelling in the little tube that carries it. The bile (in catarrhal jaundice) goes into your blood instead of into your guts, and makes you yellow all over. But when the bile goes the right way just at the right moment, from the liver to the guts, it makes the baby feel good.

Well, if you look it up in a physiology book you will be able to find out all that happens in the further digestion of the milk, but the details do not matter if you are a mother. The point is that the gurglings indicate that the period in which the child is sensitive is at an end, and the food is now really inside. From the infant's point of view this new stage must be a mystery, as physiology is beyond the infant mind. *We* know, however, that in various ways the food is absorbed from the guts, and it eventually gets distributed round the body and by means of the blood stream gets carried to every part of the tissues, which are all the time growing. In a baby these tissues are growing at a tremendous pace, and they need regularly repeated supplies.

26

The End of the Digestive Process

> Originally published in *The ordinary devoted mother and her baby* (pp. 17–21). London: C. A. Brock, 1949. Also published in *The child and the family: First relationships* (pp. 28–32). London: Tavistock, 1957; and *The child, the family, and the outside world* (pp. 40–44). Harmondsworth, UK: Penguin, 1964. Broadcast 26 October 1949, as 'The Passing of Excretions.' I. Benzie (Producer), the fourth in the series *How's the baby?* Home Service. London: British Broadcasting Corporation (see the broadcast list [CW 12:3:2]). Recorded as part of 'The Ordinary Devoted Mother and Her Baby' [CW 12:3:3].

In the last chapter [CW 3:4:25] I traced the fate of the milk as it was swallowed, digested, and absorbed. Here in the guts of the baby there is a great deal that goes on that does not concern the mother, and from the baby's point of view all this part of the process is a mystery. Gradually, however, the baby becomes involved again at the last stage, which we call excretion, and so the mother is involved too, and she can play her part best if she knows what is going on.

The fact is that the food is not all absorbed; even perfectly good breast milk leaves some kind of residue, and in any case there is the wear and tear of the guts. One way and another there is a lot left over, and it has to be got rid of.

The various things that go to make up what is going to be the motion gradually get passed on to the lower end of the guts towards the opening which is called the anus. How is this done? The stuff is moved on by a series of contraction waves which keep on going down the length of the guts. By the way, did you know that the food has to go through a narrow tube twenty feet long in a grown-up? In a baby the guts are about twelve feet long.

I sometimes have a mother say to me, 'The food went right through 'im, doctor'. It seemed to the mother that as soon as some food went into the baby it came out again at the other end. That is what it looks like, but it isn't true. The point is that the baby's guts are sensitive, and the taking of food starts up the waves of contraction in the guts; when these reach the lower end a motion is passed. Ordinarily the last part of the guts, the rectum, is more or less empty. These contraction waves get busy when there is much to be passed along, or if the baby is excited, or if the guts are inflamed by infection. Gradually, and only gradually, the infant gets some measure of control, and I want to tell you how this happens.

At first we can imagine that the rectum begins to fill simply because there is a large amount of residue waiting to pass down. Probably the actual stimulus for the bowel movement comes from the digestive process set up by the last feed. Sooner or later the rectum is filled. The infant has not known much about the stuff while it was higher up, but the filling of the rectum produces a definite sensation which is not un-pleasurable, and it makes the baby want to pass the motion right out. At first we need not expect the baby to hold it in the rectum. You know only too well that in the early stages of infant care the changing and washing of napkins looms large. If there must be clothes, then there has to be a frequent changing of napkins, otherwise the motion left for a long time in contact with the skin causes soreness. This is especially true if for some reason or other the motion has been passed on quickly and is therefore liquid. This napkin business cannot be got rid of by hasty training. If you carry on with the good work, and play for time, then things begin to happen.

You see, if the motion is held by the baby at the last stage in the rectum, it gets dried; water is absorbed from it as it waits there. The motion is then passed on as a solid thing which the baby can enjoy passing; in fact, at the moment of passing the motion there can be such an excitement just there that the baby cries from excess of feeling. You see what you are doing by leaving the matter to your baby (although helping in so far as the baby cannot manage alone)? You are giving every possible chance for him to find from experience that it feels good to collect the stuff and hold it for a while before passing it on, and even for the baby to discover that the result is interesting, and that in fact defecation can be an extremely satisfactory experience if all goes well. The establishment of this healthy attitude of the baby towards these things is the only good foundation for anything you may want to do at a later date in the way of training.

Perhaps someone told you to hold your baby out regularly after feeds from the start, with the idea of getting in a bit of training at the earliest possible moment. If you do this you should know that what you are doing is trying to save yourself the bother of dirty napkins. And there is a lot to be said for this. But the baby is not anywhere near being able to be trained yet. If you never allow for his or her own development in these matters, you interfere with the beginnings of a natural process. Also you are missing good things. For instance, if you wait you will sooner or later discover that the baby, lying over there in the cot, finds a way of letting you know that a motion has been passed; and soon you will even get an inkling that there is going to be a motion. You are now at the beginning of a new relationship with the baby, who cannot communicate with you in an ordinary grown-up way, but who has found a way of talking without words. It is as if he said, 'I think I am going to want to pass a motion; are you interested?' and you (without exactly saying so) answer 'Yes', and you let him know that if you are interested this is not because you are frightened that he will make a mess, and not because you feel you ought to be teaching him how to be clean. If you are interested it is because you love your baby in the way mothers do, so that whatever is important to the baby is also important to you. So you will not mind if you got there late, because the important thing was not keeping the baby clean, it was the answering of the call of a fellow human being.

Later on, your relationship to the infant in these terms will become richer; sometimes a baby will feel frightened of the motion that is coming, and sometimes he will feel that it is something valuable. Because what you do is based on the simple fact of your love you soon become able to distinguish between the times when you are helping your baby to be rid of bad things and the times when you are receiving gifts.

There is a practical point worth mentioning here. When a nice satisfactory motion has been passed you might think that that was the end of everything, and you pack the baby up again and get on with whatever you are doing. But the baby may show new discomfort, or may dirty the clean napkin almost immediately. It is extremely likely that a first emptying of the rectum will be followed almost immediately by a certain amount of refilling. If you are not in a hurry, and you can afford to wait, the baby will be able to pass this instalment too when the next waves of contraction come down. This might happen, and it might happen again. By not being in a hurry you leave your baby with an empty rectum. This keeps the rectum sensitive, and the next time it fills, some hours later, the baby will once more go over the whole procedure in a natural way. Mothers who are always in a hurry always have to leave their babies with something in the rectum. This will either be passed out, causing unnecessary dirtying of napkins, or else it will be held in the rectum which therefore becomes less sensitive, and the beginnings of the next experience will be interfered with to some extent. Unhurried management over a long period of time naturally lays the basis for a sense of order in the baby's relation to his excretory functions. If you are in a hurry, and cannot allow for the *total* experience, the baby will start off in a muddle. The baby who is not in a muddle will be able to follow you later on, and gradually give up some of the tremendous pleasure that belongs to the doing of a motion just exactly when the impulse comes. The baby does this not simply to comply with your wish that as few messes as possible be made, but out of a wish to wait for you, so as to get into touch with your liking to look after all that has to do with your own baby. Much later on the baby will be able to gain control down there, and to make messes when the idea is to dominate over you, and to hold things back till the convenient moment comes when the idea is to please you.

I could tell you about plenty of babies who never had a chance to find themselves in this important matter of the passing of motions. I know of a mother who practically never let any of her babies have a natural motion. She had a theory that the motion in the rectum poisons the baby in some way or other. This is simply not true, and babies and small children can hold their motions there for days without being really harmed. This mother was always interfering with each baby's rectum with soapsticks and enemas, and the result was more than chaotic. Certainly she had no hope whatever of producing happy children who could easily be fond of her.

The same general principles underly the other kind of excretion, the passing of urine.

Water is absorbed into the blood stream, and what is not needed is excreted by the baby's kidneys and passed to the bladder along with waste products dissolved in it. The baby does not know anything till the bladder begins to fill, and then there develops an urge to pass the urine out. At first this is more or less automatic, but the baby gradually finds that there is a reward for holding back a little—after holding back the baby finds it pleasurable to get rid of the water. There develops another little orgy that enriches the life of the infant, that makes life worth living, and the body worth living in.

In the course of time this discovery of the infant, that waiting pays, can be used by you, because you can get to know by signs that something may be going to happen, and you can still further enrich the baby's experience by your interest in the procedure. In time the baby will like to wait, if not too long, just in order to get the whole thing within the love relationship that exists between the two of you.

You see how it is that the baby's mother is needed for the management of the excretions, just as she is needed for the feeding? Only the mother feels it is worth while to follow the infant's needs in detail, so enabling the exciting experience of the body to become part of a love relationship between two persons, the baby and herself.

When this is what happens, and when it is kept up over a period of time, what is called training can follow without much difficulty, because the mother has earned the right to make such demands as are not beyond the infant's capacity.

Here again is an example of the way in which the foundations of health are laid down by the ordinary mother in her ordinary loving care of her own baby.

27

The Baby as a Person

Originally published in *The ordinary devoted mother and her baby* (pp. 22–26). London: C. A. Brock, 1949. Also published in *The child and the family: First relationships* (pp. 33–37). London: Tavistock, 1957; and *The child, the family, and the outside world* (pp. 75–79). Harmondsworth, UK: Penguin, 1964. Broadcast 2 November 1949, as 'No Baby Can Grow Properly Without Love'. I. Benzie (Producer), the fifth in the series *How's the baby?* Home Service. London: British Broadcasting Corporation (see the broadcast list [CW 12:3:2]). Recorded as part of 'The Ordinary Devoted Mother and Her Baby' [CW 12:3:3].

I have been wondering how to start to describe babies as persons. It is easy to see that when food goes into the baby it is digested, and some of it is distributed round the body and used for growth. Some of it is stored as energy, and some of it is got rid of in one way or another. That is looking at the baby with an interest in bodies. But if we look at the same baby, being interested in the person that is there, we can easily see that there is an imaginative feeding experience, as well as this bodily one. The one is based on the other.

I think you can get quite a lot out of thinking that all the things that you do because of your love of the baby go in just like the food. The baby builds something out of it all, and not only that, but the baby has phases of making use of you and then dropping you, just in the same way as with the food. Perhaps I can explain what I mean best by letting him suddenly grow up a little.

Here is a ten-month-old baby boy. He is sitting on his mother's knee while the mother is talking to me. He is lively and awake, and naturally interested in things. Instead of just letting everything get into a muddle I place an attractive object on the corner of the table, between where I am sitting and where the mother is sitting. The mother and I can go on talking, but out of the corner of one eye we can watch the baby. You may be sure that if he is just an ordinary baby he will notice the attractive object (let us call it a spoon), and he will reach for it. As a matter of fact, probably as soon as he has reached for it, he will suddenly be overcome with reserve. It is as if he thought, 'I had better think this thing out: I wonder what feelings mother will have on this subject. I had better hold back until I know'. So he will turn away from the spoon as if nothing were further from his thoughts. In a few moments, however, he will return to his interest in it, and he will very tentatively put a finger on the spoon. He may perhaps grasp it, and look at mother to see what he can get from her eyes. At this point I will probably have to tell mother what to do, because otherwise she will help too much, or hinder, as the case may be; so I ask her to play as small a part in what happens as possible.

He gradually finds from his mother's eyes that this new thing he is doing is not disapproved of, and so he catches hold of the spoon more firmly and begins to make it his own. He is still very tense, however, because he is not certain what will happen if he does with this thing what he wants to do so badly. He does not even know for sure what it is that he wants to do.

We guess that in the course of a little while he will discover what he wants to do with it, because his mouth begins to get excited. He is still very quiet and thoughtful, but saliva begins to flow from his mouth. His tongue looks sloppy. His mouth begins to want the spoon. His gums begin to want to enjoy biting on it. It is not very long before he has put it in his mouth. Then he has feelings about it in the ordinary aggressive way that belongs to lions and tigers, and babies, when they get hold of something good. He makes as if to eat it.

We can now say that the baby has taken this thing and made it his own. He has lost all the stillness that belongs to concentration, and wondering, and doubt. Instead he is confident, and very much enriched by the new acquisition. I would say that in imagination he has eaten it. Just as the food goes in and is digested and becomes part of him, so this which has been made his own in an imaginative way is now part of himself and can be used. How will it be used?

Well, you know the answer because this is only a special case of what is going on all the time at home. He will put it to mother's mouth to feed her, and he will want her to play at eating it. Mind you, he does not want her to bite it really, and he would be rather frightened if she actually let it go into her mouth. It's a game; it is an exercise of the imagination. He is playing, and he invites play. What else will he do? He will feed me, and he may want me to play at eating it too. He may make a gesture towards the mouth of someone on the other side of the room. Let everybody share this good thing. He has had it; why shouldn't everyone have it? He has something he can be generous with. Now he puts it inside his mother's blouse where her breast is, and then rediscovers it and takes it out again. Now he shoves it under the blotting pad and enjoys the game of losing it and finding it again, or he notices a bowl on the table and starts scooping imaginary food out of the bowl, imaginatively eating his broth. The experience is a rich one. It corresponds to the mystery of the middle of the body, the digestive processes, the time between when the food is lost by being swallowed, and when the residue is rediscovered at the lower end in the faeces and urine. I could go on for a long time describing how different babies show that they are enriched by this kind of playing.

Now the baby has dropped the spoon. I suppose his interest began to get transferred on to something else. I will pick it up and he can take it again. Yes, he seems to want it, and he takes up the game again, using the spoon as before, as an extra bit of himself. Oh, he's dropped it again! Evidently it was not quite by chance that he dropped it. Perhaps he likes the sound of the spoon as it falls on the floor. We will see. I will hand it to him again. Now he just takes it and drops it quite deliberately; dropping it is what he wants to do. Once again I give it back to him, and he practically throws it away. He is now reaching out for other interests, the spoon is finished with; we have come to the end of the show.

We have watched the baby develop an interest in something, and make it part of himself, and we have watched him use it, and then finish with it. This sort of thing is going on all the time at home, but the sequence is more obvious in this special setting, which gives time for the baby to go right through an experience.

What have we learned watching this little baby boy?

For one thing, we have witnessed a completed experience. Because of the controlled circumstances there could be a beginning, a middle, and an end to what happened; there was a total happening. *This is good for the baby.* When you are in a hurry, or are harassed, you cannot allow for *total happenings*, and your baby is the poorer. When you have time, however, as you certainly should have when you have care of a baby, you can allow for these. Total happenings enable babies to catch hold of time. They do not start off knowing that when something is on it will finish.

Do you see how the middle of things can be enjoyed (or if bad, tolerated) only if there is a strong sense of start and finish?

By allowing your baby time for total experiences, and by taking part in them, you gradually lay a foundation for the child's ability eventually to enjoy all sorts of experiences without jumpiness.

Another thing we can get out of watching that baby with the spoon. We saw how there came doubt and hesitation at the start of a new venture. We watched the child stretch out and touch and handle the spoon, and after the first simple reaction he temporarily withdrew interest. Then, by carefully sensing the feelings of his mother, he allowed interest to return. He was tense and uncertain, however, till he had actually got the spoon to his mouth and had chewed it.

At first your baby is ready to consult you, if you are there when new situations arise. So you will need to know clearly what to let the baby touch, and what not to allow. The simplest way is the best, and this is to avoid having things around that the baby must not take and mouth. You see, the baby is trying to get at the principles that underlie your decisions, so as eventually to be able to foretell what you allow. A little later words will help, and you will say 'too sharp', 'too hot', or in some other way indicate danger to the body; or you will have a way of letting it be known that your engagement ring, put on one side while you are washing, is not put there for the baby's benefit.

Do you see how you can help your baby to avoid being in a muddle about what is good and what is bad to touch? You do this simply by being clear yourself as to what you prohibit, and why; and by being there on the spot, a preventer rather than a curer. Also, you deliberately provide things that the baby will like to handle and chew.

Another thing. We could talk of what we saw in terms of skills, the baby learning to reach out and to find and to grasp, and to put an object to the mouth. I am surprised when a baby of six months goes through this whole performance. On the other hand the interests of a child of fourteen months are too varied for us to expect to see anything so clearly as we saw with our ten-month-old baby boy.

But I think the best thing we learned watching the baby was this. *We saw by what happened that he is not just a body, he is a person.*

The ages at which various kinds of skill develop are interesting to record, but there was more in this than skill. There was play. By playing, the baby showed that he had built up something in himself that could be called material for play, an inner world of imaginative liveliness, which the playing expresses.

Who can say how early there are the beginnings of this imaginative life of the infant, which enriches and is enriched by the bodily experience? At three months a baby may want to put a finger on mother's breast, playing at feeding her, while taking milk at the breast. And what about the earlier weeks? Who knows? A tiny baby may want to suck a fist or finger, while taking from breast or bottle (having cake *and* eating it, so to speak), and this shows that there is something more than just a need for the satisfaction of hunger.

But for whom am I writing? Mothers have no difficulty in seeing the person in their own babies from the start. But there are people who tell you that until they are six months old babies are nothing but bodies and reflexes. Don't be put off by people who talk like that, will you?

Enjoy finding what there is to be found, as it turns up, of the person your baby is, because the baby needs this of you. So you will be ready waiting, without hurry, fuss, or impatience, for the baby's playfulness. It is this, above all, which indicates the existence of a personal inner life in the baby. If it meets in yourself a corresponding playfulness the inner richness of the baby blossoms out, and your playing together becomes the best part of the relationship between the two of you.

28

Close-up of Mother Feeding Baby

> Originally published in *The ordinary devoted mother and her baby* (pp. 27–31). London: C. A. Brock, 1949. Also published in *The child and the family: First relationships* (pp. 38–42). London: Tavistock, 1957; and *The child, the family, and the outside world* (pp. 45–49). Harmondsworth, UK: Penguin, 1964. Broadcast 9 November 1949, as 'The Baby at Feeding Time'. I. Benzie (Producer), the sixth in the series *How's the baby?* Home Service. London: British Broadcasting Corporation (see the broadcast list [CW 12:3:2]). Recorded as part of 'The Ordinary Devoted Mother and Her Baby' [CW 12:3:3].

I have already said that the baby appreciates, perhaps from the very beginning, the *aliveness* of the mother. The pleasure the mother takes in what she does for the infant very quickly lets the infant know that there is a human being behind what is done. But what eventually makes the baby feel the person in the mother is perhaps the mother's special ability to put herself in the place of the infant, and so to know what the infant is feeling like. No book rules can take the place of this feeling a mother has for her infant's needs, which enables her to make at times an almost exact adaptation to those needs.

I will illustrate this by looking at the feeding situation, and by comparing two babies. One of them is fed by the mother at home, and the other is fed in an institution, a nice place, but a place where the nurses have a lot to do and there is no time for individual attention.

I will take the baby in the institution first. Hospital nurses who read this, and who do feed the babies in their care individually, must forgive me for using as an illustration the worst, and not the best, of what they can do.

Here then is the baby in the institution at feed-time, hardly-knowing yet what to expect. The baby that we are considering does not know much about bottles or about people, but is beginning to be prepared to believe that something satisfactory may turn up. The baby is propped up a little in the cot, and a bottle with milk is so arranged with pillows that it reaches his mouth. The nurse puts the teat into the baby's mouth, waits for a few moments, and then goes off to look after some other baby who is crying. At first things may go fairly well, because the hungry baby is stimulated to suck from the teat and the milk comes, and it feels nice; but there the thing is, sticking in the mouth, and in a few moments it has become a sort of huge threat to existence. The baby cries or struggles, then the bottle drops out, and this produces relief, but only for a little while, because soon the baby begins to want to have another go, and the bottle does not come, and then crying restarts. After a while the nurse comes back and puts the bottle in the baby's mouth again, but by now the bottle, which looks the same as it did, from our point of view, seems to the baby like a bad thing. It has become dangerous. This goes on and on.

Now let us go over to the other extreme, to the baby whose own mother is available. When I see in what a delicate way a mother who is not anxious manages the same situation I am always astounded. You see her there, making the baby comfortable, and arranging a *setting* in which the feeding may happen, if all goes well. The setting is a part of a human relationship. If the mother is feeding by the breast we see how she lets the baby, even a tiny one, have the hands free so that as she exposes her breast the texture of the skin can be felt, and its warmth—moreover the distance of her breast from the baby can be measured, for the baby has only a little bit of the world in which to place objects, the bit that can be reached by mouth, hands, and eyes. The mother allows the baby's face to touch the breast. At the beginning babies do not know about breasts being part of mother. If the face touches the breast they do not know at the beginning whether the nice feeling comes in the breast or in the face. In fact babies play with their cheeks, and scratch them, just as if they were breasts, and there is plenty of reason why mothers allow for all the contact that a baby wants. No doubt a baby's sensations in these respects are very acute, and if they are acute we can be sure they are important.

The baby first of all needs all these rather *quiet* experiences which I am describing, and needs to feel held lovingly, that is, in an alive way, yet without fuss, and anxiety, and tenseness. This is the setting. Sooner or later there will be some kind of contact between the mother's nipple and the baby's mouth. It does not matter what exactly happens. The mother is there in the situation and part of it, and she particularly likes the intimacy of the relationship. She comes without preconceived notions as to how the baby ought to behave.

This contact of the nipple with the baby's mouth gives the baby ideas!— 'perhaps there is something there outside the mouth worth going for'. Saliva begins to flow; in fact, so much saliva may flow that the baby may enjoy swallowing it, and for a time hardly needs milk. Gradually the mother enables the baby to build up in imagination the very thing that she has to offer, and the baby begins to mouth the nipple, and to get to the root of it with the gums and bite it, and perhaps to suck.

And then there is a pause. The gums let go of the nipple, and the baby turns away from the scene of action. The idea of the breast fades.

Do you see how important this last bit is? The baby had an idea, and the breast with the nipple came, and a contact was made. Then the baby was finished with the idea and turned away, and the nipple disappeared. This is one of the most important ways in which the experience of the baby we are now describing differs from that of the one that we placed in the busy institution. How does the mother deal with the baby's turning away? This baby does not have a thing pushed back into the mouth in order that sucking movements shall be started up again. The mother understands what the baby is feeling, because she is alive and has an imagination. She waits. In the course of a few minutes, or less, the baby turns once more towards where she is all the time willing to place the nipple, and so a new contact is made, just at the right moment. These conditions are repeated time and again, and the baby drinks not from a thing that contains milk, but from a personal possession lent for the moment to a person who knows what to do with it.

The fact that the mother is able to make such delicate adaptation shows that she is a human being, and the baby is not long in appreciating this fact.

I want to make rather a special thing out of the way the mother in our second illustration lets the baby turn away. It is especially here, where she takes the nipple away from the baby as the baby ceases to want it or to believe in it, that she establishes herself as the mother. This is such a delicate operation at the beginning that the mother cannot always succeed, and sometimes a baby will show a need to establish the right to the personal way by refusing food, turning the head away, or going to sleep. This is very disappointing for a mother who is longing to get on with being generous. Sometimes she cannot stand the tension in the breasts (unless someone has told her how to express milk so that she can afford to wait till the baby turns towards her). If mothers knew, however, that the turning away of the baby from the breast or from the bottle had a value, they might be able to manage these difficult phases. They would take the turning away, or the sleepiness, as an indication for special care. This means that everything must be done in the way of providing the right setting for the feed. The mother must be comfortable. The baby must be comfortable. Then there must be time to spare. And the baby's arms must be free. The baby must be able to have skin free with which to feel the skin of the mother. It may even be that a baby needs to be put naked on the mother's naked body. If there is difficulty, the one thing that is absolutely no use at all is the attempt to force the feeding. If there is a difficulty, it is only by giving the baby the setting to find the breast that there is any hope of establishing the right kind of feeding experience. Echoes of all this may appear at later stages in the infant's experiences.

While I am on this subject, I would like to talk about the position of the mother whose baby is just born. She has been through an anxious and severe experience, and she continues to need skilled help. She is still in the care of whoever has helped with the confinement. There are reasons why she is particularly liable just at this time to feel dependent, and to be sensitive to the opinions of any important woman who happens to be around, whether this be the matron of the hospital, or the midwife, or her own mother or mother-in-law. She is in a difficult position then. She has been preparing for this moment for nine months, and for reasons that I have tried to explain she is the best person to know what to do to get her baby to feed at the breast, and yet if the others who know so much are strong-minded, she can hardly be expected to fight them, certainly not until she has had two or three babies, and a lot of experience. The ideal thing, of course, is the happy relationship that often exists between maternity nurses or the midwife, and the mother.

If there is this happy relationship, the mother is given every chance to manage the first contact with the baby in her own way. The baby is beside her asleep most of the time, and she can keep on looking down into the cradle beside the bed to see whether it really is a nice human baby she has got. She gets used to her own baby's cry. If she is worried by the crying the baby is temporarily taken away while she sleeps, but is brought back. Then, when she senses that the baby begins to want food, or perhaps to want a general contact with her body, she is helped to take the baby into her arms and to nurse him. In the course of this sort of experience there starts the special contact between the baby's face, mouth, and hands, and her breasts.

One hears of the young mother who is bewildered. Nothing is explained to her; the baby is kept away in another room, perhaps along with other babies, except at feed-times. There is always a baby crying, so that the mother never gets to know the cry of her own baby. At feed-times the babies are brought in and handed to their mothers, wrapped round tightly with a towel. The mother is supposed to take this queer-looking object and breast-feed it (I say 'it' on purpose), but neither does she feel the life welling up in her breasts, nor does the baby have a chance to explore, and to have ideas. One even hears of so-called helpers who get exasperated when the baby does not start sucking, and who push the baby's nose in it, so to speak. There will be a few who have had this sort of horrid experience.

But even mothers have to learn how to be motherly by experience. I think it is much better if they look at it in that way. By experience they grow. If they look at it the other way and think that they must work hard at books to learn how to be perfect mothers from the beginning, they will be on the wrong tack. In the long run, what we need is mothers, as well as fathers, who have found out how to believe in themselves. These mothers and their husbands build the best homes in which babies can grow and develop.

29

The World in Small Doses

> Originally published in *The ordinary devoted mother and her baby* (1949). London: C. A. Brock, 1949 (32–37). Also published in *The child and the family: First relationships* (pp. 53–58). London: Tavistock, 1957; and *The child, the family, and the outside world* (pp. 69–74). Harmondsworth, UK: Penguin, 1964. Broadcast 16 November 1949, as 'Presenting the World to a Baby'. I. Benzie (Producer), the seventh in the series *How's the baby?* Home Service. London: British Broadcasting Corporation (see the broadcast list [CW 12:3:2]). Recorded as part of 'The Ordinary Devoted Mother and Her Baby' [CW 12:3:3].

If you listen to philosophical discussions you sometimes hear people using a lot of words over the business of what is real and what is not real. One person says that real means what we can all touch, see, and hear, while another says that it is only what feels real that counts, like a nightmare, or hating the man who jumps the bus queue. This sounds all very difficult. What relevance can these things have for the mother looking after her baby? I hope I will be able to explain.

Mothers with babies are dealing with a developing, changing situation; the baby starts off not knowing about the world, and by the time they have finished their job the baby is grown up into someone who knows about the world and can find a way to live in it, and even to take part in the way it behaves. What a tremendous development!

But you will know people who have difficulties in their relation to the things that we call real. They do not feel them to be real. For you and me things feel more real sometimes than at other times. Any one may have a dream that feels more real than reality, and for some people their personal imaginative world is so much more real to them than what we call the real world that they cannot make a good job of living in the world at all.

Now let us ask the question, why is it that the ordinary healthy person has at one and the same time a feeling of the realness of the world, and of the realness of what is imaginative and personal? How did it come about that you and I are like that? It is a great advantage to be like that, because if we are we can use our imagination to make the world more exciting, and we can use the things of the real world to be imaginative about. Do we just grow like that? Well, what I am saying is that we do not grow like that, not unless at the beginning each one of us has a mother able to introduce the world to us in small doses.

Now what are children like when they are two, three, or four years old? In this particular matter of seeing the world as it is, what can we say about the toddler? For the toddler, every sensation is tremendously intense. We, as grown-ups, only at special moments reach this wonderful intensity of feeling which belongs to the early years, and anything that helps us to get there without frightening us is welcome. For some it is music or a picture that gets us there, for some it is a football match, and for others it is dressing up for a dance, or getting a glimpse of the Queen as she passes in her car. Happy are those whose feet are well planted on the earth and yet who keep the capacity for enjoying intense sensations, even if only in the dreams that are dreamed and remembered.

For the little child, and how much more for the infant, life is just a series of terrifically intense experiences. You have noticed what happens when you interrupt play; in fact you like to give warning, so that if possible the child will be able to bring the play to some sort of an end and so tolerate your interference. A toy that an uncle gave your little boy is a bit of the real world, and yet if it is given in the right way at the right time and by the right person it has a meaning for the child which we ought to be able to understand and allow for. Perhaps we can remember a little toy that we had ourselves, and what it meant to us then. How drab it looks now if it is still on the mantelpiece! The child of two, three, and four is in two worlds at once. The world that we share with the child is also the child's own imaginative world, and so the child is able to experience it intensely. The reason for this is that we do not insist, when we are dealing with a child of that age, on an exact perception of the external world. A child's feet need not be all the time firmly planted on the earth. If a little girl wants to fly we do not just say 'Children don't fly'. Instead of that we pick her up and carry her around above our heads and put her on top of the cupboard, so that she feels she has flown like a bird to her nest.

Only too soon the child will find that flying cannot be done magically. Probably in dreams magical floating through the air may be retained to some extent, or at any rate there will be a dream about taking rather long steps. Some fairy story like the one about the Seven-League Boots, or the Magic Carpet, will be the grown-ups' contribution to this theme. At ten years or so the child will be practising long-jump and high-jump, trying to jump farther and higher than the others. That will be all that remains, except dreams, of the tremendously acute sensations associated with the idea of flying that came naturally at the age of three.

The point is that we don't clamp down reality on the little child, and we hope that we shall not have to clamp it down even when the child is five or six years old, because, if all goes well, by that age the child will have started a scientific interest in this thing that grown-ups call the real world. This real world has much to offer, as long as its acceptance does not mean a loss of the reality of the personal imaginative or inner world.

For the little child it is legitimate for the inner world to be outside as well as inside, and we therefore enter into the imaginative world of the child when we play the child's games and take part in other ways in the child's imaginative experiences.

Here is a little boy of three. He is happy, he plays all day long on his own or with other children, and he is able to sit up at table and eat like grown-up people. In the day-time he is getting quite good at knowing the difference between what we call real things and what we call the child's imagination. What is he like in the night? He sleeps, and no doubt dreams. Sometimes he wakes with a piercing yell. Mother jumps out of bed and goes in and turns on the light, and makes to take the child up in her arms. Is he pleased? On the contrary; he screams, 'Go away, you witch! I want my mummy'. His dream world has spread into what we call the actual world, and for twenty minutes or so the mother waits, unable to do anything, because for the child she is a witch. Suddenly he puts his arms round her neck and clings to her as if she had only just turned up, and before he is able to tell her about the broomstick he drops off to sleep, so that his mother is able to put him back in the cot and return to her own bed.

What about a seven-year-old little girl, a nice little child, who tells you that at her new school all the children are against her, and the mistress is horrid and is always picking her out, making an example of her and humiliating her? Of course you go to the school and have a talk with the teacher. I am not suggesting that all teachers are perfect; nevertheless you may find she is quite a straightforward person, and that, in fact, it distresses her that this child seems to bring troubles on herself.

Well, here again you know what children are. They are not supposed to know exactly what the world is like. They must be allowed to have what would be called delusions if we were talking about grown-ups. Probably you solve the whole problem by asking the teacher to tea. Soon you may find the child going to the other extreme, and having a very strong attachment to the teacher, even idolizing her, and now fearing the other children because of the teacher's love. In the course of time the whole thing settles down.

Now, if we look at smaller children at a nursery school it is hard to guess whether they will like their teacher from what we know about her. You might know her, and perhaps you do not think much of her. She's not attractive. She acted rather selfishly when her mother was ill, or something. What the child feels about her is not based on that sort of thing. It may be that the child becomes dependent on her, and is devoted to her, because she is reliably there and kind, and she may easily become someone who is necessary for the child's happiness and growth.

But all this comes out of the relationship that exists earlier between the mother and the infant. Here there are special conditions. The mother is sharing a specialized bit of the world with her small child, keeping that bit small enough so that the child is not muddled, yet enlarging it very gradually so that the growing capacity of the child to enjoy the world is catered for. This is one of the most important parts of her job. She does it naturally.

If we look more carefully at this we shall see that there are two things that a mother does which help here. One is that she takes the trouble to avoid coincidences. Coincidences lead to muddle. Examples would be handing a baby over to someone else's care at the same time as weaning, or introducing solids during an attack of measles, and so on. The other thing is that she is able to distinguish between fact and fantasy. This is worth looking at a bit more closely.

When the boy woke up in the night and called his mother a witch, she was quite clear that she was not a witch, and so she was content to wait until he came round. When the next day he asked her, 'Are there really witches, mummy?' she quite easily said 'No'. At the same time she looked out a story book with a witch in it. When your little boy turns away from the milk pudding you have specially prepared with the very best ingredients, and makes a face intended to convey the idea that it is poisonous, you are not upset, because you know perfectly well that it is good. You also know that just for the moment he feels that it is poisonous. You find ways round the difficulty, and quite possibly in a few minutes the pudding will be eaten with relish. If you had been uncertain of yourself you would have got all fussed up, and would have tried to force the pudding into the child's mouth to prove to *yourself* that it was good.

In all sorts of ways your clear knowledge of what is real and what is not real helps the child, because the child is only gradually getting to the understanding that the world is not as imagined, and that imagination is not exactly like the world. Each needs the other. You know that first object your baby loves—a bit of blanket or a soft toy—for the infant this is almost part of the self, and if it is taken away or washed the result is disaster. As the baby becomes able to start throwing this and other things away (expecting them to be picked up and returned, of course), you know the time is coming when you can begin to be allowed by your infant to go away and return.

I want to get back now to the beginnings. These later things are easy if the beginning happens to go well. I would like to look at the early feeding again. You remember I was describing the way in which the mother makes her breast available (or the bottle) just as the baby is preparing to conjure up something, and then lets it disappear as the idea of it fades from the baby's mind. Do you see how in doing this she is making a good start with the introduction of the world to the baby? In nine months the mother gives about a thousand feeds, and look at all the other things she does with the same delicate adaptation to exact needs. For the lucky infant the world starts off behaving in such a way that it joins up with his imagination, and so the world is woven into the texture of the imagination, and the inner life of the baby is enriched with what is perceived in the external world.

And now let us look again at the people talking about what 'real' means. If one of them had a mother who introduced the world to him when he was a baby in the ordinary good way, as you have been introducing the world to your own baby, then he will be able to see that real means two things, and he will be able to feel both kinds of reality at once. Next to him may be another person whose mother made a mess of it all, and for whom there has to be either one kind of real, or the other kind. For this unfortunate man either the world is there and everyone sees the same thing, or else everything is imaginary and personal. We can leave these two people arguing.

So a great deal depends on the way the world is presented to the infant and to the growing child. The ordinary mother can start and carry through this amazing business of introducing the world in small doses, not because she is clever, as philosophers need to be, but simply because of the devotion she feels for her own baby.

30

The Innate Morality of the Baby

> Originally published in *The ordinary devoted mother and her baby* (pp. 38–42). London: C. A. Brock, 1949. Also published in *The child and the family: First relationships* (pp. 59–63). London: Tavistock, 1957; and *The child, the family, and the outside world* (pp. 93–97). Harmondsworth, UK: Penguin, 1964. Broadcast 23 November 1949, as 'Problems of Management: Training Babies' [CW 12:4:4c]. I. Benzie (Producer), the eighth in the series *How's the baby?* Home Service. London: British Broadcasting Corporation (see the broadcast list [CW 12:3:2]). Recorded as part of 'The Ordinary Devoted Mother and Her Baby' [CW 12:3:3].

Sooner or later the question must be asked: how far should parents try to impose their standards and beliefs on the growing child? The ordinary thing would be to say that we are concerned here with 'training'. The word 'training' certainly brings to mind the sort of thing that I want to go into now, which is the business of how to get your baby to become nice and clean and good and obedient, sociable, moral, and so on. I was going to say happy too, but you cannot teach a child to be happy.

This word 'training' always seems to me to be something that belongs to the care of dogs. Dogs do need to be trained. I suppose we can learn something from dogs, in that if you know your own mind your dog is happier than if you do not; and children, too, like you to have your own ideas about things. But a dog doesn't have to grow up eventually into a human being, so when we come to your baby we have to start again, and the best thing is to see how far we can leave out the word 'training' altogether.

There's room for the idea that the sense of good and bad, like much else, comes naturally to each infant and child provided certain conditions of environmental care can be taken for granted. But it is a complex matter, this process of development from impulsiveness and claiming to control everyone and everything, to an ability to conform. I cannot tell you how complex it is. Such development takes time. Only if you feel it is worth while will you allow opportunity for what has to happen.

I am still talking about infants, but it is so very difficult to describe what is happening in the first months in infant terms. To make it easier, let us look now at a boy of five or six drawing. I shall pretend he is conscious of what is going on, though he is not really. He is making a picture. What does he do? He knows the impulse to scribble and to make a mess. That is not a picture. These primitive pleasures have to be kept fresh, but at the same time he wants to express ideas, and also to express them in such a way that they may possibly be understood. If he achieves a picture he has found a series of controls that satisfies him. First of all there is a piece of paper of a particular size and shape which he accepts. Then he hopes to use a certain amount of skill that has come of practice. Then he knows that the picture when it is finished must have balance—you know, the tree on either side of the house—this is an expression of the fairness which he needs and probably gets from the parents. The points of interest must balance, and so must the lights and shades and the colour scheme. The interest of the picture must be spread over the whole paper, and yet there must be a central theme which knits the whole thing together. Within this system of accepted, indeed self-imposed, controls he tries to express an idea, and to keep some of the freshness of feeling that belonged to the idea when it was born. It almost takes my breath away to describe all this, yet your children achieve it quite naturally if you will give them half a chance.

Of course, as I said, he does not know all those things in a way that would make it possible for him to talk about them. Still less does an infant know what is going on within.

The baby is rather like this older boy, only at first it is much more obscure. The pictures don't actually get painted, in fact of course they are not pictures at all, but they are little contributions to society which only the mother of the baby is sensitive enough to appreciate. A smile can contain all this, or a clumsy gesture of the arm, or a sucking noise indicating readiness for a feed. Perhaps there is a whimpering sound by which the sensitive mother knows that if she comes quickly she may be able to attend personally to a motion which otherwise becomes just a wasted mess. This is the very beginning of cooperation and social sense, and is worth all the trouble it involves. How many children who wet the bed for some years after they could get up, and save a lot of washing, are going back in the night to their infancy, trying to go over their experience again, trying to find and correct something that was missing. The thing missing in that case was the mother's sensitive attention to signals of excitement or distress which would have enabled her to make personal and good what otherwise had to be wasted, because there was no one there to participate in what happened.

Just as the baby needs to link his physical experiences to a loving relationship with the mother, so he needs this relationship as a framework for his fears. These fears are primitive in nature, and are based on the infant's expectation of crude retaliations. The infant gets excited, with aggressive or destructive impulses or ideas, which he shows as screaming or wanting to bite, and immediately the world seems to be full of biting mouths and hostile teeth and claws and all kinds of threats. In this way the infant's world would be a terrifying place were it not for the mother's general protective role which hides these very great fears that belong to the infant's early experience of living. The mother (and I'm not forgetting the father) alters the quality of the small child's fears by being a human being. Gradually the mother, and others, are recognized by the infant as human beings. So instead of a world of magical retaliations, the infant acquires a parent who understands, and who reacts to the infant's impulses, and who can be hurt or made angry. When I put it this way you will see immediately that it makes an immense difference to the infant whether the retaliatory forces become humanized or not. For one thing, the mother knows the difference between actual destruction and the intention to destroy. She says 'Ow!' when she gets bitten. But she is not disturbed at all by recognizing that the baby wants to eat her. In fact, she feels that this is a compliment, and the way the baby shows excited love. And of course, she is not too easy to eat. She says 'Ow!' but that only means that she felt some pain. A baby can hurt the breast, especially if teeth unfortunately appear early. But mothers do survive, and babies have a chance to gain reassurance from the survival of the object. You give babies something hard, something which has good survival value, like a rattle or a bone ring, because you know that it is a relief for the baby to be able to bite all out.

In these early stages what is adaptive or 'good' in the environment is building up in the infant's storehouse of experiences as a self quality, indistinguishable at first from the infant's own healthy functioning. And while the baby is consciously aware of each failure of reliability, the storing of the 'good' experiences is a process that is not a matter of consciousness.

There are two ways in which a child can be introduced to standards of cleanliness and morality, and later to religious and political beliefs. One is for the parents to implant such standards and beliefs, to force the baby or the child into accepting them, making no attempt to integrate them with the developing personality. Sadly, there are children whose development is so unsatisfactory that this is the only way for them.

The second way is to allow and encourage the innate tendencies towards morality. Because of the mother's sensitive ways, which belong to the fact of her love, the roots of the infant's personal moral sense are preserved. We have seen how the baby hates to waste an experience, and much prefers to wait, and bear frustration of primitive pleasures, if waiting adds the warmth of a personal relationship. And we have seen how the mother helps to provide the framework of a loving relationship for the infant's feelings of activity and violence. In the process of integration, impulses to attack and destroy, and impulses to give and share are related, one lessening the effect of the other. Coercive training fails to make use of this child's integrative process.

What I am describing here is in fact the gradual build-up in the child of a capacity to feel a sense of responsibility, which at base is a sense of guilt. The environmental essential here is the continued presence of the mother or mother-figure over the period of time in which the child is accommodating the destructiveness that is part of his or her make-up. This destructiveness becomes more and more a feature in the experience of object relationships, and the phase of development to which I am referring lasts from about six months to two years after which the child may have made a satisfactory fusion of the idea of destroying the object with the fact of loving the same object. The mother is needed over this time and she is needed because of her survival value. She is an environment mother and at the same time an object mother, the object of excited loving. The child gradually comes to integrate these two aspects of the mother and to be able to love and to be affectionate with the mother at the same time. This involves the child in a special kind of anxiety which is called a sense of guilt. The infant gradually becomes able to tolerate feeling anxious (guilty) about the destructive elements in instinctual experiences, because he knows that there will be opportunity for repairing and rebuilding.

The balance implied here gives a deeper sense of right and wrong than any merely imposed parental standards. What it does owe to the mother is the reliable environment provided by her love. We can see the capacity for a sense of guilt disappearing, along with the loss of confidence in the reliability of the environment, as when a mother has to be away from her infant, or when she is ill, or perhaps preoccupied.

We can if we like think of the child as developing an internal good mother, who feels it is a happy achievement to get any experience within the orbit of a human relationship. When this has begun to happen, the mother's own sensitivity can become less intense. At the same time she can begin to reinforce and enrich the child's developing morality.

Civilization has started again inside a new human being, and the parents should have some moral code waiting for their child when, much later, he starts looking for one. One function of this will be to humanize the child's own cripplingly fierce morality, his hatred of compliance at the expense of a personal way of life. It is good for this fierce morality to be humanized, but it must not be killed—as it can be by parents understandably putting too great a value on peace and quiet. Compliance brings immediate rewards and adults only too easily mistake compliance for growth.

# Weaning

> Originally published in *The ordinary devoted mother and her baby* (pp. 43–47). London: C. A. Brock, 1949. Also published in *The child and the family: First relationships* (pp. 64–68). London: Tavistock, 1957; and *The child, the family, and the outside world* (pp. 80–84). Harmondsworth, UK: Penguin, 1964. Broadcast 30 November 1949. I. Benzie (Producer), the ninth and final talk in the series *How's the baby?* Home Service. London: British Broadcasting Corporation (see the broadcast list [CW 12:3:2]). Recorded as part of 'The Ordinary Devoted Mother and Her Baby' [CW 12:3:3].

You know me well enough by now not to expect me to tell you exactly how and when to wean; there are more good methods than one, and you can get advice from your Health Visitor or clinic. What I want to do is to talk about weaning in a general way, to help you to see what you are doing, whichever way you do it.

The fact is that most mothers don't have any difficulty. Why is this?

The main thing is that the feeding itself has gone well. The baby really has had something to be weaned from. You cannot deprive people of something they have never had.

I can distinctly remember on one occasion, as a little boy, being allowed to eat as much of raspberries and cream as I could possibly take. It was a wonderful experience. Now I can enjoy memories of that one experience better than I enjoy eating raspberries. Perhaps you can remember something like that?

So the basis of weaning is the good feeding experience. In an ordinary nine months at the breast a baby has had it a thousand or so times, and this gives plenty of good memories, or material for good dreams. But it is not the thousand times, it is also the way the baby and the mother were brought together. The mother's sensitive adaptation (as I have said so often) to the infant's needs started off the idea of the world as a good place. The world went to meet the infant, and so the infant could go out to meet the world.

The mother's cooperation with the baby at the beginning led naturally on to the baby's cooperation with the mother.

If you believe, as I do, that the baby has ideas right from the start, the feeding times were often pretty terrible, disrupting the quiet of sleep or of waking contemplation. Instinctual demands can be fierce and frightening, and at first can seem to the infant like threats to existence. Being hungry is like being possessed by wolves.

By nine months the baby has become used to this sort of thing, and has become able to hold together even while these instinctual urges hold sway. The baby has even become able to acknowledge the urges as a part of what it means to be a person alive.

As we look at the infant developing into a person, we can see how the mother is gradually perceived in the quiet times as a person too, as something attractive and valued exactly as she appears. How awful then to be hungry, and to feel oneself ruthlessly attacking this same mother. No wonder infants often lose appetite. No wonder some infants fail to allow the breasts to the mother, but separate off the mother who is loved as whole and beautiful from the things (the breasts) that are the objects of excited attack.

Adults find it difficult to let themselves go when they are excited about each other, and this causes much misery, and makes for unsuccessful marriages. The basis for eventual health in this and in many other respects is the whole experience of being carried through infancy by the ordinary good mother who is not afraid of her infant's ideas, and who loves it when her baby goes at her all out.

Perhaps you see why it really is a richer experience for a mother to feed by the breast, and for a baby to be fed at the breast? Everything can be done as well by bottle, and often it is best to go on to the bottle, which may be easier for the baby precisely because it is less exciting. But the breast-feeding experience carried through and terminated successfully is a good basis for life. It provides rich dreams, and makes people able to take risks.

But all good things must come to an end, as the saying is. It is part of the good thing that it ends.

In the last chapter [CW 3:4:30] I described a baby who caught hold of a spoon. He took it, he mouthed it, he enjoyed having it to play with and then he dropped it. So the idea of the ending can come from the baby.

It is plain that at seven, eight, or nine months a baby is beginning to be able to play games of throwing things away. It is a very important game, and it can even be exasperating, because someone has to be all the time bringing back the things thrown down. Even in the street, when you come out of the shop you find the baby has thrown out of the pram on to the pavement a teddy-bear, two gloves, a pillow, three potatoes, and a piece of soap. Probably you find someone picking everything up, because the baby obviously expects this.

By nine months most babies are pretty clear about getting rid of things. They may even wean themselves.

In weaning, the aim really is to use the baby's developing ability to get rid of things, and to let the loss of the breast be not just simply a chance affair.

But we must look to see why a baby should ever be weaned at all. Why not go on for ever? Well, I think I have to say that it would be sentimental never to wean. It would be unreal somehow. A wish to wean must come from the mother. She must be brave enough to stand the baby's anger and the awful ideas that go with anger, and just to do what rounds off the job of good feeding. No doubt the baby who has been successfully fed is happy to be weaned in due course, especially as there goes with this a vast extension of the field of experience.

Naturally, when weaning-time comes you will be already introducing other things. You will have provided hard things, rusks and so on, for the baby to chew, and you will have substituted broth or something for one of the breast feeds. You will have put up with a possible refusal of anything new, and found that, by waiting and then going back to the thing that had been refused, you may be rewarded by an acceptance of it. There is usually no need for a sudden change-over from all breast to no breast at all. When (through illness or some other bad chance) the sudden change-over has had to be made, you will have expected difficulties.

If you know that the reactions to weaning are complex you will naturally avoid handing your baby over to someone else's care just as you wean. It would be a pity to wean at the same time as you move from one home to another, or when you go to stay with your aunt. Weaning is one of those experiences that the baby can grow on, if you provide a stable setting for the experience. If you cannot do this, then weaning can be a time when difficulties start.

Another thing, you may easily find that your baby thrives on being weaned in the day, but perhaps for the last feed the breast is the only good thing. You see, your baby is growing up, but his forward march is not maintained all the time. You will find this all along. You will be quite happy if your child is as old as his age some of the time; perhaps he will be beyond his age at certain moments. But every now and again he will be just a baby, even a tiny baby. And you go to meet these changes.

Your older boy is dressing up and bravely fighting enemies. He is ordering everyone about. He bumps his head on the table as he stands up and then suddenly he is a baby, with his head on your lap, sobbing. You expect this, and you expect your baby of twelve months to be only six months old at times. It is all part of your skilled job, knowing just how old your child is at any one moment.

So you may be going on with a breast feed in the evening after you have weaned in the day. But sooner or later you will have to wean altogether, and if you know what you intend to do it is easier for the child than if you cannot make up your mind.

Let me look and see now what reactions you may expect to the weaning which you so bravely do. It may be, as I have said, that the baby does a self-weaning act, and so you do not notice any trouble. Even here there may be some lessening of the zest for food.

Very often, when the weaning is done it is done gradually, and in a stable setting, and no special trouble arises. The infant obviously loves to have the new experience. But I do not want you to think it is very unusual if there are reactions to weaning, even severe ones. A baby who has been doing well may react by losing eagerness for food, or by painfully refusing food, showing a longing for it by irritability and crying. It would be harmful to force food on the baby at this stage. For the time being everything has gone bad from his point of view and you cannot get round this. You can only wait, being ready for a gradual return of feeding.

Or the baby may start to wake screaming. You just help on the waking-up process. Or things may go well, but nevertheless you notice a change towards sadness in the child, a new note in the crying, perhaps going over into a musical note. This sadness is not necessarily bad. Don't just think sad babies need to be jogged up and down till they smile. They have something to be sad about, and sadness comes to an end if you wait.

The baby is sad at times like the weaning-time because circumstances have made anger come and spoil something that was good. In the baby's dreams the breasts are no longer good, they have been hated, and so now they are felt to be bad, even dangerous. That is why there is a place for the wicked woman in the fairy stories who gives poisoned apples. For the newly-weaned infant it is the really good mother whose breasts have become bad, and so there has to be time allowed for recovery and readjustment. But an ordinary good mother does not shirk even this. Often in the twenty-four hours she has to be the bad mother for a few minutes, and she gets used to this. In time she is seen as the good mother again. Eventually the child grows up and gets to know her just as she really is, neither ideal nor indeed a witch.

So, there is a wider aspect of weaning—weaning is not only getting a baby to take other foods, or to use a cup, or to feed actively using the hands. It includes the gradual process of disillusionment, which is part of the parents' task.

The ordinary good mother and father do not want to be worshipped by their children. They endure the extremes of being idealized and hated, hoping that eventually their children will see them as the ordinary human beings they certainly are.

32

Young Children and Other People

Originally published in *Young Children*, 1949, 1(3), 36. Also published in *The child and the family: First relationships* (pp. 92–99). London: Tavistock, 1957; and *The child, the family, and the outside world* (pp. 103–110). Harmondsworth, UK: Penguin, 1964.

The emotional development of an infant starts at the beginning of his life. If we are to judge the way in which a human being deals with his fellow creatures, and see how he builds up his personality and life, we cannot afford to leave out what happens in the earliest years, months, and even weeks and days of his life. When we approach the problems of adults, for instance those associated with marriage, we are, of course, confronted with a great deal that belongs to later development. Nevertheless, in the study of any one individual we find the past as well as the present, the infant as well as the adult. Feelings and thoughts which can conveniently be called sexual appear at an early age, much earlier than was allowed for in the philosophy of our grandparents, and in a sense the whole range of human relationships is there from the start.

Let us see what happens when healthy small children play at fathers and mothers. On the one hand we can be sure that sex comes into the game, although very often not by direct representation. It is possible to detect many symbols of adult sex behaviour, but it is not with this that I am concerned at the present moment. More important from our point of view is that these children are enjoying in their play something which is based on their ability to feel identified with their parents. Obviously they have observed a great deal. One can see in their games that they are building a home, arranging the house, taking joint responsibility for the children, even maintaining a framework in which the children in this game can discover their own spontaneity. (For children become frightened of their own impulses if left entirely on their own.) We know this is healthy; if children can play together like this they will not need later on to be taught how to build a home. They know the essentials already. Putting it the other way round, is it possible to teach people how to build a home if they have never had it in them to play fathers and mothers? I should think probably not.

While we are glad to see children thus able to enjoy games which show their ability to become identified with the home and with the parents, and with a mature outlook and a sense of responsibility, these are not things that we want our children to achieve all day long. Indeed, it would be alarming if they did so. We expect the same children who play this game in the afternoon to be just greedy children at tea-time, jealous of each other at bed-time, naughty and defiant the next morning; for they are still children. If they are lucky their real home exists. In the setting of their real home, they can go on discovering their own spontaneity and individuality, letting themselves go, as a story-teller does, surprising himself at the ideas that turn up as he warms to his task. In real life they can use their own real parents, although in the game they seek in turns to be the parents themselves. We welcome the appearance of this game of home-building along with all the other games of teachers and pupils, doctors, nurses, and patients, bus drivers and passengers.

We can see the health in it all. But by the time children have reached this stage at which they play games, we can easily understand that they have already been through many complex processes of development, and these processes are, of course, not ever actually completed. If children need an ordinary good home with which to become identified, they also deeply need a stable home and a stable emotional environment in which they can have the opportunity to make steady and natural progress, in their own time, through the very early stages of development. By the way, it is not necessary for parents to know all that goes on in the minds of their small children, any more than they need know all about anatomy and physiology in order to give their children physical health. It is essential for them, however, to have the imagination to recognize that parental love is not merely a natural instinct within themselves, but it is something which a child absolutely needs of them.

The baby is in a bad way who is cared for by a mother who, though well-meaning, believes that babies are little more at the beginning than a bundle of physiology and anatomy and conditioned reflexes. No doubt the baby will be well fed, and he may achieve physical health and growth, but unless his mother can see the human being in the new-born infant, there is but little chance that mental health will be soundly based in such a way that the child in later life can have a rich stable personality that can not only adapt to the world, but also be part of the world which demands adaptation.

The trouble is that the mother naturally tends to be afraid of her great responsibility, and she easily flies to the textbooks and the rules and regulations. The proper care of an infant can only be done from the heart; perhaps I should say that the head cannot do it alone, but can do it only if feelings are free.

Giving food is only one of the ways in which a mother makes herself known to her infant, but it is an important one. I wrote earlier that the child who has been sensitively fed at the beginning and sensitively managed in other ways has really got beyond any answer that can be given to our philosophical conundrum, 'Is that object over there really there, or is it only imagined?' Whether the object is real or illusory has become relatively unimportant to him because he has found a mother who has been willing *to provide him with the illusion,* and to provide it unfailingly and for a long enough period so that the gulf that there can be between what can be imagined and what is actually to be found has been reduced for this child personally as much as it is possible for it to be reduced.

Such a child has established at the end of his nine or so months a good relationship to something outside himself which he is coming to recognize as his mother, a relationship which is able to survive all possible frustrations and complications and even loss by separation. The baby who has been fed mechanically and insensitively and with no one wanting actively to adapt to the needs of that particular infant is at a great disadvantage, and if such a baby can conceive of a devoted mother at all such a mother must remain an imaginary idealized figure.

We may easily find a mother who is unable to live in the world of the infant, who must live in the mother's world. Such a child may make very good progress from the point of view of the superficial observer. It may not be until adolescence or even later that he at last makes appropriate protest, and either breaks down or finds mental health only in defiance.

In contrast, the mother who actively adapts in a rich way gives her baby a basis for making contact with the world, and more than that, gives a richness to the baby's relationship with the world which can develop and come to fruition as maturity follows in the course of time. A not unimportant part of this initial relationship of the baby with the mother is the inclusion in it of powerful instinctual drives; the survival of the baby and the mother teaches the baby through experience that instinctual experiences and excited ideas can be allowed, and that they do not necessarily destroy the quiet type of relationship, friendship, and sharing.

It should not be concluded that every baby who is sensitively fed and managed by a devoted mother is necessarily bound to develop complete mental health. Even when the early experiences are good, everything gained has to be consolidated in the course of time. Nor should it be concluded that every baby who is brought up in an institution, or by a mother who is unimaginative or too frightened to trust her own judgement, is destined for the mental hospital or Borstal. Things are not so simple as this. I have deliberately simplified the problem for the sake of clarity.

We have already seen that the healthy little child who is born into good conditions, whose mother has treated him as a person in his own right from the start, is not just nice, and good, and compliant. The normal child has a personal view of life from the beginning. Healthy babies often have quite strong feeding difficulties; they may be defiant and wilful in regard to their excretions; they protest often and vehemently with screaming, they kick their mothers and pull their mothers' hair, and they try to gouge their eyes out; in fact they are a nuisance. But they display spontaneous and absolutely genuine affectionate impulses, a hug here and a little bit of generosity there; through these things the mothers of such infants find reward.

Somehow the textbooks seem to like good, compliant, clean children, but these virtues are only of value when the children develop them in the course of time, because of their growing ability to become identified with the parental side of home life. This is rather like the natural progression in a child's artistic efforts, which was described in an earlier chapter.

Nowadays we so often speak of the maladjusted child, but the maladjusted child is one to whom the *world* has failed to adjust adequately at the beginning and in the early stages. The compliance of an infant is a terrible thing. It means that the parents are buying convenience at a heavy price, which will have to be paid over and over again either by them, or by society if the parents cannot stand the racket.

I should like to mention a difficulty in this matter of the earliest relationship between the mother and the infant which concerns any prospective mother. At the time of the birth of the baby and for the few days afterwards, the doctor must be an important person for her, the one who is responsible for what goes on, and in whom she has confidence. There is nothing more important at such a time than for the mother to know her doctor, and the nurse who works with the doctor. Unfortunately it cannot be assumed that the doctor who is so very skilled in regard to physical health and physical disease and with the whole problem of the management of childbirth is equally well informed in regard to the emotional tie between the baby and the mother. There is so much for a doctor to learn that he can hardly be expected to be an expert on the physical side and also to be right up to date with the latest that there is to be known about the psychology of mothers and their babies. It is always possible, therefore, that an excellent doctor or nurse may interfere, without meaning to do any harm at all, in this delicate matter of the first contact between mother and baby.

The mother indeed does need the doctor and the nurse, and their skill, and the framework which they provide enables her to put her worries aside. Within that framework, however, she needs to be able to find her infant and to enable her infant to find her. She needs to be able to let this happen in a natural way, not according to any rules that can be found in books. Mothers need not feel ashamed to find they are specialists just at this point where the doctor and the nurse are only in a position to assist.

There can be observed a general cultural tendency away from direct contact, away from the clinical, away from what used to be called vulgar, that is to say naked, natural, and real, and there is a tendency towards whatever is at one remove from actual physical contact and interchange.

There is another way in which the infant's emotional life forms the basis for the emotional life of the individual at a later stage. I have spoken about the way in which instinctual drives enter the relationship of the infant to the mother right from the beginning. Along with these powerful instincts are the aggressive elements, and also there is all the hate and anger that arise from frustration. The aggressive element in, and associated with, the excited love impulses makes life feel very dangerous, and because of this most individuals become to some extent inhibited. It is perhaps profitable to look at this part of the problem a little more closely.

I would say that the most primitive and early impulses are felt ruthlessly. If there is a destructive element in the early feeding impulse the infant is at first not concerned with the consequences. I am, of course, talking about the ideas, and not just about the actual physical processes which we can watch with our eyes. At first the infant is carried away by impulses, and only very gradually there comes the realization that the thing attacked in an excited feeding experience is a vulnerable part of the mother, the other human being who is so much valued as a person in the quiet intervals between excitements and orgies. The excited infant violently attacks the mother's body in fantasy although the attack that we see is but feeble; satisfaction comes with the feeding experience, and for the time being the attack ceases. Every physical process is enriched by fantasy, which steadily develops definiteness and complexity as the baby grows. In the baby's fantasy the mother's body was torn open so that the good things could be got at and incorporated. How important it is, therefore, for a baby to have his mother consistently looking after him, looking after him over a period of time, surviving his attacks, and eventually there to be the object of the tender feeling and the guilt feeling and sense of concern for her welfare which come along in the course of time. Her continuing to be a live person in the baby's life makes it possible for the baby to find that innate sense of guilt which is the only valuable guilt feeling, and which is the main source of the urge to mend and to re-create and to give. There is a natural sequence of ruthless love, aggressive attack, guilt feeling, sense of concern, sadness, desire to mend and build and give; this sequence is the essential experience of infancy and early childhood and yet it cannot become a real thing unless the mother, or someone doing her job for her, is able to live through the phases with the infant, and so to make possible the integration of the various elements.

And here is yet another way of stating some of the things that the ordinary good mother is doing for her infant. Without undue difficulty and without knowing what she is doing, the average good parent is all the time helping the child to distinguish between the actual happenings and what goes on in the imagination. She is sorting out for the infant the actual from the enriching fantasy. We say she is being objective. In the matter of aggression this is particularly important. A mother protects herself from being bitten badly and she prevents the two-year-old child from hitting the new baby on the head with a poker, but at the same time she recognizes the tremendous force and reality of the destructive and aggressive *ideas* that belong to the child who is behaving tolerably well, and she is not alarmed by ideas. She knows that ideas must be there, and when they gradually appear in play or in dreams she is not surprised, and she even provides stories and storybooks which carry on the themes that arise spontaneously in the child mind. She does not try to prevent the child from having ideas of destruction, and in that way she enables innate guilt to develop in its own way. It is innate guilt that we hope will turn up as the infant develops, and for which we are willing to wait; imposed morality bores us.

The period in which one is called on to be a mother or father is certainly a time of self-sacrifice. The ordinary good mother knows without being told that during this time nothing must interfere with the continuity of the relationship between the child and herself. Does she know that when she is acting quite naturally in this way, not only is she laying the foundation of the mental health of her child, but also the child cannot achieve mental health without having at the beginning just that experience which she is taking so much trouble to provide?

33

Stealing and Telling Lies

Originally published in *The child and the family* (1957). London: Tavistock, 1957 (pp. 117–120). Also published in *The child, the family, and the outside world* (pp. 161–166). Harmondsworth, UK: Penguin, 1964.

The mother who has had several healthy children will know that each one of them presented acute problems every now and again, especially when two, three, and four years old. One child had a period of night-screaming of very severe intensity so that the neighbours thought that she was being ill-treated. Another one absolutely refused to be trained to be clean. Another one was so clean and good that the mother was worried lest the child should be completely lacking in spontaneity and personal enterprise. Yet another of her children was liable to terrific temper tantrums, perhaps with head banging and the holding of breath, until the mother was at her wit's end, and the child was blue in the face and as near to having a fit as possible. A long list could be made of this sort of thing happening naturally in the course of family life. One of these uncomfortable things that happen, and one that sometimes gives rise to special difficulties, is the habit of stealing.

Little children quite regularly take pennies out of their mothers' handbags. Usually there is no problem here whatever. The mother is quite tolerant of the way the child carries on, turning out the contents of her bag, and generally messing things up. She is rather amused, when she troubles to notice it. She may even have two bags, one of which the child never gets to at all, while another more workaday one is available for the little child's exploration. Gradually the child just grows out of this and nothing more is thought of it. The mother quite rightly feels that this is healthy and a part of the child's initial relation to herself, and so to people in general.

We can easily see why it is, however, that occasionally one finds a mother really worried when her little child takes things that belong to her, and hides them. She has had experience of the other extreme, the thieving older child.

There is nothing more disturbing to the happiness of a household than the presence in it of an older child (or grown-up for that matter) who is liable to steal. Instead of the general trusting of everyone, and a free and easy way of leaving things all over the place, there has to be a specialized technique designed to protect important possessions such as money, chocolates, sugar, etc. In this case there is someone ill in the house. Many people get a very nasty feeling when they think of this. They feel uneasy when they are confronted with thieving just as they do when the word masturbation is mentioned. Apart from their having met with thieves, people may find themselves very definitely upset at the very thought of thieving, because of battles they themselves have fought over their own thieving tendencies in their own childhood. It is because of this uncomfortable feeling about out-and-out thieving that mothers sometimes worry unnecessarily about the quite normal tendency of little children to take things from their own mothers' possessions.

After a moment's thought, it will be seen that in an ordinary household, one in which there is no ill person who could be called a thief, actually quite a lot of stealing goes on; only it is not called stealing. A child goes into the larder and takes a bun or two, or helps himself to a lump of sugar out of the cupboard. In a good home no one calls the child who does this a thief. (Yet the same child in an institution may be punished and branded because of the rules that happen to obtain there.) It may be necessary for parents to make rules in order to keep the home a going concern. They may have to make a rule that whereas the children can always go and take bread, or perhaps a certain kind of cake, they may not take special cakes, and may not eat sugar from the store-cupboard. There is always a certain amount of to-and-fro about these things, and life in a household to some extent consists in the working out of the relation between the parents and the children in these and similar terms.

But a child who, say, regularly goes and steals apples, and quickly gives them away without himself enjoying them, is acting under a compulsion, and is ill. He can be called a thief. He will not know why he has done what he has done, and if pressed for a reason he will become a liar. The thing is, what is this boy doing? (Certainly the thief may be a girl, but it is clumsy to use both pronouns each time.) *The thief is not looking for the object that he takes. He is looking for a person. He is looking for his own mother, only he does not know this.* To the thief it is not the fountain pen from Woolworths, or the bicycle from the neighbour's railings, or the apple from the orchard, that can give satisfaction. A child who is ill in this way is incapable of enjoying the possession of things stolen. He is only acting out a fantasy which belongs to his primitive love impulses, and the best he can do is to enjoy the acting out, and the skill exercised. The fact is that he has lost touch with his mother in some sense or other. The mother may or may not still be there. She may even be there, and a perfectly good mother, and able to give him any amount of love. From the child's point of view, however, there is something missing. He may be fond of his mother and even in love with her, but, in a more primitive sense, for some reason or other she is lost to him. The child who is thieving is an infant looking for the mother, or for the person *from whom he has a right to steal*; in fact, he seeks the person from whom he can take things, just as, as an infant and a little child of one or two years old, he took things from his mother simply because she *was* his mother, and because he had rights over her.

There is one further point; *his own mother is really his, because he invented her*. The idea of her arose gradually out of his own capacity to love. We may know that Mrs So-and-so, who has had six children, at a certain time gave birth to this baby Johnny, and that she fed him and looked after him, and then eventually had another child. From Johnny's point of view, however, when he was born this woman was something he created; by actively adapting herself to his needs, she showed him what it would be sensible to create, as it was actually there. What his mother gave to him of herself had to be conceived of, had to be *subjective* for him before *objectivity* began to mean anything. Ultimately, in the tracing down of thieving to its roots, it can always be found that the thief has a need to re-establish his relation to the world on the basis of a re-finding of the person who, because she is devoted to him, understands him and is willing to make an active adaptation to his needs; in fact, to give him the illusion that the world contains what he can conceive of, and to enable him to place what he conjures up just where there actually is a devoted person in external 'shared' reality.

What is the practical application of this? The point is that the healthy infant in each one of us only gradually becomes able to perceive objectively the mother whom at first he created. This painful process is what is called disillusionment, and there is no need actively to disillusion a small child; rather can it be said that the ordinary good mother holds back disillusionment, and allows it only in so far as she feels the infant can take it, and welcome it.

A two-year-old child who is stealing pennies from mother's handbag is playing at being a hungry infant who thought he created his mother, and who assumed that he had rights over her and her contents. Disillusionment can come only too quickly. The birth of a new baby, for instance, can be a terrible shock just in this particular way even when the child is prepared for his or her advent and even when there is good feeling towards the new baby. The sudden access of disillusionment in respect of a little child's feeling that he created his own mother which the advent of the new baby can cause, easily starts a phase of compulsive stealing. Instead of playing at having full rights over his mother, the child may be found to be compulsively taking things, especially sweet things, and hiding them, but without really getting satisfaction from having them. If parents understand what this phase of a more compulsive type of stealing means they will act sensibly. They will tolerate it, for one thing, and they will try to see that the child whose nose has been put out of joint can at least rely on a certain quantity of special personal attention, at a certain time each day; and the time for starting the weekly penny may have arrived. Above all, parents who understand this situation will not come down like a ton of bricks on the child and demand confession. They will know that if they do so the child will certainly start lying as well as thieving, and it will be absolutely their fault.

These are common matters in ordinary healthy households, and in the vast majority of cases the whole thing is got through sensibly, and the child who is temporarily under compulsion to steal things recovers.

There is a vast difference, however, according to whether parents understand enough about what is happening to avoid unwise action, or whether they feel they must 'cure' the thieving in its early stages, in order to prevent the child from becoming a confirmed thief at a later date. Even when things eventually go well the amount of unnecessary suffering which children undergo through mismanagement of this sort of detail is tremendous. The essential suffering is sufficient indeed. It is not only in respect of thieving. In all sorts of ways children who have suffered some too great or sudden access of disillusionment find themselves under a compulsion to do things without knowing why, to make messes, to refuse to defecate at the correct moment, to cut the heads off the plants in the garden, etc.

Parents who feel they must get to the bottom of these acts, and who ask children to explain why they have done what they have done, are vastly increasing the children's difficulties, which are already intense enough just then. A child cannot give the real reason, not knowing it, and the result may be that, instead of feeling almost unbearable guilt as a result of being misunderstood and blamed, he will become split in his person; split into two parts, one terribly strict, and the other possessed by evil impulses. The child then no longer feels guilty, but is instead being transformed into what people will call a liar.

The shock of having one's bicycle stolen is not, however, mitigated by the knowledge that the thief was unconsciously looking for his mother. This is altogether another kettle of fish. Revenge feelings in the victim can certainly not be ignored, and any attempt to be sentimental about delinquent children defeats its own aim by raising the tension of general antagonism towards criminals. Magistrates in a juvenile court cannot only think of the thief as ill, and cannot ignore the anti-social nature of the delinquent act, and the irritation which this must engender in the localized bit of society which is affected. Indeed we are putting a tremendous strain on society when we ask the courts to recognize the fact that a thief is ill, so that treatment rather than punishment may be prescribed.

There is of course much stealing which never comes into the courts, because it is dealt with satisfactorily in the home of the child by ordinary good parents. One can say that a mother feels no strain when her small child is stealing from her, as she would never dream of calling this stealing, and she easily recognizes that what the child is doing is an expression of love. In the management of the four- and five-year-old child, or the child who is passing through a phase in which there is a certain amount of compulsive stealing, there is of course some strain on the parents' tolerance. We should give these parents anything that we can give in the way of understanding of the processes involved, in order to help them to carry their own children through to social adjustment. It is for this reason that I have tried to put down one person's point of view, deliberately simplifying the problem in order to present it in a form that can be understood by the good parent or teacher.

34

The Impulse to Steal

Originally published in *The child and the outside world* (pp. 176–180). London: Tavistock, 1957.

It seems to me that there is something that the ordinary parent wants to know about thieving. A statement is needed which joins up the ordinary primitive love impulses of the little child with the compulsive acts of the older child, and of the adult. Of course, any explanation that can be made in a few words must be too simple. For instance, when an older child has a compulsion to steal there may very likely be a hallucinated dominant person, or voice, that directs him, and this sort of complexity has to be left out, if a general statement is to be formulated. On the understanding that a great deal is being left out, I find it useful to put the psychology of stealing in the following way.

Simplified Statement of the Impulse to Steal

There are degrees of stealing.

When a child takes something and enjoys it we do not find ourselves wanting to use the word thief. If a child goes over the wall and takes a ripe apple and eats it and enjoys it, we feel that he is very much like any other boy, and also that he is like the small child who reaches for something on the table which has an exciting colour or shape, regardless of whether it has been offered to him or not. The older child who gets over into the orchard and takes green apples, eats them rather quickly, and then gets stomach ache, is obviously acting a little under the stress of anxiety. This is the very slightest degree of thieving. If he is sick afterwards, this may be due to the sourness of the apples, or to guilt, or maybe to both these things. This is a little nearer to thieving.

A child who, time after time, goes and steals apples, and quickly gives them away without himself enjoying them, is acting under a compulsion, and is ill. He can be called a thief. He will not know why he has done what he has done, and if pressed for a reason he will become a liar. The thing is, what is this boy doing? (Certainly the thief may be a girl, but it is clumsy to use both pronouns each time.) *The thief is not looking for the object that he takes. He is looking for a person. He is looking for his own mother, only he does not know this.* To the thief it is not the fountain pen from Woolworths, or the bicycle from the neighbour's railings, or the apple from the orchard, that can give satisfaction. A child who is ill in this way is incapable of enjoying the possession of things stolen. He is only acting out a fantasy which belongs to his primitive love impulses, and the best he can do is to enjoy the acting out, and the skill exercised. The fact is that he has lost touch with his mother in some sense or other. The mother may or may not still be there. She may even be there, and a perfectly good mother, and able to give him any amount of love. From the child's point of view, however, there is something missing. He may be fond of his mother and even in love with her, but, in a more primitive sense, for some reason or other she is lost to him. The child who is thieving is an infant looking for the mother, or for the person *from whom he has a right to steal*; in fact, he seeks the person from whom he can take things, just as, as an infant and a little child of 1 or 2 years old, he took things from his mother simply because she was his mother, and because he had rights over her.

There is one further point; *his own mother is really his, because he invented her.* The idea of her arose gradually out of his own capacity to love. We may know that Mrs So-and-so, who has had six children, at a certain time gave birth to this baby Johnny, and that she fed him and looked after him, and then eventually had another child. From Johnny's point of view, however, when he was born this woman was something he created; by actively adapting herself to his needs, she showed him what it would be sensible to create, as it was actually there. What his mother gave to him of herself had to be conceived of, had to be *subjective* for him before *objectivity* began to mean anything. Ultimately, in the tracing down of thieving to its roots, it can always be found that the thief has a need to re-establish his relation to the world on the basis of a refinding of the person who, because she is devoted to him, understands him and is willing to make an active adaptation to his needs; in fact to give him the illusion that the world contains what he can conceive of, and to enable him to place this that he conjures up just where there actually is a devoted person in external 'shared' reality.

What is the practical application of this? The point is that the healthy infant in each one of us only gradually becomes able to perceive objectively the mother whom at first he created. This painful process is what is called disillusionment, and there is no need actively to disillusion a small child; rather can it be said that the ordinary good mother holds back disillusionment, and allows it only in so far as she feels the infant can take it, and welcome it.

A two-year-old child who is stealing pennies from mother's handbag is playing at being a hungry infant who thought he created his mother, and who assumed that he had rights over her and her contents. Disillusionment can come only too quickly. The birth of a new baby, for instance, can be a terrible shock just in this particular way even when the child is prepared for his or her advent and even when there is good feeling towards the new baby. The sudden access of disillusionment in respect of a little child's feeling that he created his own mother which the advent of the new baby can cause, easily starts a phase of compulsive stealing. Instead of playing at having full rights over his mother, the child may be found to be compulsively taking things, especially sweet things, and hiding them, but without really getting satisfaction from having them. If parents understand what this phase of a more compulsive type of stealing means they will act sensibly. They will tolerate it, for one thing, and they will try to see that the child whose nose has been put out of joint can at least rely on a certain quantity of special personal attention, at a certain time each day; and the time for starting the weekly penny may have arrived. Above all, parents who understand this situation will not come down like a ton of bricks on the child and demand confession. They will know that if they do so the child will certainly start lying as well as thieving, and it will be absolutely their fault.

These are common matters in ordinary healthy households, and in the vast majority of cases the whole thing is got through sensibly, and the child who is temporarily under compulsion to steal things recovers.

There is a vast difference, however, according to whether parents understand enough about what is happening to avoid unwise action, or whether they feel they must 'cure' the thieving in its early stages, in order to prevent the child from becoming a confirmed thief at a later date. Even when things eventually go well the amount of unnecessary suffering which children undergo through mismanagement of this sort of detail is tremendous. The essential suffering is sufficient indeed. It is not only in respect of thieving. In all sorts of ways children who have suffered some too great or sudden access of disillusionment find themselves under a compulsion to do things without knowing why, to make messes, to refuse to defæcate at the correct moment, to cut the heads off the plants in the garden, etc.

Parents who feel they must get to the bottom of these acts, and who ask children to explain why they have done what they have done, are vastly increasing the children's difficulties, which are already intense enough just then. A child cannot give the real reason, not knowing it, and the result may be that, instead of feeling almost unbearable guilt as a result of being misunderstood and blamed, he will become split in his person; split into two parts, one terribly strict, and the other possessed by evil impulses. The child then no longer feels guilty, but is instead being transformed into what people will call a liar.

The shock of having one's bicycle stolen is not, however, mitigated by the knowledge that the thief was unconsciously looking for his mother. This is altogether another kettle of fish. Revenge feelings in the victim can certainly not be ignored, and any attempt to be sentimental about delinquent children defeats its own aim by raising the tension of general antagonism towards criminals. Magistrates in a juvenile court cannot only think of the thief as ill, and cannot ignore the anti-social nature of the delinquent act, and the irritation which this must engender in the localised bit of society which is affected. Indeed we are putting a tremendous strain on society when we ask the courts to recognise the fact that a thief is ill, so that treatment rather than punishment may be prescribed.[1]

There is of course much stealing which never comes into the courts, because it is dealt with satisfactorily in the home of the child by ordinary good parents. One can say that a mother feels no strain when her small child is stealing from her, as she would never dream of calling this stealing, and she easily recognises that what the child is doing is an expression of love. In the management of the four- and five-year-old child, or the child who is passing through a phase in which there is a certain amount of compulsive stealing, there is certainly some strain on the parents' tolerance. We should give these parents anything that we can give in the way of understanding of the processes involved, in order to help them to carry their own children through to social adjustment. It is for this reason that I have tried to put down one person's point of view, deliberately simplifying the problem in order to present it in a form that can be understood by the good parent or teacher.

Summary of Views Expressed

The infant who quite ordinarily and healthily claims possession of his mother, and who purloins whatever attracts him, is basking in the *illusion* that he created whatever interests him in the world's shop window. The young child who quite commonly does a bit of compulsive stealing from mother's handbag, and from the food cupboard, is reacting to a jerk forward in the painful process of *disillusionment*.

The thief, an ill person, is most of the time hopeless about the world and its relation to himself. Periodically, however, he gets a wave of hope, and this takes the form of an attempt to *get behind the disillusionment process*; the infant self, with memories of basking in illusion and in subjectivity unchallenged, comes to life, and for a brief spell inhabits the child's person. The result from our point of view is that this person, child, adolescent or adult, acts as one possessed, possessed by one aspect of his infant self, compelled to steal to make contact with society.

Note

1. See 'Some Psychological Aspects of Juvenile Delinquency' [CW 3:1:7].

Sex Education in Schools

Originally published in *Medical Press*, 1949, 222(5761). Also published in *The child and the outside world: Studies in developing relationships* (pp. 40–44). London: Tavistock, 1957; and *The child, the family, and the outside world* (pp. 216–220). Harmondsworth, UK: Penguin, 1964.

Children cannot be classed together and described all in a bunch. Their needs vary according to their home influences, the kind of children they are, and their health. However, in a brief statement on this subject of sex education it is convenient to speak generally, and not to try to adapt the main thesis to individual requirements.

Children need three things at the same time:

(1) They need persons around them in whom they can confide simply by virtue of the fact that they are trustworthy human beings with ordinary capacity for human friendship.
(2) They need instruction in biology along with other school subjects—it is assumed that biology means the truth (in so far as it is known) about life, growth, propagation, and the relation of living organisms to environment.
(3) They need continued steady emotional surroundings in which they themselves can discover each in his or her own way the upsurging of sex in the self, and the way in which this alters, enriches, complicates, and initiates human relationships.

Quite another thing is the lecture on sex, given by a person who comes to a school, delivers a talk, and then goes away. It would seem that people with an urge to teach sex to children should be discouraged. Besides, what cannot be done by the school staff cannot be tolerated by the staff either. There is something better than knowledge about sex, and that is the discovery of it by the individual.

In boarding-schools the existence of married staff with growing families in the school surround provides a natural and favourable influence, more stimulating and instructive than many lectures. In day schools the children are able to be in touch with the growing families of relations and neighbours.

The trouble about lectures is that they bring something difficult and intimate into children's lives at moments that are chosen by chance rather than by the accumulation of need in the child.

A further disadvantage of sex talks is that they seldom give a true and complete picture. For instance, the lecturer will have some bias, such as feminism, the idea that the female is passive and the male active, a flight from sex play to mature genital sex, a false theory of mother-love that leaves out the hard features and leaves only sentimentality, and so on.

Even the best sex talks impoverish the subject, which when approached from within, by experiment and experience, has the potential of infinite wealth. But it is only in an atmosphere created by the maturity of the adults that healthy adolescents can discover in themselves the body-and-soul longing for union with body and soul. In spite of these important considerations it seems that there must be room for the real experts who make a special study of sexual function and of the presentation of this sort of knowledge. Would it not be a solution to invite the experts to talk to school staffs and to develop discussions of the subject in an organized way by the teachers? The staff would then be free to act according to their own personal way in their contacts with the children, yet with a firmer foundation of knowledge of facts.

Masturbation is a sexual by-product of great importance in all children. No talk on masturbation can cover the subject, which in any case is so personal and individual that only the private talk with a friend or confidant has value. It is no use telling children in groups that to masturbate is not harmful, because perhaps for one of the group it *is* harmful, compulsive, and a great nuisance, in fact, evidence of psychiatric illness. For the others it may be harmless, and even not any trouble at all, and it is then made complex by being referred to, with the suggestion that it might be harmful. Children do, however, value being able to talk to someone about all these things, and it should have been the mother who was free to discuss absolutely anything that the child can conceive of. If mother could not do this, then others must be available, perhaps even a psychiatric interview needs to be arranged; but the difficulties are not met by sex instruction in class. Moreover, sex instruction scares away the poetry and leaves the function and sex parts high and dry and banal.

It would be more logical to point out in the art class that ideas and imaginative flights have bodily accompaniments, and that these need to be revered, and attended to, as well as ideas.

There is one obvious difficulty for those who have adolescents in their care. It is no use whatever if those who talk about allowing children to discover themselves and each other sexually are blind to the existence of the liability of some of the girls to become pregnant. This problem certainly is a real one, and has to be faced, because the illegitimate child has an unhappy position, and has a much greater task than the ordinary child if he is to make the grade and eventually become a social being; indeed unless adopted at a very early stage, the illegitimate child is unlikely to come through without scars, and perhaps ugly ones. Everyone who manages adolescents must cope with this problem according to his or her own convictions, but public opinion ought to take into account the fact that in the best type of management risks are taken and accidents do occur. In free schools, where there is practically no ban on sex, the illegitimate child is surprisingly rare, and when pregnancies do occur it is usual to find that one at least of the partners is a psychiatric case. There is the child, for instance, who, unconsciously fearing and fleeing from sex play, jumps right over to a spurious sexual maturity. Many children who have had no satisfactory infantile relation to their own mothers reach to inter-personal relationships for the first time in the sexual relationship, which is therefore extremely important to them, although from the onlookers' point of view insecurely mature, because not derived gradually from the immature. If there is a big proportion of such children in a group, sexual supervision must obviously be strict, because society cannot take more than a certain number of illegitimates. On the other hand, in most groups of adolescents the majority are more or less healthy, and in that case the question has to be asked, is their management to be based on what healthy children need or on society's fear of what may happen to a few anti-social or ill members?

Adults hate to think that children ordinarily have a very strong social sense. In the same way adults hate to think that little children have early guilt feelings, and quite regularly parents implant morality where a natural morality could have developed, and would have become a stable and pro-social force.

Ordinary adolescents do not want to produce illegitimate children, and they take steps to see that this does not happen. Given opportunity, they grow in their sex play and sex relationships to the point where they realize that the having of babies is what the whole thing is leading up to. This may take them years. But ordinarily this development comes, and then these new members of human society begin to think in terms of marriage, and of the setting up of the framework in which new babies and children can be.

Sex instruction has very little to do with this natural development which each adolescent must make for himself or herself. A mature and unanxious and unmoralistic environment helps so much that it can almost be said to be necessary. Also the parents and teachers need to be able to stand the surprising antagonism adolescents may develop towards adults, especially towards those who want to help at this critical time of growth.

When the parents are not able to give what is needed, the school staff or the school itself can often do a great deal to make up for this deficiency, but by example and by personal integrity and honesty and devotion and being on the spot to answer questions, and not by organized sex instruction.

For younger children the answer is biology, the objective presentation of nature, with no bowdlerization. At first most little children like to keep and to learn about pets and to collect and understand the ways of flowers and insects. Somewhere in the period before adolescence they can enjoy progressive instruction in the ways of animals, their adaptation to environment, and their ability to adapt environment to themselves. In among all this comes the propagation of the species, and the anatomy and physiology of copulation and pregnancy. The biological instructor that children value will not neglect the dynamic aspects of the relationship between the animal parents and the way family life develops in the evolutionary series. There will not be much need for conscious application of what is taught in this way to human affairs, because it will be so obvious. It is more likely that the children will by subjective elaboration see human feelings and fantasies into the affairs of animals than that they will blindly apply the so-called animal instinctual processes to the affairs of the human race. The teacher of biology, like the teacher of any other subject, will need to be able to direct the pupils towards objectivity and the scientific approach, expecting this discipline to be very painful to some of the children.

The teaching of biology can be one of the most pleasant and even the most exciting of tasks for the teacher, chiefly because so many children value this introduction to the study of what life is about. (Others, of course, come at the meaning of life better through history, or the classics, or in their religious experiences.) But the application of biology to the personal life and feelings of each child is altogether another matter. It is by the delicate answer to the delicate question that the linking up of the general to the particular is done. After all, human beings are not animals; they are animals plus a wealth of fantasy, psyche, soul, or inner world potential or whatever you will. And some children come at the soul through the body and some come to the body through the soul. Active adaptation is the watchword in all child care and education.

To sum up, full and frank information on sex should be available for children, but not as a thing so much as a part of the children's relationship to known and trusted people. Education is no substitute for individual exploration and realization. True inhibitions are resistant to education, and in the average case for which psychotherapy is not available these inhibitions are best dealt with through the understanding of a friend.

36

Enuresis: Notes for a Lecture to the Tavistock Children's Department

This manuscript was annotated with the following remark by Robert Tod, dated 29 October 1979: 'This paper contains notes compiled by Donald Winnicott of a paper he gave to the staff of the Tavistock Clinic Children's Department in about 1949'.[i]

1. Descriptive.
2. Physical Aspects.
3. Normal urinary function
   (a) In own right.
   (b) With elements displaced from
      1. Salivation.
      2. Oral function.
      3. Anal function.
      4. Genital function.

---

[i] The Tavistock Clinic was established by Dr Hugh Crighton-Millar in 1920. It was opened as a response to the effects of the First World War, which had left many men permanently scarred by the brutality of battle. The effects of emotional trauma—'shell shock'—were not widely understood or treated.

Following major advances in treatment and training between 1932 and 1939, many of those trained at the Tavistock went on to occupy leading positions in the fields of psychiatry and child guidance in the UK and overseas. During the Second World War, the Clinic moved from Tavistock Square to Hampstead and the greater part of the trained staff joined the armed forces as psychiatric specialists. The war-time experiences they encountered were to influence the Clinic for the remainder of the century. In the postwar period, research and development at the Tavistock had a radical impact on several aspects of medical practice, including GP training and practice, child care in hospital, and health and social policy.

In July 1948, the Tavistock Clinic became part of the UK National Health Service. It moved to its current position in Belsize Lane in 1967.

4. Urination expressing
   (a) Love.
   (b) Aggression.
5. Enuresis in relation to masturbation.
6. Enuresis as conscious defiance.
7. Enuresis as S.O.S. for environmental change.
8. Enuresis as an anti-social act, related to stealing and messing.
9. Enuresis related to
   (a) The flow of tears.
   (b) Sadness.
   (c) Depression.
10. Urgency and frequency of micturition with or without incontinence in
    (a) Excitement.
    (b) Anxiety.
    (c) Hypermania.
11. Unconscious micturition associated with repressed fantasy with anaesthesia of the urinary apparatus with denial of depression.
12. Enuresis related to the bridge-building which enables there to be contact between the inner world and internal relationships, between fantasy and fact, perhaps indicating lack of a person in the environment willing to communicate in fantasy terms with the child.

More Primitive Phenomena

1. Enuresis in states of depersonalisation.
2. Enuresis as a part function in states of unintegration of the personality.
3. The bladder as an internalised chamber pot.
4. The bladder as an internalised breast.

PART 5

1950

1

Letter to Clare Britton

[Excerpt] Originally published in S. Grolnick, L. Barkin, & W. Muensterberger (Eds.), *Between Fantasy and Reality: Transitional Objects and Phenomena*. New York: Aronson, 1978; also published in C. Winnicott, R. Shepherd, & M. Davis (Eds.), *Psychoanalytic explorations* (p. 16–17). London: Karnac.

Clare Britton (1906–1984) was a social worker and psychoanalyst who worked with Winnicott on the Oxfordshire evacuation programme during the war. Britton was appointed the head of the first training course for social workers at the London School of Economics and later became Director of Child Care Studies at the Home Office. She married Donald Winnicott in 1951.

Early 1950

Last night I got something quite unexpected, through dreaming, out of what you said. Suddenly you joined up with the nearest thing I can get to my transition object: it was something I have always known about but I lost the memory of it, at this moment I became conscious of it. There was a very early doll called Lily belonging to my younger sister and I was fond of it, and very distressed when it fell and broke. After Lily I hated *all* dolls. But I always knew that before Lily was a quelquechose of my own. I knew retrospectively that it must have been a doll. But it had never occurred to me that it wasn't just like myself, a person, that is to say it was a kind of other me, and a not-me female, and part of me and yet not, and absolutely inseparable from me. I don't know what happened to it. If I love you as I loved this (must I say?) doll, I love you all out. And I believe I do. Of course I love you all sorts of other ways, but this thing came new at me. I felt enriched, and felt once more like going on writing my paper on transition objects (postponed to October). (You don't mind do you—this about you and the T.O.?)

2

Aggression in Relation to Emotional Development

Originally published in *Collected papers: Through paediatrics to psycho-analysis* (pp. 204–218). London: Tavistock, 1958.

The first part of this paper was a contribution to a Symposium with Anna Freud, given to the Royal Society of Medicine, Psychiatry Section, 16 January 1950. The second section was given to a private group in January 1955, and the third section to a private group in November 1954. An early draft of this paper, dated December 1947 and probably written for a symposium at the Royal Society of Medicine (see letter to Anna Freud, [CW 3:3:5]), included several additional paragraphs, which have been reproduced in the footnotes.

I. Contribution to Symposium

The main idea behind this study of aggression is that if society is in danger, it is not because of man's aggressiveness but because of the repression of personal aggressiveness in individuals.

In a study of the psychology of aggression a severe strain is imposed on the student, for the following reason. In a total psychology, being-stolen-from is the same as stealing, and is equally aggressive. Being weak is as aggressive as the attack of the strong on the weak. Murder and suicide are fundamentally the same thing. Perhaps most difficult of all, possession is as aggressive as is greedy acquisition; indeed acquisition and possession form a psychological unit, either is incomplete without the other. This is not saying that acquiring and possessing are good or bad.

These considerations are painful, because they draw attention to dissociations that are hidden in current social acceptance; they cannot be left out of a study of aggression. Also, the basis for a study of actual aggression must be a study of the roots of aggressive intention.

Prior to integration of the personality there is aggression.[1] A baby kicks in the womb; it cannot be assumed that he is trying to kick his way out. A baby of a few weeks thrashes away with his arms; it cannot be assumed that he means to hit. A baby chews the nipple with his gums; it cannot be assumed that he is meaning to destroy or to hurt. At origin aggressiveness is almost synonymous with activity; it is a matter of part-function.

It is these part-functions that are organized by the child gradually, as he becomes a person, into aggression. In illness a patient may display activities and aggressiveness not fully meant. Integration of a personality does not arrive at a certain time on a certain day. It comes and goes, and even when well attained it can be lost through unfortunate environmental chance. Nevertheless, purposive behaviour is eventually arrived at if there is health. In so far as behaviour is purposive, aggression is meant. Here immediately comes the main source of aggression, instinctual experience. Aggression is part of the primitive expression of love. A description of this in oral terms is appropriate since I am studying the first love impulses.

Oral erotism gathers to itself aggressive components, and in health it is oral love that carries the basis of the greater part of actual aggressiveness— that is, aggression intended by the individual and felt as such by the people around.

All experience is both physical and non-physical. Ideas accompany and enrich bodily function, and bodily functioning accompanies and realizes[2] ideation. Also, of the sum of ideas and of memories it must be said that these gradually separate out into that which is available to consciousness, that which is available to consciousness only in certain circumstances, and that which is in the repressed unconscious, unavailable because of intolerable affect.

I am aware that I am mixing the theme of actual aggressiveness with that of aggressive impulse. I do feel, however, that the one cannot be studied without the other. No one act of aggression can be fully understood as an isolated phenomenon; and in fact the study of any one act of a child involves consideration of the following:

The child in his environment, with adults caring for him.
The child mature according to his chronological and emotional age.
The child who, although mature according to his age, contains within himself all degrees of immaturity reaching right back to the primary state.
The child as an ill person, having fixations at immature levels.
The child in a relatively unorganized emotional state, still liable with more or less ease to regression and to spontaneous recovery from regression.

AGGRESSION AT VARIOUS STAGES

It would be helpful if we could start at the beginning of the individual's life, but here there is much that is not known with certainty. A complete study would trace aggressiveness as it appears at the various stages of ego development:

Early	Pre-integration	
	Purpose without concern	
Intermediate	Integration	
	Purpose with concern	
	Guilt	
Total personal	Inter-personal relationships	
	Triangular situations, etc.	
	Conflict, conscious and unconscious	

What I attempt here is mainly a development of the second of these three themes, the intermediate.[3]

PRE-CONCERN

It is necessary to describe a theoretical stage of unconcern or ruthlessness in which the child can be said to exist as a person and to have purpose, yet to be unconcerned as to results. He does not yet appreciate the fact that what he destroys when excited is the same as that which he values in quiet intervals between excitements. His excited love includes an imaginative attack on the mother's body. Here is aggression as a part of love.[4,i]

One can see some degree of this appearing as a dissociation between quiet and excited aspects of the personality, so that children who are ordinarily nice and lovable will 'act out of character' and do aggressive things to people they love, not feeling fully responsible for their actions.

If aggression is lost at this stage of emotional development there is also some degree of loss of capacity to love, that is to say, to make relationships with objects.

STAGE OF CONCERN

Now comes the stage described by Melanie Klein as the 'depressive position' in emotional development. For my purpose I will call this the Stage of

---

[i] [1947:] In practice aggression becomes controlled by the child himself. Babies do not regularly bite the breast even when they have teeth, although it is quite certain they have it in them to do so. They have ideas. They can bite on substitute hard objects and conceive of and seek indestructible objects for reassurance. Also they begin to split their objects into good and bad, that is into those that they wish to protect and those they feel should be destroyed.

Concern. The individual's ego integration is sufficient for him to appreciate the personality of the mother figure, and this has the tremendously important result that he is concerned as to the results of his instinctual experience, physical and ideational.

The stage of concern brings with it the capacity to feel guilty. Henceforth some of the aggression appears clinically as grief or a feeling of guilt or some physical equivalent, such as vomiting. The guilt refers to the damage which is felt to be done to the loved person in the excited relationship. In health the infant can hold the guilt, and so with the help of a personal and live mother (who embodies a time factor) is able to discover his own personal urge to give and to construct and to mend. In this way much of the aggression is transformed into the social functions, and appears as such. In times of helplessness (as when no person can be found to accept a gift or to acknowledge effort to repair) this transformation breaks down, and aggression reappears. *Social activity cannot be satisfactory* except it be based on a feeling of *personal* guilt in respect of aggression.

ANGER

In my description there now comes a place for anger at frustration. Frustration, which is inevitable in some degree in all experience, encourages the dichotomy: 1. innocent aggressive impulses towards frustrating objects, and 2. guilt-productive aggressive impulses towards good objects. Frustration acts as a seduction away from guilt and fosters a defence mechanism, namely, the direction of love and hate along separate lines. If this splitting of objects into good and bad[5] takes place, there is an easing of guilt feeling; but in payment the love loses some of its valuable aggressive component, and the hate becomes the more disruptive.[ii]

GROWTH OF INNER WORLD

The psychology of the infant from now on becomes more complicated. The individual child becomes concerned not only with the effect on his mother of his impulses, but he also notes the results of his experiences in his own self. Instinctual satisfactions make him feel good, and he perceives intake and output in a psychological as well as in a physical sense. He becomes filled with what he feels to be good, and this initiates and maintains his confidence in himself and in what he feels he may expect from life. At the same time he has

---

[ii] [1947:] It will be noted that the basis for theft has now been stated, namely the purposive aim of taking the good things from the mother's body. That is to say, like other forms of aggression, theft is at origin a part of the love impulse. Every thief is unconsciously looking for the mother from whom he can claim the right to "steal" in the act of loving her.

to reckon with his angry attacks, as a result of which he feels he becomes filled with what is bad or malign or persecuting. These evil things or forces, being inside him, as he feels, form a threat from within to his own person, and to the good which forms the basis of his trust in life.

He now starts a life-long task of management of his inner world, a task which, however, cannot be started until he is well lodged in his body and able to differentiate between what is inside himself and what is external, and between what is actual and what is his own fantasy. His management of the external world depends on his management of his inner world.

An extremely complex series of defence mechanisms develops, which should be examined in any attempt to understand aggression in a child who has reached this stage of emotional development. It will be impossible here to do more than enumerate some of the ways in which this part of human psychology is relevant to the present theme.

First I will describe the return from introversion, since this is an important and common source of actual aggression.

In health the child's interest is directed both towards external reality and towards the inner world, and he has bridges between the one world and the other (dreams, play, etc.). In ill-health the child may re-arrange his relationships so that the good is concentrated within and the bad is projected. He now lives in his inner world. He may be said to have become introverted (or pathologically introverted).

A recovery from pathological introversion involves a new turning out into what is for such a child an external world full of persecutors, *and at this point in his recovery the child regularly becomes aggressive.* This is an important source of aggressive *behaviour.* If in a child's recovery from introversion the attack-in-defence is mishandled by those in charge, the child easily slips back into introversion. Apart from illness, some degree of this state of affairs is met daily in the life of any small child, and the concept is by no means a purely theoretical one. An individual is in a sensitive state on coming round after a period of concentration on a personal task.

It must be remembered that in childhood we are watching the human being only gradually becoming able to distinguish between the subjective and objective. A state of what looks like delusional madness easily appears through the child's projection of inner world experience. Even the healthy child of two or three commonly wakes in the night and feels he is in a world which (from our point of view) is his own inner world, not the external reality that we can share with him. In daytime small children become deluded in their play activities and, in fact, children can be found to be living chiefly in their inner world when apparently to us they are in our world. This need not be unhealthy, but in the management of such a child we cannot expect to meet with logic, which applies only to external or shared reality. A large proportion even of adults never achieve a reliable capacity for objectivity, and those who are most reliably objective are often comparatively out of touch with their own inner world's richness.

Three other examples will be given of the way in which the child's management of his own inner world explains aggressive behaviour.

In the child's fantasy the inner world is localized primarily in the belly or secondarily in the head or some other specific bodily area.

A child who has reached a certain degree of personality organization meets with an experience such that it is beyond his power to deal with it by identification. For instance, his parents quarrel in front of him at a time when he is fully occupied over some other problem. He manages only by taking the whole experience into himself in order to master it. It can then be said that a fixed state of parents quarrelling is living inside him, and a quantity of energy is thenceforth directed towards the control of the internalized bad relationship. Clinically he becomes tired, or depressed, or physically ill. At certain times the internalized bad relationship takes over, and then the child behaves as if 'possessed' by the quarrelling parents. We see him as compulsively aggressive, nasty, unreasonable, deluded.[6]

Alternatively the child with introjected quarrelling parents periodically engineers quarrelling in the people around him, then using the real external badness as a projection of what was 'bad' within. In such a case, there may easily be times of madness with true hallucination of quarrelling voices or people.

In the child's management of his inner world and in the attempt to preserve in it what is felt to be benign, there are moments when he feels that all would be well if a unit of malign influence could be eliminated. (This is equivalent to the scapegoat idea.)

Clinically there appears a dramatization of ejection of badness (kicking, passage of flatus, spitting, etc.). Alternatively the child is accident-prone, or there is a suicide attempt—with the aim to destroy the bad within the self; in the total fantasy of the suicide there is to be a survival, with the bad elements destroyed, but survival may not occur.

The management of inner world phenomena, felt by the child to be in the belly (or head, etc.), from time to time presents so great a difficulty that the child puts on a comprehensive control—with depressive mood as the clinical result. This leads to a state of inner deadness which is intolerable. The complementary state of mania is liable to occur. In this the inner world liveliness takes over and activates the child, who may clinically be violently aggressive, without obvious external stimulus for anger. These phases of mania are not the same as that which is called the manic defence, in which there is a denial of inner deadness by artificial activity (the so-called manic defence against depression, Klein). The clinical result of the manic defence is not an aggressive outburst, but a state of common anxious restlessness, hypomania, in which there is mild aggression in the form of untidiness, messiness, irritability with lack of constructive perseverance.

In health, the individual can store badness within for use in an attack on external forces that seem to threaten what is felt to be worth preserving. Aggression then has social value.

The value of this (as compared with maniacal or delusional aggression) lies in the fact that objectivity is preserved, and the enemy can be met with economy of effort. The enemy then does not need to be loved in order to be attacked.[iii]

SUMMARY

The foregoing mainly describes the relation of aggression to what I have called the *intermediate* stage of emotional development. This stage precedes the *total personal*, with its interpersonal relationships and the triangular situations of the Oedipus complex, and it follows on after the *early* stages of ruthlessness, and of the era before purpose and before the integration of the personality.

Aggression that belongs to the stage that I have called *total personal* is already familiar to the present generation through the accepted work of Freud.

[iii] [1947:] *Aggression in the Relationship Between Mature Persons*
Only after all this are we prepared to consider the more mature child whose instinctual drives have come to include the genital organization. But the story is the same, with the accent on genital rather than on oral experience. At the same time the child's own idea of his personality becomes more capable of description in the familiar terms of behaviour enriched by phantasy, conscious and unconscious, instead of in less familiar terms of management of internal and external reality.

Now inter-personal relationships can be studied along with rivalries, jealousies and death wishes. But these matters are not so difficult to grasp in these times when the once revolutionary theories of Freud are generally accepted, at least as ideas.

It is but seldom that actual aggressive behaviour can be explained on a basis of mature emotional development with genital organization completed. The problem remains, however, would there be wars if all men and women were emotionally mature? Would adolescents, if mature for their age, need to fight to kill, or to possess? Would mature adults require their adolescent children to risk death in the initiation rite? Possibly. In considering this we must be prepared to consider the value of war, not only to study the causes of war in order to be able to end wars.

In practice a human being is only to some extent and in certain circumstances a being dominated by a simple genital organization, the rest of the psyche can never be ignored; and society itself which cannot marry or propagate, is almost entirely moulded on the pregenital organizations of individuals, and on the child's conception of himself that I have tried to indicate by outline in this paper.

For social health, what is needed is the personal maturity of individuals, from which the rest follows. For bringing about this personal maturing of individuals environmental conditions of love and stability are absolutely essential.

in My theme is not exhausted. Two examples of important themes not dealt with, yet vital to an understanding of actual aggressivity:

> A powerful background to social unrest is the resentment felt by children and adults when they come to recognize that in the early stages of their personal development they were dependent, doubly dependent because blissfully unaware of the fact, on their mother's care. It is both men and women who develop this hate of the providers of essentials and the democratic idea is in part an attempt to get behind this memory of dependence.

in The hate of external reality itself on account of its disillusioning power.

Important sources of aggression date from the *very early* stages of the development of the human being, and some of these will be traced in the next part of this chapter.

II. Very Early Roots of Aggression

In its simplest form the question that we ask is: does aggression come ultimately from anger aroused by frustration, or has it a root of its own?

The answer is necessarily highly complex unless a deliberate effort is made to cut through the great mass of clinical fact that goes to make up our daily analytic practice. If we do this, however, we run the risk of being accounted unaware of what we have in fact deliberately ignored.

We can say that in the primitive love impulse we shall always be able to detect reactive aggression, since in practice there is no such thing as a complete id satisfaction. Is it necessary therefore to attempt to dissect down? I think it is necessary because of the confusion that results from failure to do so. This is especially true in view of the fact that the primitive love impulse is operative at a stage when ego growth is only starting, when integration, for instance, is not an established fact. There is a primitive love that is operative when there is not yet a capacity for taking responsibility. In this era there is not even ruthlessness; it is a pre-ruth era, and if destruction be part of the aim in the id impulse, then destruction is only incidental to id satisfaction. Destruction only becomes an ego responsibility when there is ego integration and ego organization sufficient for the existence of anger, and therefore of fear of the talion. However early anger and fear can be detected, there is still room for recognition of those ego developments before which it is not sensible to talk of the individual's anger.

Hate is relatively sophisticated and cannot be said to exist in these early stages. It is necessary therefore to examine aggression apart altogether from the reactive aggression that inevitably follows the id impulse because of failure of id experience due to the operation of the reality principle.

It is convenient then to say that the primitive love impulse (id) has a destructive quality, though it is not the infant's aim to destroy since the impulse is experienced in the pre-ruth era.

From this assumption it is possible to go into the matter of the root of the destructive element in the primitive love (id) impulse.

To simplify matters, the variable factor of birth trauma can be left out, and a normal or non-traumatic birth can be taken for granted. By normal here I mean that the birth is felt by the infant to be the result of his own effort. Neither delay nor precipitation interfered with this (see Birth Memories, Birth Trauma, and Anxiety [CW 3:4:8]).

The early id experiences bring into play a new element for the baby, instinctual crises, characterized by a preparatory period, a climax, and a period following some degree of satisfaction. Each of these three phases brings its own problems for the infant.

Our task is to examine the pre-history of the aggressive element (destructive by chance) in the earliest id experience. We have at hand certain elements which date from at least as early as the onset of foetal movements—namely motility. No doubt a corresponding element on the sensory side must eventually be added. Can this motility that dates from intra-uterine life, and that persists in infancy (and indeed throughout life), be linked up with the activity inherent in id experience proper? Indeed, is this activity to be classified as an id or an ego element? Or is it better to allow an undifferentiated ego-id phase (Hartmann, 1952) and to leave aside the attempt to classify motility on the ground that it appears before ego-id differentiation?

Each infant must be able to pour as much as possible of primitive motility into the id experiences. Here no doubt comes the truth of the need the infant has for the frustrations of reality—since id satisfaction if it could be complete and without hindrance would leave the infant with that which is derived from the motility root unsatisfied (Riviere, 1936).

In the pattern of id experience that belongs to any one infant there is x per cent of primitive motility included in the id experience. There is then $(100 - x)$ per cent left over for use in other ways—and here indeed is a reason for the vast difference in the experience of various individuals in regard to their aggressiveness. Here also is the origin of one kind of masochism (see later).

It is profitable to examine the patterns that evolve round this matter of motility (Marty et Fain, 1955).

In one pattern, the environment is constantly discovered and rediscovered because of motility. Here each experience within the framework of primary narcissism emphasizes the fact that it is in the centre that the new individual is developing, and contact with environment is *an experience of the individual* (in its undifferentiated ego-id state, at first). In the second pattern the environment impinges on the foetus (or baby) and instead of a series of individual experiences there is a series of *reactions to impingement*. Here then develops a withdrawal to rest which alone allows of individual existence. Motility is then only experienced as a reaction to impingement.

In a third pattern, which is extreme, this is exaggerated to such a degree that there is not even a resting place for individual experience, and the result is a failure in the primary narcissistic state to evolve an individual. The 'individual' then develops as an extension of the shell rather than of the core, and as an extension of the impinging environment. What there is left of a core is hidden away and is difficult to find even in the most far-reaching analysis. The individual then *exists by not being found*. The true self is hidden, and what we have to deal with clinically is the complex *false self* whose function is to keep this true self hidden. The false self may be conveniently society-syntonic, but the lack of true self gives an instability which becomes more evident the more society is deceived into thinking that the false self is the true self. The patient's complaint is of a sense of futility.

The first pattern is what we call healthy. It depends for its formation on good-enough mothering, with love expressed (as at first it can only be expressed) in physical terms. The mother holds the baby (in womb, or in arms) and through love (identification) knows how to adapt to ego needs. Under these conditions, and under these alone, the individual may start to exist, and starting to exist to have id experiences. The stage is set for the maximum of infusion of motility into id experiences. There is a fusion of the x per cent of motility potential with erotic potential (with x quantitatively high). Nevertheless even here there is $(100 - x)$ per cent of motility potential left out of the pattern of fusion, and available for pure motility use.

It must be remembered that the fusion allows of experience *apart from the action of opposition* (reaction to frustration). That which is fused with the erotic potential is satisfied in instinctual gratification. By contrast, the $(100 - x)$ per cent unfused motility potential *needs to find opposition*. Crudely, it needs something to push against, unless it is to remain unexperienced and a threat to well-being. In health, however, by definition, the individual can enjoy going around looking for appropriate opposition.

In the second and third patterns it is only through environmental impingement that the motility potential becomes a matter of experience. Here is illhealth. To a lesser or a greater degree, the individual *must* be opposed, and only if opposed does the individual tap the important motility source. This is satisfactory while environment consistently impinges, but:

> Environmental impingement must continue.
> Environmental impingement must have a pattern of its own, else chaos reigns since the individual cannot develop a personal pattern.
> This means dependence, out of which the individual might not grow.
> Withdrawal becomes an essential feature in the pattern. (Except in the extreme degree, with true self hidden; then even withdrawal is not available as a primitive defence.)

When the second and third patterns are operative there can be no health, and no treatment is of avail unless it changes the basic pattern in the direction of the pattern I have described first. Patients who have developed according to the second and third patterns do, however, come to analysis, and they may seem at first to be able to make especially good use of the analyst's work done on the false assumption that the patient really exists.

Here is a special comment on the positive value of the neurotic patient's resistances. The fact of these resistances, which can be analysed, gives a good prognosis. The absence of resistances leads to a diagnosis of disturbance in the early patterning of the kind I have described.

It would follow from these considerations that it is not possible to bring about a higher degree of fusion of motility and erotic potentials by analysis except in those who are normal by this method of classification. Where the first pattern is not established there cannot be a fusion except in a secondary way, through the 'erotization' of aggressive elements. Here is a root for compulsive sadistic trends, which can turn round into masochism. The individual feels real only when destructive and ruthless. He tries to bring about relationships through interplay with another individual by finding an erotic component to fuse with the aggression which is not in itself much more than pure motility. Here the erotic achieves fusion with motility, whereas in health it is more true to say that motility fuses with the erotic.

It is probable that in the perversions two kinds of masochism can be distinguished; one kind comes from a sadism which is an erotization of a crude motility urge, and the other kind is a more direct erotization of the passive of active motility; and it would appear that the development is directed one way or the other according to whether the first partner was masochistic or sadistic. The partnership produces a relationship which is valued the more because relationships were feeble when developed out of the erotic life, owing to relative lack of fusion of motility elements into the erotic life.

The sense of real comes especially from the motility (and corresponding sensory) roots, and erotic experiences with a weak infusion of the motility element do not strengthen the sense of reality or of existing. In fact such erotic experiences may be avoided precisely because they lead the subject to a sense of not existing, that is to say, in individuals whose early pattern is not of the variety that I have placed first in my description.

We are left with the conclusion that a great deal happens prior to the first feed, even if ego organization is immature. The summation of motility experiences contributes to the individual's ability to start to exist, and out of primary identification to repudiate the shell and to become the core. The good-enough environment makes this development possible. Only if the early environment is good enough does it make sense for us to discuss the early psychology of the human infant, since, *unless the environment has been good enough, the human being has not become differentiated, and has not come up as a subject for discussion in terms of normal psychology.* Where the individual does exist, however, we may say that one main way in which the ego and id, now differentiated, maintain a relationship, and keep a relationship in spite of the difficulties that belong to the operation of the reality principle, is through the fusion of a high proportion of primary motility potential in with erotic potential.

From these there follow other ideas that concern the problem of the external nature of objects. This subject is discussed in the third part of this chapter.

III. The External Nature of Objects

In psycho-analytic practice, when an analysis has gone a long way, the analyst gets a privileged view of the early phenomena of emotional growth.

I have recently been struck by the following idea, derived from clinical work, that when a patient is engaged in discovering the aggressive root the analyst is more exhausted by the process, one way or another, than when the patient is discovering the erotic root of the instinctual life.

Immediately it will be observed that the material that concerns me here is that which is associated in our minds with the word 'de-fusion'. We assume a fusion of aggressive and erotic components in health, but we do not always give proper significance to the pre-fusion era, and to the task of fusion. We may easily take fusion too much for granted, and in this way we get into futile arguments as soon as we leave the consideration of an actual case.

It must be conceded that the task of fusion is a severe one, that even in health it is an uncompleted task, and that it is very common to find large quantities of unfused aggression complicating the psychopathology of an individual who is being analysed.

In analysis, if this be true, we have to deal with separate expressions of the aggressive and erotic components, and to hold each separately for the patient who, in the transference, cannot achieve a fusion of the two. In severe disorders that involve failure at the point of fusion, we find the patient's relationship to the analyst aggressive and erotic in turn. And it is here that I am claiming that the analyst is more likely to be tired by the former than by the latter type of partial relationship.

The immediate conclusion to be drawn from this observation is that in the early stages, when the *Me* and the *Not-Me* are being established, it is the aggressive component that more surely drives the individual to a need for a *Not-Me* or an object that is felt to be *external*. The erotic experiences can be completed while the object is subjectively conceived or personally created, or while the individual is near to the narcissistic state of primary identification of earlier date.

The erotic experiences can be completed by anything that brings relief to the erotic instinctual drive, and that allows of forepleasure, rising tension of general and local excitement, climax and detumescence or its equivalent, followed by a period of lack of desire (which may itself produce anxiety because of the temporary annihilation of the subjective object created through desire). On the other hand, the aggressive impulses do not give any satisfactory experience unless there is opposition. The opposition must come from the environment, from the *Not-Me* which gradually comes to be distinguished from the *Me*. Erotic experience can be said to exist in the muscles and other tissues involved in effort, but this erotism is of a different order from that of the instinctual erotism associated with specific erotogenic zones.

Patients let us know that the aggressive experiences (more or less de-fused) feel real, much more real than do the erotic experiences (also de-fused). Both are real, but the former carry a feeling of real, which is greatly valued. The fusion of the aggression along with the erotic component of an experience enhances the feeling of the reality of the experience.

It is true that to some extent aggressive impulses can find their opposition without external opposition; this is displayed normally in the fish-movements of the spinal column that date from prenatal life, and abnormally in the to-and-fro (futile) movements of ill infants (rocking, or tension denoting a magical internal and invisible to-and-fro movement). In spite of those considerations can one not say that in normal development opposition from outside brings along the development of the aggressive impulse?

In normal birth the opposition encountered provides a type of experience which gives effort a head-first quality. Although birth is often not normal, so that it becomes a vast complication, and although birth may take place by breech instead of by head, there seems to be a general validity in the association between pure effort and a head-first relationship to opposition. This could be tested out by observation on infants who are making an effort to feed—according to my theory they can be helped by a degree of opposition to the top of the head.

This idea is usually expressed in the following terms: 'An infant does not thrive on perfect adaptation to need. A mother who fits in with a baby's desires too well is not a good mother. Frustration produces anger and this helps the infant to gain enhanced experience'. This is true and not true. In so far as it is untrue, it neglects two factors—one is that the infant does need perfect adaptation at the theoretical start, and then needs a carefully graduated failure of adaptation; the other is that this statement leaves out of consideration the lack of fusion of the aggressive and the erotic roots of experience, whereas in theory at least, the de-fused state (or the fore-fusion state) must be studied.

Those who make the statement more or less as quoted here only too easily assume that aggression is a reaction to frustration, that is to say, to frustration during erotic experience, during a phase of excitement with instinctual tension rising. That there is anger at frustration in such phases is only too obvious, but in our theory of the earliest feelings and states we need to be prepared for aggression that *precedes* the ego integration that makes anger at instinctual frustration possible, and that makes the erotic experience an experience.

It can be said that each baby has a potential of zonal erotic instinct, that this is biological, and that the potential is more or less the same for each baby. By contrast the *aggression component must be extremely variable*; by the time that we observe a baby's anger at frustration at a feeding delay a great deal has happened that has made the baby's aggressive potential great or little. To get to something in terms of aggression corresponding to the erotic potential it would be necessary to go back to the impulses of the foetus, to that which makes for movement rather than for stillness, to the aliveness of tissues and to the first evidence of muscular erotism. We need a term here such as life force.

No doubt the life-force potential of each individual foetus is more or less the same, just as is the erotic potential of each baby. The complication is that the amount of aggressive potential an infant carries depends on the amount of opposition that has been met with. In other words, opposition affects the conversion of life force into aggression potential. Moreover, excess of opposition introduces complications that make it impossible for the existence of an individual who, having aggressive potential, could achieve its fusion with the erotic.

It is not possible to go further with this argument without considering in detail the fate of the life force of the (prenatal) infant.

In health the foetal impulses bring about a discovery of environment, this latter being the opposition that is met through movement, and sensed during movement. The result here is an early recognition of a *Not-Me* world, and an early establishment of the *Me*. (It will be understood that in practice these things develop gradually, and repeatedly come and go, and are achieved and lost.)

In ill-health at this very early stage it is the environment that impinges, and the life force is taken up in reactions to impingement—the result being the opposite to the early firm establishment of the *Me*. In the extreme there is very little experience of impulses except as *reactions*, and the *Me* is not established. Instead we find a development based on the experience of reaction to impingement, and there comes into existence an individual that we call false because the personal impulsiveness is missing. In this case there is no fusion of the aggressive and erotic components, since the *Me* is not established when erotic experiences occur. The infant does indeed live, because of being seduced into erotic experience; but separately from the erotic life, which never feels real, is a purely aggressive reactive life, dependent on the experience of opposition.

It has been necessary, in this description, to discuss two extremes in the attempt to lead the way to a description of the common state in which *some degree of lack of fusion* has been a feature. The personality comprises three parts: a true self, with *Me* and *Not-Me* clearly established, and with some fusion of the aggressive and erotic elements; a self that is easily seduced along lines of erotic experience, but with the result of a loss of sense of real; a self that is entirely and ruthlessly given over to aggression. This aggression is not even organized to destruction, but it has value to the individual because it brings a sense of real and a sense of relating, but it is only brought into being by active opposition, or (later) persecution. It has no root in personal impulse, motivated in ego spontaneity.

The individual may achieve a false fusion of the aggressive and erotic by converting this pure de-fused aggression into masochism, but for this to occur there must be a reliable persecutor, and the reliable persecutor is a sadistic lover. In this way masochism can be primary to sadism. However, in following the development of an emotionally *healthy* human being we see sadism as primary to masochism. In health sadism implies successful fusion, that which is absent in the conditions in which masochism develops straight out of the pattern of reactive aggression, unfused.

The main conclusion to be made out of these considerations is that confusion exists through our using the term aggression sometimes when we mean spontaneity. The impulsive gesture reaches out and becomes aggressive when opposition is reached. There is reality in this experience, and it very easily fuses into the erotic experiences that await the new-born infant. I am suggesting: *it is this impulsiveness, and the aggression that develops out of it, that makes the infant need an external object,* and not merely a satisfying object.

Many infants, however, have a massive aggressive potential that belongs to reaction to impingement, that becomes activated by persecution: in so far as this is true the infant welcomes persecution, and feels real in reacting to it. But this represents a false mode of development since the infant needs continued persecution. The quantity of this reactive potential is not dependent on biological factors (which determine motility and erotism) but is dependent on the chance of early environmental impingement, and therefore, often, on the mother's psychiatric abnormalities, and the state of the mother's emotional environment.

In adult and mature sexual intercourse, it is perhaps true that it is not the purely erotic satisfactions that need a specific object. It is the aggressive or destructive element in the fused impulse that fixes the object and determines the need that is felt for the partner's actual presence, satisfaction, and survival.

Notes

1. I would now link this idea with that of motility (cf. Marty et Fain, 1955).
2. cf. Sechehaye's term: 'symbolic realization'.
3. In Part II of this chapter, I attempt to deal with the theme of aggression relative to the early stages of ego development.
4. This has been called 'pre-ambivalent', but this term avoids the issue of the integration of part-object and whole object, breast and mother who holds and cares.
5. I should now say 'idealized and bad' instead or 'good and bad' (1957).
6. This state of affairs is related to that which Anna Freud has termed 'identification with the aggressor' (1937). The work of Melanie Klein introduced us to the concept of the omnipotent control of inner phenomena as a defence.

3

Letter to *The Times*

NEGLECTED CHILDREN

Originally published in *The Times,* issue 51603, p. 5; also published in Rodman, F. R. (Ed.), *The spontaneous gesture. Selected letters of D. W. Winnicott* (Letter 16, p. 21). Cambridge, MA: Harvard University Press, 1987.

31 January 1950

Sir: The most important element in our country at any one moment is the ordinary home in which ordinary parents are doing an ordinary good job, starting off infants and children with that basis for mental health which enables them eventually to become part of the community. Nothing must be allowed to interfere with this, which is not only good but also a delicate matter and easily disturbed. It is indeed deplorable that there are homes in which children are neglected or cruelly treated, and organizations such as the National Society for the Prevention of Cruelty to Children which help such children need our support in their difficult task. If, however, by supplementation of those voluntary bodies by some Government department improved access to bad homes should involve the slightest degree of intrusion on the ordinary common good home, more harm than good will be done. Nothing could be more disastrous than the extension of interference by militant sentimentalists who will make parents afraid to be natural.

The danger is that workers with official backing will fear to enter into suspected homes because of the legal safeguards which protect the home from State interference, or else the legal safeguards themselves will have to be diminished and the privacy of the ordinary good home will be lost. Moreover, from the published accounts no one would be able to guess that there is a serious shortage of trained workers so that the implementation of the new Act which has resulted from the valuable Curtis Report cannot be effectual for many years. The cry about children badly treated in their own homes comes from very easily roused pity and not from any knowledge of the actual situation in respect of persons able to do this work well.

I am yours, etc.
D. W. Winnicott

4

Letter to Otho W. S. Fitzgerald

Originally published in Rodman, F. R. (Ed.), *The spontaneous gesture. Selected letters of D. W. Winnicott* (Letter 15, pp. 19–20). Cambridge, MA: Harvard University Press, 1987.

Otho Fitzgerald (1908–2000) was the medical superintendent at Shenley Hospital near St Albans, UK. The hospital was founded as a progressive mental health institution in 1934. Along with the Cassel Hospital, Winnicott would sometimes use Shenley when hospitalisation of his analytic patients became necessary.

3 March 1950

Dear Dr Fitzgerald:

Thank you for your letter.[i] The real trouble with the psychoanalysts is that they are all working very long hours doing analyses and bearing quite heavy clinical burdens and also teaching those of the people being analysed who are candidates. The strain on the senior members at the present moment is terrific owing to the fact that it takes so long to create an experienced psycho-analyst, and since the war there has been a huge influx of candidates. While deploring this I do personally feel that it has to be accepted because with all the faults, some of them very obvious, which belong to the psycho-analytic society, there is this thing about it—that a consolidated scientific group is building which will be a very important factor in general psychiatric education eventually. What will be most likely to seduce members from these activities at the present time I am not certain. Certainly most of us would feel it to be a waste of time to sit on planning committees arranging some kind of teaching which would be a compromise between what are called various schools of thought.

---

[i] Fitzgerald had written to Winnicott to request suggestions for bringing together psychiatrists, psychotherapists, and psychoanalysts.

In my opinion it is the psycho-analytic group which must eventually include what is good in all the other groups, and thinking of the future it is more important that the Society should concern itself with the research which will resolve the disagreements amongst its members than that it should try to be friendly all round. I am afraid that none of the other groups is capable of growing in the same way and eventually including what is valuable in the Freudian group, with the possible exception of the Jungians. In my personal opinion even in this case of the Jungians there is insufficient common ground to enable their society to keep out a lot of psycho-therapists who, while starting off as talented and even brilliant people, have a lack of experience of the psychiatric discipline.

In America I feel the whole thing is quite different, partly because the word psycho-analyst has a much more diffuse meaning, and also because the financial situation is different over there. It is extremely difficult for a senior analyst to earn a good living at present owing to the fact that as a senior analyst most of his patients are candidates, and these are chosen not because of their wealth but because of their suitability.

A further point is that Americans seem to be able to work all day and most of the night although I think this has the drawback of giving them insufficient time to live and think and feel.

At this point in the letter there should come a practical suggestion about the 'key which will unlock the barriers between psycho-analysts and organically-minded psychiatrists'. I shall want more time before I can say anything about this. What I would do, however, is to make a negative contribution and say that the trouble really is that the unconscious has to be believed in before the psycho-analysts can start talking, and there are comparatively few psychiatrists who can take what has to be said. It is much easier to talk to post-graduate teachers, for instance, or to ordinary medical students, about the unconscious, than to talk to psychiatrists. The fact that I am writing this to you shows that I know there are exceptions. I shall be writing again, I hope.

Yours sincerely,
D. W. Winnicott

5

Childhood Psychosis

Originally published as an editorial leader article in the *British Medical Journal*, 1950, 1(4659), 944–945, and therefore not attributed to Winnicott.

At first glance the words 'psychosis in childhood' would seem to describe clear-cut and accepted conditions. The paediatrician is aware of the rare juvenile G.P.I., of the commoner post-encephalitic mental states, and of mental states secondary to growing intracranial tumour. Also he may have studied mental defect and so know that defectives are specially apt to have regression phases, manic-depressive swings of mood, and withdrawal states. Neurology carries him thus far. Beyond this paediatricians as well as psychiatrists have drawn attention to the fact that organized mental illnesses, illnesses that are well known as types of insanity in adults, are not in fact confined to the adult population. The insanities can be demonstrated in adolescents, and indeed in younger children and even in the very young. Depression phases are common and severe depression moods not rare. Manic-depressive swing of mood is to be found in the hotch-potch that is called delinquency, this not being a diagnosis so much as a reference to the fact that the juvenile court is apt to take part in directing management of the child. From time to time the papers report attempts of children to commit suicide, and the children's doctor hears of many cases of suicidal attempts which do not reach the papers. Moreover, schizoid cases of all kinds and degrees are to be found by those who look for them in any out-patient department, and from time to time frank schizophrenics appear in the hospital wards—children who seem mad, who are odd, who are withdrawn, whose behaviour is bizarre, or who act as if they were 1 year old instead of 7 or 8. By the uninitiated these children are easily classified wrongly as mentally defective—wrongly because in fact they have normal brains. On the other hand, because of these children's capacity to change in relation to environment, physicians may fail to recognize the seriousness of the condition.

Several papers[1-7] have been published in recent years on psychotic disorders in children, but sooner or later the worker in this field is driven to consider the whole theory of the emotional development of the individual. This, of course, is an enormous subject on its own, and it is not surprising that the paediatrician, already a specialist, hesitates before embarking on the study of a new specialty whose dimensions are of the order of those of physiology. It seems to be inevitable, therefore, that when it comes to the intimate study of a psychotic child paediatrics and psychology part company: this is a pity, because it is only by comparing the emotional development of the psychotic child with healthy emotional development that progress can be made. Lack of precise knowledge is the reason for the widely differing accounts of the frequency of child psychosis given by various observers.

Bradley[8] has surveyed the literature of schizophrenia in childhood, and deliberately gives the impression that this is a moderately rare condition. Child psychiatrists are well aware, however, that once a clinic is known to be interested in this problem the cases tend to arrive in quantities. Moreover, apart from the clearly recognized syndrome, there is immediately a great increase of the number of cases that can be classified as psychotic rather than neurotic if the latent psychosis in much of the psychosomatic disorder of childhood is taken into consideration. In fact according to modern psychological theory there is no clear-cut line between psychotic illness and unorganized disturbances which have a psychotic quality; and more stress is laid now than formerly on the relation between the various kinds of psychological disturbance and the various stages of normal emotional development of the infant and of the child.

At the conclusion of a paper describing a series of cases of child psychosis Kanner[9] wrote: 'We must, then, assume that these children have come into the world with innate inability to form the usual, biologically provided affective contact with people, just as other children come into the world with innate physical or intellectual handicaps.... Here we seem to have pure-culture examples of inborn autistic disturbances of affective contact'. The case histories, however, are so faithfully rendered that the lack in early infancy of the straightforward devotion of a mother can be seen in nearly all the children. Even when the possibility of an inborn factor is allowed there is still plenty of room for research into the effect of the very early environment. This is relatively seldom discussed, for the simple reason that knowledge about what an infant needs at the very earliest stages is only just being gained. In a recent lecture Winnicott[10] made an attempt to state the early infant mother relationship in terms which can be understood at the same time by paediatricians and by psychiatrists, whether psychiatrists of children or of adults. He assumes the correctness of the theory that the foundation of mental health, so far as the development of psychoses is concerned, is laid down by the mother, who supplies a specialized relationship which is called 'being devoted to her own infant'. This is similar to the theory that the foundation of health, so far as the development of neuroses is concerned, is laid down by the mother and the father, who build a home environment for the toddler. It is an extension backwards of the well-accepted theory that without a good home a child starts with a serious handicap, especially as it affects his ability to become at one and the same time an individual and a member of society.

Much research remains to be done on the meaning of the word psychosis as opposed to neurosis, as well as on the relation of all kinds of psychological disturbances to the stages of emotional development through which every child must pass on the road towards emotional maturity. About twenty years ago it was held that neurosis in adults was a regression to a period of early childhood, with its fears, phobias, and anxieties unjustified by reality. This is no longer considered to be a correct statement, since it is possible to distinguish a neurotic small child from a normal one. Similarly, at the present time psychotic illness is often described as a regression to an infantile level of emotional development. This again is likely to prove incorrect, since it is possible to distinguish between an infant whose emotional development is proceeding naturally and one whose development shows psychotic features. There are two complicating factors. One is the relatively weak organization of the infant's personality; because of this whatever is gained can easily be lost by untoward circumstances. The other is that healthy emotional development is not by any means exactly correlated with physical health. For instance, the foundations of mental health may be less soundly laid in an infant who is taking everything that is given him and is bursting with physical well-being, than in another infant who is refusing food, not gaining weight satisfactorily, and is a cause of anxiety.

When a serious attempt is made to give personal treatment to a psychotic child the psycho-analyst will find that he is dealing with things which the treatment of non-psychotic cases has already made familiar. It is simply a matter of the accent, and there is no essential difference between adult and child. In neurosis the accent is on the unconscious or repressed conflicts in the whole person, especially the conflict of love and hate, with its origin in early childhood. Depression again is an experience of a whole person, though in analysis the accent is on guilt rather than anxiety, and the therapist finds himself reaching to the beginnings in infancy of the individual's sense of concern, and to the early stages of his ability to feel that what he loves must be protected from himself because of his destructive impulses and ideas.[11] In schizophrenia all these factors appear to some extent, but the main abnormality is that the personality itself is deranged.[12] The accent is on the splitting of the personality rather than on the repression or forgetting of a painful conflict by the whole person. Also there is likely to be found a very carefully organized introversion with an artificial arrangement of relationships, so that all the friendly things are within and the hostile things without. In some cases the analyst finds a most deceptive false integration into the personality of the mother, with lack of real personal sense of self.

The psychotic child needs a specialized environment more or less continuously over a period of time, and for this reason the study of the child should be undertaken at home, provided it is not only a good home but also capable of making an active adaptation to the particular child's needs. Alternatively the child should be admitted to a small hostel which deliberately aims at active adaptation. There is little to be said for the treatment of a psychotic child in a hospital ward. The study of childhood psychosis is extremely important, not primarily because certain psychotic children may be successfully treated, but because of the light such study must eventually throw on the psychogenesis of the highly organized psychoses of adults and also on the problem of healthy emotional development.

Notes

1. Creak, E. M., and Shorting, B. J., *J. Ment. Sci.*, 1944, 90, 365.
2. Little, H. M., *Penn. Med. J.*, 1947, 51, 174.
3. Rapaport, J., *Nerv. Child.*, 1942, 1, 188.
4. Despert, J. L., ibid., 1942, 1, 199.
5. Cottington, F., ibid., 1942, 1, 172.
6. Bruch, H., and Cottington, F., ibid., 1942, 1.
7. Bradley, C., ibid., 1942, 1, 141.
8. *Schizophrenia in Childhood.* 1941, New York.
9. *Nerv. Child.*, 1943, 2, 217.
10. *Brit. J. Med. Psychol.*, 1948, 21, 229 [CW:3:3:2].
11. Klein, M., *Contributions to Psycho-analysis,* 1921–45, pp. 282–310.
12. Klein, M., *Int. J. Psycho-Anal.,* 1946, 3 and 4, p. 99. ('Notes on Some Schizoid Mechanisms').

6

Letter to P. D. Scott

Originally published in Rodman, F. R. (Ed.), *The spontaneous gesture. Selected letters of D. W. Winnicott* (Letter 17, pp. 22–23). Cambridge, MA: Harvard University Press, 1987.

Peter D. Scott (1914–77) was a consultant psychiatrist at the Maudsley Hospital in London and the psychiatrist in charge of a London County Council remand home.

11 May 1950

Dear Dr Scott:

I think your students are trying to tell you something that I really have said. You will understand that I am extremely keen on penal reform and what I am saying when talking to students is part of the effort towards penal reform. The point that your students refer to is not one that I have made carefully in a published paper although I have often spoken about it. In any case it is very easily misunderstood.

My idea is that any kind of sentimentality is worse than useless. The difficulty is not so much in the feeling that the public has about any one anti-social act. Through identification with the criminal or the anti-social person the public is often extremely sympathetic, and guilty on behalf of the criminal. Nevertheless there is, I am sure, a very real thing which we could call the unconscious revenge reservoir of a community. It would be possible to pass Acts of Parliament which ignore this revenge reservoir. In the extreme of this there would be incidents in which what is called lynch law would come into operation. In fact I would say that the function of judicial procedure is primarily one of preventing lynch law and it does this firstly by taking over responsibility for revenge and secondly by allowing for the cooling of tempers and the operation of objectivity.

I think that it is extremely difficult to get general recognition of this function of judicial procedure, especially amongst the legal profession, who tend to think of the law as a 'thing', or at best, an ass, and who fail to see in the judicial procedure expression of their own deep-seated feelings.

Holding these views, I feel that there is a great danger that the reforms which we are trying to bring about will be introduced by cold methods and then swept away by a wave of reaction. The judicial procedure must preserve its function.

Within this framework, I believe that there is room for the advances which psychiatry is beginning to be able to make, although only just beginning. The public in this country is prepared, according to my view, for a certain amount of treatment of antisocial persons instead of punishment. This feeling, I would say, would eventually go into reverse, should it turn out that in actual fact very few criminals can be successfully treated. There is no doubt whatever that even if our knowledge of the psycho-pathology of criminology were to be completed tomorrow, there would still be a very great number of years before psychotherapists could be properly trained in numbers sufficient to make a practical difference to the problem. But we know that there is so much that we are only just beginning to know, so that in actual fact most of the treatment of the criminal is a matter of research.

The upshot of all this is in my opinion that the psychiatrist's job includes that of reminding the judges and those responsible for judicial procedure that their primary function is to express unconscious public revenge in the most civilised way. The psychiatrist is then in a position to give his opinion about a criminal, and it seems to me that we are not far off a state of affairs in which we can say that every criminal is ill. It is for the doctor to say this. It is not for the doctor to say what the public needs in the way of revenge. After judicial procedure has terminated there is room for any amount of research, if the psychiatrists can be used that way, on the treatment of all types of anti-social persons. It seems to me that there are certain types of crime in which our society is ready to treat rather than punish—homosexuality, for instance, and the perversions in general; attempted suicide; infanticide. The application of all this to anti-social behaviour in children is too big a subject to deal with in a letter.

You will realise I hope that I am a bit of an amateur when I am applying psychoanalysis to this subject, but as you were referring to my views I have tried to explain them.

I am trying to remind myself of having met you or your work but so far without success.

I am enclosing a copy of a letter which I wrote to the *Times* in August last year,[i] and should be grateful if you would return this when you have finished with it.

Yours sincerely,
D. W. Winnicott

---

[i] 'Punishment and Crime: A Psychologist's View', letter to *The Times*, 10 August 1949 [CW 3:4:16]

7

Letter to *The Times*

MALADJUSTED CHILDREN: DAMAGING EFFECT OF DELAY

Originally published in *The Times*, issue 51690, p. 5.

13 May 1950

Sir: All those who are clinically involved in this subject recognize the very urgent need for a vast increase of hostel accommodation. The first reason is that the immediate problem in the home is acute. Often it can be said that if a child is not quickly removed, the home will degenerate and the child will become involved in the courts. A waiting period is often disastrous.

After a child has been deemed maladjusted and has been placed, there is the secondary problem, how best to arrange for the child's management. It is often forgotten that these children are many of them extremely ill and not able to respond quickly to good management. The environment has failed to adjust to such children in the early stages when sensitive management lays down the foundation for subsequent mental health, and a corrective environment cannot cure this situation except by operating over a long period, and then by no means always successfully. This work depends entirely on the people who undertake it. These people require understanding support, they need to be protected from the burden arising from excessive load, and they need to be protected from administrative procedure. They also need to be able to talk over the cases with psychiatrists who have theoretical knowledge but who are not involved emotionally.

In regard to the suggestion in your leading article that a careful investigation of hostels dealing with maladjusted children should be set up, any investigation must reveal a good deal of failure because of the inherent factors and also because of the overload which is imposed on those who do this exacting work. The first need is for a very great increase of hostel provision as this would enable the dangerous waiting period to be eliminated and also would gradually lead to an end of the overloading which makes this work futile. Above all there must be recognition that failure in a proportion of cases arises out of the serious mental state of the individual children, and is no reflection on the policy of providing hostels which are needed for dealing with the crises of which workers in the field are much more aware than are administrators and investigators.

I am yours, &c.,
D. W. WINNICOTT

8

Review: *The Infancy of Speech and the Speech of Infancy*
BY LEOPOLD STEIN (LONDON: METHUEN, 1949)

Review originally published in *British Journal of Medical Psychology*, 1950, 23, 120–121.

In this inquiry into the origin of speech, the author studies the history of the problem and then makes a bold attempt at reconstructing primeval speech under the guidance of such psycho-biological trends as can still be detected in the utterances of man's forerunners, primitive races, the child, and of civilized peoples.

He helps the reader by describing the world during the time that it has been populated, for about 1,000,000 years. In demonstrating man's activities from early palaeolithic times, under the guidance of archaeological findings, he tries to depict the sociopsychological traits of successive racial groups and their languages as embedded in their attitudes. The author shows no reluctance to fill in gaps in this picture by his own fantasies.

He postulates three rungs of meaning. At the lowest rung the sounds are simply a part of behaviour and expressive of the emotional relation of the individual to his own personal state and to the environment. At the second rung, emotional language begins to be used by the individual as a tool for a purpose. At the third rung, which takes us to the top of the ladder, language, as apart from thought-action, is employed and developed in a more or less deliberate effort to extend the range of social intercourse by putting 'labels' on objects, ideas and feelings.

There is an immense amount of learning displayed in the 200 pages in which the author develops this theme, so that the book has a great interest for the general reader as well as for the speech therapist. Perhaps the most valuable part is the descriptive enumeration of the types of sound utterance which the various races integrate, each in its own way, into a language. The author must be congratulated on having condensed into a book what must constitute almost a life time of reading and clinical work and thought.

Letter to Roger Money-Kyrle

Roger Money-Kyrle (1898–1980) was a British psychoanalyst and follower of Melanie Klein.

10 July 1950

Dear Money-Kyrle,

I am definitely intending to have the article[i] ready by September 1st. Thank you very much for your letter, although I can think of better things that you might be doing in a boat at Henley.

I very much look forward to reading your book on Psychology and Politics.[ii]

Yours ever,
D. W. Winnicott

---

[i] See also CW 3:4:10, CW 3:4:12, CW 3:4:13, CW 3:5:11, and CW 3:5:13 for Winnicott's correspondence with Money-Kyrle regarding a possible article for Melanie Klein's Festschrift.

[ii] Money-Kyrle, *Psychoanalysis and Politics* (1951).

10

The Deprived Child and How He Can Be Compensated for Loss of Family Life

Originally published in *The family and individual development* (pp. 132–145). London: Tavistock, 1965.

Given as a lecture to the Nursery School Association, July 1950.

By way of introduction to the subject of providing for the child who has been deprived of family life, let us remember this: that the chief concern of a community should be for its healthy members. It is the usual run of good homes that need priority, for the simple reason that the children who are being nurtured in their own homes are the ones that reward; it is the care of these children that pays the dividends.

Two things follow, if this be accepted. First, provision for the ordinary home of a basic ration of housing, food, clothing, education, and recreation facilities, and what could be called cultural food, has first claim on our attention. Second, we must see that we never interfere with a home that is a going concern, not even for its own good. Doctors are especially liable to get in the way between mothers and infants, or parents and children, always with the best intentions, for the prevention of disease and the promotion of health; and doctors are by no means the only offenders in this respect. For example:

> A mother who had been divorced asked me for advice in the following situation. She had a six-year-old daughter, and a religious organization with which the father of this child was connected wished to take the child away from the mother and put her in a boarding school—for holidays as well as term-time—because this organization did not approve of divorce. The fact that the child was quite settled and secure with the mother and her new husband was to be ignored, and a state of deprivation was to be created for this child because of a principle: a child must not live with a divorced mother.

A great number of deprived children are in fact engineered in one way or another, and the remedy lies in avoidance of bad management.

Nevertheless, I have to face up to the fact that I am myself a deliberate home-breaker, like many others. We are all the time sending children away from their homes. In my clinic alone we have cases every week in which it is urgently necessary to get the child away from home. It is true that such children are seldom under the age of four. Everyone working in this field knows the type of case in which, for one reason or another, a state of affairs has arisen of such a nature that, unless the child is removed within a few days or weeks, the home will break up or the child will certainly get to the courts. Often one can predict that the child will do well away from home or that the home will do well with the child away. There are many distressing cases that mend themselves if one can immediately bring about these separations, and it would be a great pity if all that we are doing to avoid the unnecessary destruction of good homes should in any way weaken the efforts of the authorities that are responsible for the provision of short-term and long-term accommodation for the kind of children that I am considering here.

When I say that in my clinic we have these cases each week, I am implying that in the great majority of cases we manage to help the child in the setting which already exists. This is of course our aim, not only because it is economical but also because when the home is good enough the home is the proper place for the child to grow up in. The vast majority of the children who need psychological help are suffering from disturbances in respect of *internal* factors, disturbances in the emotional development of the individual, disturbances which are largely inherent because life is difficult. These disturbances can be treated with the child at home.

Assessment of Deprivation

In order to discover how we can best help a deprived child we first have to determine what amount of normal emotional development was made possible in the beginning by a good-enough environment ((i) infant-mother relationship, (ii) triangular father-mother-child relationship); and then in the light of this to try to assess the damage done by the deprivation, when it began and as it subsequently persisted. The history of the case is therefore important.

The following six categories may be found useful as a way of classifying cases of broken home:

(a) Ordinary good home, broken by an accident to one or both parents.
(b) Home broken by the separation of the parents, who are good as parents.
(c) Home broken by the separation of the parents, who are not good as parents.

(d) Home incomplete, because there is no father (child illegitimate). The mother is good; grandparents may take over parental role, or help to some extent.
(e) Home incomplete, because there is no father (child illegitimate). The mother is not good.
(f) There never was a home.

In addition, cross-classifications will be made:

(a) according to the age of the child; and the age at which a good-enough environment ceased;
(b) according to the child's nature and intelligence;
(c) according to the child's psychiatric diagnosis.

We avoid making any assessment of the problem on the basis of the child's symptoms, or the nuisance value of the child, or the feelings roused in us by the child's plight. These considerations lead us astray. Often the history is lacking or deficient in essential parts. Then, and in fact commonly, the only way to determine the fact of an early good-enough environment is to supply a good environment and see what use the child can make of it.

Here special comment is needed on the meaning of the words 'what use the child can make of a good environment'. A deprived child is ill, and it is never so simple a matter that environmental readjustment will bring about a changeover in the child from ill to healthy. At best, the child who can benefit from a simple environmental provision begins to get better, and as the change takes place from ill to less ill the child becomes increasingly able to be angry about the past deprivation. Hate of the world is there somewhere, and health has not arrived unless the hate has been felt. In a small proportion of cases the hate is felt, and even this small complication can cause difficulties. However, this favourable result comes about only if everything is relatively available to the child's *conscious* self, and this is but seldom the case. To some extent, or to a very great extent, the feelings belonging to the environmental failure are not available to consciousness. Where deprivation occurs on top of a satisfactory early experience something like this *can* happen and the hate appropriate to the deprivation can be reached. The following example illustrates this kind of situation:

> Here is a girl of seven. Her father died when she was three but she negotiated this difficulty all right. The mother cared for her excellently and married again. This remarriage was successful and the child's stepfather was very fond of her. All was well until the mother became pregnant. At this point the father completely changed in his attitude to the stepdaughter. He became orientated towards his own baby and withdrew affection from the stepchild. After the birth of the baby things got worse, and the mother

was in a position of divided loyalties. The child could not thrive in this atmosphere but, removed to a boarding school, she may quite possibly be able to do well and even to understand the difficulty that occurred in her own home.

On the other hand, the next case shows the effects of an unsatisfactory early experience:

> A mother brings her little boy of two and a half. He has a good home but he is only happy when having the personal attention of his mother or father. He cannot leave his mother and therefore cannot play on his own, and the approach of strangers is felt by him to be terrifying. What has gone wrong in this case, considering that the parents are ordinary normal people? The fact is that the boy was adopted at five weeks, and already by that time he was ill. There is some evidence that the matron of the home in which he was born made a special pet of him, since she seems to have tried to hide him from these parents who were looking for an infant to adopt. The transfer at five weeks caused a severe upset in the emotional development of the infant, and the adopting parents are only beginning to be able gradually to overcome the difficulties—which they certainly did not expect, taking over a baby at so early a date. (They had in fact tried very hard to get a baby even earlier, in the first week or two of the infant's existence, because they were aware of the complications that could arise.)

We have to know what sort of things happen in the child when a good setting is broken up and also when a good setting has never existed, and this involves a study of the whole subject of the emotional development of the individual. Some of the phenomena are well-enough known: hate is repressed or the capacity to love people is lost. Other defensive organizations become set up in the child's personality. There may be regression to some early phases of the emotional development which were more satisfactory than others, or there may be a state of pathological introversion. Much more commonly than is generally thought, there is a splitting of the personality. In the simplest form of this splitting, the child presents a shop-window or out-turned half, built up on a basis of compliance, and the main part of the self containing all the spontaneity is kept secret and is all the time involved in hidden relationships to idealized fantasy objects.

Although it is difficult to make a simple and clear statement of these phenomena, an understanding of them is necessary if we are to see what are the favourable signs in the case of deprived children. If we do not understand what is there when the child is very ill, we cannot see, for instance, that a depressed mood in a deprived child may be a favourable sign, especially when not accompanied by strong persecution ideas. A simple depressed mood indicates at any rate that the child has retained unity of personality and has a sense of concern, and is indeed taking responsibility for all that has gone wrong. Also, antisocial acts, such as bed-wetting and stealing, indicate that at any rate momentarily there can be hope—hope of rediscovering a good-enough mother, a good-enough home, a good-enough inter-parental relationship. Even anger may indicate that there is hope, and that for the moment the child is a unit and able to feel the clash between what is conceivable and what is actually to be found in what we call shared reality.

Let us consider the meaning of the antisocial act, for instance, stealing. When a child steals, what is sought (by the total child, i.e. the unconscious included) is not the object stolen; what is sought is the person, the mother, from whom the child has the right to steal because she is the mother. In fact every infant at the start can truly claim the right to steal from the mother because the infant invented the mother, thought her up, created her out of an innate capacity to love. By being there the mother gave her infant, gradually, bit by bit, the person of herself as material for the infant to create into, so that in the end his subjective self-created mother was quite a lot like the mother we can agree about. In the same way, the child who wets the bed is looking for the mother's lap that is meet to be wetted in the early stages of the infant's existence.

The antisocial symptoms are gropings for environmental recovery, and indicate hope. They fail not because they are wrongly directed, but because the child is unconscious of what is going on. The antisocial child needs therefore a specialized environment that has a therapeutic aim, and that can give a reality response to the hope that is expressed in the symptoms. This has to be spread over a long period, however, to become effectual as a therapeutic, since, as I have said, much is unavailable to the child as conscious feeling and memory; and also the child has to gain great confidence in the new environment, in its stability and its capacity for objectivity, before the defences can be given up—defences against intolerable anxiety that is always liable to be reactivated by new deprivation.

We know, then, that the deprived child is an ill person, a person with a past history of traumatic experience, and a personal way of coping with the anxieties roused; and a person with a capacity for recovery greater or less according to the degree of loss of consciousness of the appropriate hate and of the primary capacity to love. What practical measures can be undertaken to help such a child?

Providing for the Deprived Child

Obviously someone has to care for the child. The community no longer denies responsibility for children who are deprived; indeed, the swing is right in the other direction today. Public opinion demands that the best that is possible shall be done for the child whose own family life is lacking. Many of our troubles at the present time come from the practical difficulties that arise in the application of the principles deriving from the new attitude.

It is not possible to do the right thing for a child by passing a law or by setting up administrative machinery. These things are necessary but are only the first miserable stage. In every case a proper management of a child involves *human beings,* and these human beings have to be of the right kind; and there is a distinct limit to the number of such people who are immediately available. This number is much increased if in the administrative machinery there is a provision for *intermediate* persons, who can on the one hand deal with the overriding authorities and on the other hand keep in touch with the persons actually doing the work, appreciating their good points, acknowledging success where it occurs, enabling the educative process to leaven and make interesting the job, discussing failures and the reasons for failure, and being available to give relief where necessary by removal of a child from a foster home or hostel, perhaps at short notice. The care of a child is very much a whole-time process, and leaves the person who is doing the work with little emotional reserve for coping with administrative procedure or with the wide social issues represented in certain cases by the police. Conversely, the person who is able to keep one eye firmly on administration or on the police is unlikely to be first-rate in the care of a child.

Coming now to more specific matters, it is necessary to keep in mind the psychiatric diagnosis of every child for whom provision has to be made. As I have pointed out, this diagnosis can be made only after a carefully taken history or perhaps after a period of observation. The point is that a child deprived of family life can have had a good start in infancy and can even have had the beginnings of a family life. The foundation of the mental health of the child may in such a case have been well laid down, so that the illness secondary to the deprivation supervenes on health. On the other hand, another child, not perhaps looking worse, has no healthy experience which can be rediscovered and reactivated by the child in a new environment; and, further than that, there may have been such a poor or complex management of early infancy that the foundations for mental health in terms of personality structure and reality sense may be deficient. In such extreme cases the good environment has to be created for the first time, or a good environment may have no chance at all because the child is fundamentally unsound, perhaps with the addition of a hereditary tendency to insanity or instability. In the extreme cases the child is insane, although this word is not used in respect of children.

It is important to recognize this part of the problem, otherwise those who are assessing results will be surprised to find that with the very best management there are always failures, and always children who grow up eventually to become insane or at best antisocial.

The diagnosis of the child having been made, in terms of the presence or absence of positive features in the early environment and the child's relation to it, the next thing to consider is procedure. I want to emphasize here (and I write as a psycho-analyst of children) that the clear principle of the management of the deprived child is not the provision of psychotherapy. Psychotherapy is something which eventually, one hopes, may be added in some instances to whatever else is done. At the present time, generally speaking, personal psychotherapy is not practical politics. The essential procedure is the provision of an alternative to the family. We can classify what we provide in the following way:

(i) Foster parents, who wish to give the child a family life like that which the child could have been provided with by the actual parents. It is generally acknowledged that this is the ideal, but one must quickly add that it is essential that children sent to foster parents must be children who can respond to something so good. This practically means that they must have had something of a good-enough family life somewhere in their past and have been able to respond to it. In this foster home they have a chance to rediscover something they have had and have lost.

(ii) Next come the small homes in the care, if possible (but not necessarily), of married wardens, each home containing children in various age groups. Such small homes can conveniently be grouped together, with advantages both from the administrative point of view and from the point of view of the children, who acquire cousins, so to speak, as well as siblings. Here again, the best is being attempted, and therefore it is essential that children who cannot benefit from something so good shall be kept away. One unsuitable child can spoil the good work of a whole group. It must be remembered that good work is emotionally more difficult than less good work, and only too easily, if there is a failure, those in charge give up the best and slip over into the easier and less valuable types of management.

(iii) In the third category the groups are larger. The hostel perhaps contains eighteen. The wardens can keep in personal touch with all the children but they have assistants, and the management of the assistants is an important part of their job. Loyalties are divided and the children have opportunity for putting the grown-ups against each other and playing on latent jealousies. We are already in the direction of the less good management. On the other hand, we are also in the direction of the type of management that can deal with the less satisfactory type of deprived child. The way in which things are worked is less personal, more dictatorial, and the demands made on each child are less. A child in such a home is less in need of a previous good experience which can be revived. In such homes there is less need than there is in the small homes for the child to grow towards the ability to identify with the home while retaining personal impulsiveness and spontaneity. The intermediate thing is good enough in the larger homes, that is to say, a merging of identity with the other children in the group. This involves both loss of personal identity and loss of identification with the total home setting.

(iv) Next in our classification comes the larger hostel, in which the wardens are mainly engaged in the management of the staff and only indirectly concerned with the minute-to-minute management of the children. Here there are advantages in that a larger number of children can be accommodated. The fact that there is a larger staff means that there is more opportunity for discussion among the staff; there are also advantages for the children in that there can be teams competing with each other. I think it can be claimed that this hostel is further in the direction of the type of management that can cope with the more ill children, i.e. those whose good experiences at the beginning were small. The rather impersonal chief can be in the background as a representative of authority which such children need; which they need because within themselves they are incapable of holding both the spontaneity and the control at the same time. (Either they must be identified with authority and turn into miniature gauleiters, or else they must be impulsive, relying entirely on external authority for control.)

(v) Beyond this is the still larger institution which does its best for children under impossible conditions. For some time there will have to be such institutions. They have to be run by dictatorship methods, and what is good for the individual child has to be subordinated on account of the limitations of that which society can provide immediately. Here is a good form of sublimation for potential dictators. One can even find other advantages in this undesirable state of affairs, for, the accent being on dictatorship methods, quite hopelessly difficult children can be managed in such a way that they do not get into trouble with society over long periods. Really ill children can be happier here than in better homes, and they can become able to play and learn, so much so that the uninformed observer must be impressed. It is difficult in such institutions to recognize the children who become ripe to be removed to a more personal type of management, where their growing capacity to identify with society without losing their own individuality can be catered for.

The Deprived Child

THERAPEUTICS AND MANAGEMENT

I now want to contrast the two extremes of management, the one being the foster home and the other the large institution. In the former, as I have said, the aim is truly therapeutic. It is hoped that the child will recover in the course of time from the deprivation which, without such management, would not only leave a scar but would actually leave crippling. If this is to happen, much more is needed than the child's response to the new environment.

At first the child is apt to make a quick response and those concerned are apt to think that their troubles are over. When the child gains confidence, however, there follows a growing capacity for anger with the previous environmental failure. It is unlikely, of course, that what happens will exactly look like this, especially since the child is not conscious of the main revolutionary changes which are taking place. The foster parents will find that they themselves periodically become the target of the child's hate. They will have to take over the anger which is beginning to be able to be felt and which belongs to the failure in the child's own home. It is very important for foster parents to understand this, otherwise they get disheartened; and child care officers must know about it, otherwise they will blame foster parents and believe the children's stories about ill treatment and starvation. If the foster parents receive a visit from an officer who is looking for signs of trouble, they may become over-anxious, and this makes them try to seduce the child into being friendly and happy, thus depriving the child of a most important part of recovery.

Sometimes a child will very cleverly bring about specific ill treatment, in an attempt to bring into the actual present a badness that can be met by hate; the cruel foster parent is then actually loved because of the relief that the child feels through transformation of 'hate versus hate' locked up within into hate meeting external hate now. Unfortunately at this point the foster parents are liable to become misunderstood in their social group.

There are ways out. For instance, some foster parents will be found to work on the rescue principle. For them the child's parents were hopelessly bad, and they say so over and over again out loud to the child, and thus they divert the child's hate from themselves. This method may work fairly well but it ignores the reality situation, and in any case disturbs something which is a feature in deprived children, that they tend to idealize their own home such as it is. No doubt it is more healthy when the foster parents can take the periodical waves of negative feeling and survive them, reaching each time to a new, more secure (because less idealized) relation to the child.

In contrast, the child in the big institution is *not* being managed with the aim of curing him of his illness. The aims are, first, to provide housing and food and clothing for children who are neglected; second, to devise a type of management in which the children live in a state of order rather than chaos; and third, to keep as many of the children as possible from a clash with society until they must be let loose on the world somewhere about the age of sixteen. It is no good mixing things up and pretending that at this end of the scale an attempt is being made to create normal human beings. A strict management in such cases is essential, and if to this can be added some humanity so much the better.

It must be remembered that even in very strict communities, as long as there is consistency and fairness the children can discover humanity among themselves, and they can even come to value the strictness because of the fact that it implies stability. Understanding men and women working this kind of system can find ways of introducing more humane moments. Something can be done, for instance, by selecting suitable children for regular contacts with reliable aunt and uncle substitutes in the outside world. People can be found who will write on the child's birthday, and who will ask the child home to tea three or four times a year. These are only examples but they show the sort of thing that can be done and that is done without disturbance of the strict setting in which the children live. It has to be remembered that if the strict setting is the basis, then it is disturbing to the children if this strict setting has exceptions and loopholes. If there has to be a strict setting, then let it be consistent, reliable, and fair, so that it can have positive value. Besides, there will always be those children who abuse privileges, and then the children who could use them will have to suffer.

In this type of large institution, for the sake of peace and quiet, the accent is put on management on behalf of society. Within this framework the children must lose their own individuality to a greater or lesser extent. (I am not ignoring the fact that in the intermediate institutions there is room for a gradual growth of the children who are healthy enough to grow, so that they become increasingly able to identify with society without loss of identity.)

There will still be some children who, because they are what I want to call mad (although one must not use such a word), are failures even if dictated to. For such children there must be the equivalent of the mental hospital which caters for adults, and I think we have not yet determined what is the best that society can do for these extreme cases. Such children are so ill that those who are looking after them easily recognize that when they begin to become antisocial this means that they are beginning to get better.

I conclude this section by referring two matters which are of great importance in a consideration of the needs of the deprived child.

IMPORTANCE OF CHILD'S EARLY HISTORY

The first of these very much concerns the child care worker, especially in her capacity of boarding out and of keeping a watchful eye on the new situation. If I were a child care officer, as soon as a child came into my care I would immediately want to collect together every particle of information that could be found about that child's life up to the present moment. This is always urgent because the passage of every day makes it less easy for anyone to come by the essential facts. How distressing it was in the second world war, when the failures of the evacuation scheme were being dealt with, and there were children about whom one could never find out anything!

We know how normal children sometimes say as they are going to bed, 'What did I do today?', and then the mother says, 'You woke up at half past six, and you played with your teddy, singing nursery rhymes until we woke, and then you got up and went out into the garden, and then you had breakfast, and then . . .', and so on, until the whole scheme of the day has been integrated from outside. The child has all the information there but likes to be helped to be aware of it all. This feels good and real and helps the child to distinguish reality from the dream and from imaginative play. The same thing writ large would be represented by the way the ordinary parent has of going over the past life of the child, including what the child only just remembers and also what the child does not know anything about.

The lack of this simple thing is a serious loss for the deprived child. At any rate there should be someone who has gathered together whatever is available. In the very favourable case the child care officer will be able to have a long interview with the actual mother, letting her gradually unfold the whole history from the moment of birth, even perhaps giving important details about her experiences during pregnancy and the experiences leading up to conception, which may or may not have determined much of her attitude to the child. Often, however, the worker will have to go here and there and everywhere to collect information; even the name of a friend that the child had in the institution before last may be valuable. There will follow the task of organizing a contact with the child, when the social worker gains the child's confidence. Some way may be found of letting the child know that here or in a file in the office of the children's officer there is the saga of the child's life as lived hitherto. The child may not want to be told anything for the time being, but later on details may be needed. It is particularly the illegitimate and the child with a broken home who eventually need to be able to get to the facts—that is, if health is to be reached, and I assume that in the case of the fostered child the aim is to produce a healthy child. The child at the other extreme, managed by dictatorial methods in a large group, is less likely to become well enough to assimilate the truth about the past.

Because this is so, and because there is an acute shortage of workers, the start should be made at the more normal end. Even so, child care workers are likely to feel that, much as they would like to do this kind of thing, it is impossible because of their case load. My point is that child care workers must decide absolutely that they will not take more cases than they can manage. There is no half and half business about the care of children. It is a matter of dealing with a few children well and handing the others over to the large institution with dictatorial methods until society can manage something better. Good work has to be personal, or it is cruel and tantalizing both to the child and to the child care worker. *The work is only worth doing if it is personal and if those who are doing the work are not overburdened.*

It must be remembered that if child care workers accept too much work they will be bound to have failures, and eventually statisticians will come along and prove that the whole thing is wrong, and that the dictatorial methods are more effectual in providing factories with workers, and homes with domestic servants.

TRANSITIONAL PHENOMENA

The other point that I wish to make can be got at again by first looking at the normal child. How is it that ordinary children can be deprived of their homes and of all that is familiar to them without becoming ill? Every day children go into hospital and come out again, not only physically mended but also undisturbed and even enriched by the new experience. Over and over again children go away to stay with aunts and uncles, and in any case they go away with their parents from familiar surrounding to strange ones.

This is a very complex subject, which we may approach in the following way. Let us think of any child whom we know well, and ask ourselves what it is that the child takes to bed to help in the transition from waking to dream life: a doll; several dolls perhaps; a teddy; a book; a bit of mother's old dress; a corner of an eiderdown; a bit of old blanket; or it may be a handkerchief which was substituted for a napkin at a certain stage in the infant's development. In some cases it may be that there was no such object, but the child simply sucked what was available, a fist, and then the thumb or two fingers; or perhaps there was a genital activity to which the word masturbation is more easily applied; or the child may lie on the tummy or make rhythmic movements, showing the orgiastic nature of the experience by sweating in the head. In some cases from early months the infant will have demanded nothing less than the personal appearance of a human being, probably the mother. There is a wide range of possibilities which can be commonly observed. Among the various dolls and teddies belonging to a child, there may be one particular, probably soft, object that was introduced to the infant at about ten, eleven, or twelve months, which the infant treats in a most brutal as well as a most loving manner, and without which the infant could not conceive of going to bed; this thing would certainly not have to be left behind if the child had to go away; and if it were lost it would be a disaster for the child and therefore for those caring for him or her. It is unlikely that such an object would ever be given away to another child, and in any case no other child would want it; eventually it becomes smelly and filthy and yet one dare not wash it.

I call this thing a transitional object. By this means I can illustrate that one difficulty every child experiences is to relate subjective reality to shared reality which can be objectively perceived. From waking to sleeping the child jumps from a perceived world to a self-created world. In between there is a need for all kinds of transitional phenomena—neutral territory. I would describe this precious object by saying that there is a tacit understanding that no one will claim that this real thing is a part of the world, or that it is created by the infant. It is understood that both these things are true: the infant created it and the world supplied it. This is the continuation forward of the initial task which the ordinary mother enables her infant to undertake, when by a most delicate active adaptation she offers herself, perhaps her breast, a thousand times at the moment that the baby is ready to create something like the breast that she offers.

Most of the children who come into the category of the maladjusted either have not had an object of this kind, or they have lost it. There must be someone for the object to stand for, which means that the condition of these children cannot be cured simply by giving them a new object. A child may, however, grow to such confidence in the person who is caring for him or her that objects that are deeply symbolical of that person will appear. This will be felt as a good sign, like being able to remember a dream, or to dream of a real event.

All these transitional objects and transitional phenomena enable the child to stand frustrations and deprivations and the presentation of new situations. Do we make sure in our management of deprived children that we respect such transitional phenomena as do exist! I think that if we look at the use of toys, of auto-erotic activities, of bedtime stories and nursery rhymes in this way, we can see that, by means of these things, children have got a capacity for being deprived to some extent of what they are used to and even of what they need. A child removed from one home to another or from one institution to another may manage or may not manage according to whether a bit of cloth or a soft object can go with him or her from one place to the other; or whether there are familiar rhymes to be said at bedtime that link the past with the present; or whether the auto-erotic activities can be respected and tolerated and even valued because of their positive contribution. Surely with children whose environments are disturbed these phenomena have a special importance, and the study of them should enable us to increase our capacity to give help to these human beings who are being bandied about before they have been able to accept that which we accept only with the greatest difficulty: that the world is never as we would create it and that the best that can happen for any one of us is that there shall have been sufficient overlap of external reality and what we can create. We accept the idea of an identity between the two as an illusion.

It may be hard for people who have had fortunate environmental experiences to understand these things; nevertheless, the infant or the little child who is being moved about from one place to another is coping with exactly this problem. If we deprive a child of the transitional objects and disturb the established transitional phenomena, then the child has only one way out, which is a split in the personality, with one half related to a subjective world and the other reacting on a compliance basis to the world which impinges. When this split is formed and the bridges between the subjective and the objective are destroyed, or have never been well formed, the child is unable to operate as a total human being.

To some extent this state of affairs can always be found in the child who comes under our care because of being deprived of family life. In the children that we hope to send to foster parents or to the small sensitive hostel there will certainly be found in every case some degree of this splitting. The subjective world has the disadvantage for the child that although it can be ideal it can also be cruel and persecutory. At first the child will translate whatever is found in these terms, and either the foster home is wonderful and the real home is bad, or vice versa. In the end, however, if all goes well, the child will be able to have a fantasy of good and bad homes and to dream and talk about them and to draw them, and at the same time to perceive the real home provided by the foster parents as it is actually.

The actual foster home has the advantage of not swinging violently from good to bad and from bad to good. It remains more or less just middlingly disappointing and middlingly reassuring. Those who are managing deprived children can be helped by recognizing that each child does to some extent bring a capacity for accepting a neutral territory, localized in some way or other into masturbation or the use of a doll or the enjoyment of a nursery rhyme or something like that. So, from the study of what normal children enjoy, we can learn what these deprived children absolutely need.

Letter to Roger Money-Kyrle

Roger Money-Kyrle (1898–1980) was a British psychoanalyst and follower of Melanie Klein.

8 August 1950

Dear Money-Kyrle,

I have now had two or three days free from patients. This has enabled me to start to get down to the idea of the article for Melanie Klein's book.[i]

The result of all this is that I realise that the subject is probably beyond me. When I originally suggested it I did not think I would be the one to do it and I think it will take me a couple of years to work it out.

It might turn out that the paper I am preparing for October on Transition Phenomena will be suitable for the book, but it will be too late I expect.

It is disappointing that I am not able to have something in this book but probably the disturbances in my private affairs along with rather a trying year in respect of clinical load (apart altogether from the suicide) accounts for my defaulting. I shall continue to work on the theme of the Classification of Environment and I believe that this could not be done before Melanie Klein's theories had been developed.

With good wishes,
Yours very sincerely,
D. W. Winnicott

Dictated but not read.

---

[i] See also the letters to Money-Kyrle [CW 3:4:10; CW 3:4:12; CW 3:4:13; CW 3:5:9; CW3:5:1].

12

Letter to Hannah 'Queen' Henry

Originally published in Rodman, F. R. *Winnicott: Life and work* (pp. 67–68). Cambridge, MA: Perseus, 2003. Hannah Henry was a close friend of Winnicott's from 1926 until his death. Winnicott stayed with Henry, known as 'Queen', in Suffolk on his separation from his first wife, Alice, in 1949.

30 October 1950

Dear Queen,

It was good to hear from you. So there you are now at Aldeburgh complete with old women who are so happy with you, according to their capacity to be happy anywhere.

Do you know I've been ill again? Had a second attack 8 wks ago, and have only now been able to get back here from Plymouth. Sisters nursed me back to health. I've a few weeks now for convalescence, and its suiting me to be here.[i]

I had meant to write & tell you the sad news that I've abandoned Alice. The Winnicott firm has dissolved. It came to that. I'm not trying to get out of the fact that I'm just being horrid.

It seemed to me clear that we were doing each other harm, & that the future held nothing better for us in our relationship, only worse. This is awful when one remembers how much Alice & I have experienced together, and have as common memories. Nevertheless, when two people live together, either the body warms or cools when there is contact, and for me there had come a feeling of strain that is indescribable. For Alice too I'm sure there should eventually be relief.

There is a third person, someone who has a different effect on me, but I don't really believe I'd have allowed this to mark things up if I had not been bothered by certain dominating trains of thought in Alice that wrecked my

---

[i] Winnicott may already have had as many as three coronaries by this point.

relation to Alice. The strange thing is that I'm awfully fond of Alice, deeply attached, always shall be, but can't bear the idea of a return to actually living with her.

I think you ought to know these things, as I believe you are fond of both of us, and many of our friends are deeply distressed to find I'm not the ideal dear boy they thought I was. I wouldn't like you to hear about it by chance.

Sorry this is all about me, or us—I'm sorry too that you won't ever be visited again by Alice-and-Donald. I think each of us will continue to be very fond of you in our separate ways.

My love to you.
Donald

Alice is still at No. 7 yet, when not at New Quay.
Remember the war visits? Sleep on kitchen floor etc.?

13

Letter to Roger Money-Kyrle

Roger Money-Kyrle (1898–1980) was a British psychoanalyst and follower of Melanie Klein.

16 November 1950

Dear Money-Kyrle,

Many thanks for your letter. I would so very much like to contribute to the Klein number of the journal and so to the book,[i] and I will try, but I simply cannot promise; you must not count on me.

In regard to the Environmental paper, which I am as keen on as ever, I feel it is unlikely that I shall be ripe for so difficult a statement by May. I would very much like to have something to contribute which is a definite development of Melanie Klein's work and I am not sure at the moment of the subject I can usefully tackle. The only thing you can do is to go on asking me, and if I possibly can I shall submit something.

In a conversation with Melanie Klein I found that she was quite in favour of a statement on the Environmental Factor although I think she feels that what has to be said has been already said perhaps with too great emphasis (Bowlby etc.). She may be right, but it seems to me that those who have said what has to be said have not done what could be done in the way of classification, and have put wrong emphasis etc. We shall see.

I am very much better but not quite back at work yet.

With best wishes,
Yours sincerely,
D. W. Winnicott

---

[i] See also letters to Money-Kyrle [CW 3:4:10; CW 3:4:12; CW 3:4:13; CW 3:5:9; CW 3:5:11].

14

Knowing and Learning

Originally published in *The child and the family: First relationships*. (pp. 69–73). London: Tavistock, 1957. Also published in C. Winnicott, R. Shepherd, & M. Davis (Eds.), *Babies and their mothers* (pp. 15–21). Reading, MA: Addison-Wesley, 1987; and *Winnicott on the child* (pp. 19–23). Cambridge, MA: Perseus, 2002. Broadcast 22 March 1950, as 'Knowing and learning how to be a mother'. I. Benzie (Producer), as the seventh of an eight-part series *How's the baby?* Home Service. London: British Broadcasting Corporation. (see the broadcast list [CW 12:3:2]). Recorded as part of 'The ordinary devoted mother and her baby' [CW 12:3:3].

There is much for a young mother to learn. She gets told useful things by experts, about the introduction of solids into the diet, about vitamins, and about the use of the weight chart: and then sometimes she gets told about quite a different kind of thing, for instance, about her reaction to her infant's refusal of food.

It seems to me to be important for you to be quite clear about the difference between these two types of knowledge. What you do and know, simply by virtue of the fact that you are the mother of an infant, is as far apart from what you know by learning as is the east from the west coast of England. I cannot put this too strongly. Just as the professor who found out about the vitamins that prevent rickets really has something to teach you, so you really have something to teach him about the other kind of knowledge, that which comes to you naturally.

The mother who breast-feeds her baby simply does not have to bother about fats and proteins while she is thoroughly caught up in the management of the early stages. By the time she weans at nine months or so and the baby is making fewer demands on her, she is becoming free to study facts and advice which doctors and nurses offer. Obviously there is a great deal that she could not know intuitively, and she does want to be told about the giving of solids, and about how to use the sort of foods that are available in such a way that the baby will be able to grow and keep healthy. But she must wait for such instruction until she is in a state of mind to receive it.

We can easily see that years of brilliant research have gone into the doctor's bit of advice about vitamins, and we can look with awe at the scientist's work and at the self-discipline that such work entails, and be grateful when, by the results of scientific research, a great deal of suffering can be avoided, perhaps by some quite simple advice like adding a few drops of cod-liver oil to the diet.

At the same time the scientist, if he cares to do so, may look with awe at the mother's intuitive understanding, which makes her able to care for her infant without learning. In fact, the essential richness of this intuitive understanding, I would say, is that it *is* natural and unspoiled by learning.

The difficult task, in preparing a series of talks and books on infant care, is to know how to avoid disturbance of what comes naturally to mothers while getting them informed accurately as to the useful facts that emerge from scientific research.

I want you to be able to feel confident about your capacity as mothers, and not feel that because you could not know about vitamins, you also could not know about, for instance, how to hold your infant.

How to hold your infant; that would be a good example for me to follow up.

The phrase 'holding the baby' has a definite meaning in the English language; someone was co-operating with you over something, and then waltzed off, and you were left 'holding the baby'. By this we can see that everybody knows that mothers naturally have a sense of responsibility, and if they have a baby in their arms they are involved in some special way. Of course, some women get left holding the baby literally, in the sense that the father is unable to enjoy the part he has to play, and unable to share with the mother the great responsibility which a baby must always be to someone.

Or perhaps there is no father. Ordinarily, however, the mother feels supported by her husband and so is free to be a mother properly, and when she holds her baby she does it naturally, and without thinking it out. Such a mother will be surprised if I talk about such a thing as holding a baby as a skilled job.

When people see a baby they love to be able to be allowed to experience just this thing, of holding the baby in their arms. You don't let people hold your baby if you feel it means nothing to them. Babies are very sensitive indeed to the way they are held, so that they cry with one person and rest contented with another, even when they are quite tiny. Sometimes a little girl will ask to hold a newly-arrived baby brother or sister, and this is a big event. The wise mother will remember not to give the child the whole responsibility, and will be there all the time if she lets this happen, ready to take the baby back into her own safe keeping. The wise mother will certainly not just take it for granted that an older sister is safe with the baby in her arms. This would be to deny the meaning of it all. I know people who can remember throughout their lives the awful feeling of holding the baby brother or sister, and of the nightmare of not feeling safe. In the nightmare the baby is dropped. The fear which can turn up in the nightmare as doing harm in practice makes the big sister catch hold of the baby too tightly.

All this leads on to what you do yourself quite naturally because of your devotion to your baby. You are not anxious and so are not gripping too tight. You are not afraid you will throw the baby on to the floor. You just adapt the pressure of your arms to the baby's needs, and you move slightly, and you perhaps make some sounds. The baby feels you breathing. There is warmth that comes from your breath and your skin, and the baby finds your holding to be good.

Of course there are all kinds of mothers, and there are some who are not quite so happy about the way they hold their babies. Some feel a bit doubtful; the baby seems happier in the cot. There may be something left over in such a mother of the fear which she had to deal with when she was a little girl, when her mother let her hold a newborn baby. Or she may have had a mother who was not very good at this sort of thing herself, and she is afraid of passing on to her baby some uncertainty, belonging to the past. An anxious mother uses the cot as much as possible, or even hands the baby over to the care of a nurse, carefully chosen because of the natural way she handles babies. There is room for all kinds of mothers in the world, and some will be good at one thing and some good at another. Or shall I say some will be bad at one thing and some bad at another? Some are anxious holders.

It may be worth while looking even a little more closely at this business, because if you do handle your baby well I want you to be able to know that you are doing something of importance. This is a little part of the way in which you give a good foundation for the mental health of this new member of the community.

Look at it imaginatively.

Here is the infant right at the beginning (from what happens at the beginning we can see what happens, over and over again, later on). Let me describe three stages in the infant's relation to the world (represented by your arms and your breathing body), leaving out hunger and anger, and all the great upheavals. First stage: the infant is self-contained, a live creature, yet surrounded by space. The infant knows of nothing, except of self. Second stage: the infant moves an elbow, a knee, or straightens out a little. The space has been crossed. The infant has surprised the environment. Third stage: you who are holding the infant jump a little, because the door bell rang, or the kettle boiled over, and again the space has been crossed. This time the environment has surprised the infant.

First, the self-contained infant is in the space that is maintained between the child and the world, then the infant surprises the world, and thirdly, the world surprises the infant. This is so simple that I think it will appeal to you as a natural sequence, and therefore a good basis for the study of the way you hold your infant.

This is all very obvious, but the trouble is that if you do not know these things you may easily let your immense skill get wasted, because you will not see how to explain to neighbours, and to your husband, how necessary it is for you, in your turn, to have a space to yourself in which you can start your infant off with a sound basis for life.

Let me put it this way. The baby in the space becomes ready, in the course of time, for the movement that surprises the world, and the infant who has found the world in this way becomes, in time, ready to welcome the surprises that the world has in store.

The baby does not know that the space around is maintained by you. How careful you are that the world shall not impinge before the infant has found it! By a live and breathing quietness you follow the life in the infant with the life in yourself, and you wait for the gestures that come from the infant, gestures that lead to your being discovered.

If you feel heavy with sleep, and especially if you are in a depressed mood, you put the infant in a cot, because you know that your sleeping state is not alive enough to keep going the infant's idea of a space around.

If I have referred specially to tiny infants, and your management of them, this does not mean that I am not also referring to older children. Of course most of the time the older child has passed through to a much more complex state of affairs, and is not in need of the very special management which comes naturally to you when you are holding your baby who is only a few hours old. But how often it happens that the older child, just for a few minutes, or for an hour or two, needs to go back, and to go over the ground again that belongs to the earliest stages. Perhaps your child has had an accident, and comes to you crying. It may be five or ten minutes before there is a return to play. In the meantime you have had the child in your arms, and you have allowed for just this same sequence that I have been talking about. First of all, the quiet yet live holding, and then the readiness for the child to move and to find you, as the tears clear away. And at length you are able, quite naturally, to put the child down. Or a child is unwell, or sad, or tired. Whatever it is, for a little while the child is an infant, and you know that time has to be given so that there can be a natural return from essential security to ordinary conditions.

Of course I might have chosen many other examples of the way in which you have knowledge, simply because you are specialists in this particular matter of the care of your own children. I want to encourage you to keep and defend this specialist knowledge. It cannot be taught. Then you can learn things from other kinds of specialist. Only if you can keep what is natural in you is it safe for you to learn anything that doctors and nurses can teach you.

It might be thought that I have been trying to teach you now how to hold your baby. This seems to me to be far from the truth. I am trying to describe various aspects of the things you do naturally, in order that you may be able to recognise what you do, and in order that you may be able to get the feeling of your natural capacity. This is important, because unthinking people will often try to teach you how to do the things which you can do better than you can be taught to do them. If you are sure of all this, you can start to add to your value as a mother by learning the things that can be taught, for the best of our civilisation and culture offers much that is of value, if you can take it without the loss of what comes to you naturally.

15

Instincts and Normal Difficulties

> Originally published in *The child and the family: First relationships* (pp. 74–78). London: Tavistock, 1957. Also published in *The child, the family, and the outside world* (pp. 98–102). Harmondsworth, UK: Penguin, 1964. Broadcast 29 March 1950, as 'Symptoms of illness.' I. Benzie (Producer), as the final part of the series *How's the baby?* Home Service. London: British Broadcasting Corporation. (see the broadcast list [CW 12:3:2]). Recorded as part of 'The ordinary devoted mother and her baby' [CW 12:3:3].

When it comes to illness, talks and books are rather misleading. What a mother needs for her ill child is a doctor who can see and examine the baby and have a discussion with her. But the common troubles of ordinary healthy children are a different matter, and I think mothers find it rather helpful when it is pointed out to them that their well children are not to be expected to go straight ahead without giving any cause for worry and anxiety.

Ordinary healthy children undoubtedly do present all kinds of symptoms.

What is it that causes these troubles in infancy and early childhood? If we take it for granted that your management has been skilled and consistent, so that you can be said to have laid down the foundations for the health of this new member of society satisfactorily, what is it that determines that the child still presents problems? The answer is, I think, chiefly to do with the matter of instincts. It is about this that I wish to write now.

It may be that just for the moment your child is lying quietly over there sleeping, or cuddling something, or playing, in one of those quiet periods that you welcome. But you know only too well that in health there are recurring excitements. You can either look at it one way and say that the child gets hungry, that the body has needs, or instincts, or else you look at it another way, and say that the child begins to have exciting ideas. These exciting experiences play a very important part in the child's development, promoting as well as complicating growth.

During excitement the child has impelling needs. Often you are able to satisfy them. The needs, however, can be very great indeed, at certain moments, and some of them cannot be satisfied fully.

Now some of these needs (hunger for example) are universally recognized and easy to bring to your notice. The nature of other kinds of excitement is less widely understood.

The fact is that any part of the body may be excited at one time or another. The skin, for instance. You have seen children scratching their faces, or scratching the skin in other places, the skin itself becoming excited, and developing some kind of rash. And there are certain parts of the skin that are more sensitive than others, especially at certain times. You can go over the whole of the body of the child and think out the various ways in which excitement becomes localized. We certainly cannot leave out the sexual parts. These things are very important to the infant, and they make up the high lights of the waking life of infancy. Exciting ideas go along with the bodily excitements, and you will not be surprised if I say that these ideas not only have to do with pleasure, they also have to do with love, if the baby is developing well. Gradually the infant becomes a person capable of loving persons, and feeling loved as a person. There is a very powerful bond between the baby and the mother and father and other people around, and the excitements have to do with this love. In the form of some bodily excitement, love periodically becomes acutely felt.

The ideas that go with the primitive love impulses are predominantly destructive, and are nearly related to those of anger. The result for the baby feels good, however, if the activity leads to instinctual gratifications.

You can easily see that during such periods there is inevitably a great deal of frustration, and this leads in health to anger, even rage. You will not think your infant is ill if from time to time you are presented with a picture of rage, which you learn to distinguish from sadness, fear, and pain. In rage the infant's heart is beating faster than it will ever beat again. In fact, as many as 220 heart beats a minute can be counted, if you want to listen. Anger means that the child has got as far as believing in something and in someone to be angry with.

Now, a risk is taken whenever emotions are fully felt, and these experiences of excitement and rage must often be very painful; so you will find your perfectly normal child trying to discover ways of avoiding the most intense feelings. One way of avoiding feelings is by a damping down of instinct—for instance, the infant becomes unable to let the full extent of the excitement of feeding take place. Another way is accepting certain kinds of food but not other kinds. Or other people may give the feed, but not the mother. Every possible variation can be found, if one knows enough children. This is not necessarily illness; it is simply that we see little children discovering all sorts of techniques for managing feelings which are intolerable. They have to avoid a certain amount of natural feelings because these are too intense, or else because the full experience brings about painful conflicts.

Feeding difficulties are common in normal children, and it often happens that mothers have to put up with very disappointing months, and even years, in which a child wastes all their ability to provide good food. Perhaps a child only takes routine food, and anything prepared with special care or delicacy is rejected. Sometimes mothers have to let children refuse food altogether for quite a long time, for if they try to force it in such circumstances they only increase the child's resistance. If they wait, however, and do not make a 'thing' out of it, at some time or other the child will start eating again. One can well imagine a mother who is not experienced being worried during such a period, and needing a doctor or a nurse to reassure her that she is not neglecting her child, or doing harm.

Infants periodically have various kinds of orgy (not only feeding orgies), and these orgies are natural, and very important to them. Their excretory processes are particularly exciting to them, and the sexual parts of their bodies even more so, at appropriate moments, as they grow. It is of course easy to see the boy's erection, and difficult to know what the little girl baby feels sexually.

By the way, you will have noticed that babies do not start off thinking the same as you do about what is nice and what is nasty. Stuff that is got rid of with excitement and pleasure is likely to be felt to be good, and even good to eat, and good to smear the cot and the walls with. That may be a nuisance, but it is natural, and you will not mind too much. You will be contented to wait for more civilized sentiments to turn up of their own accord. Sooner or later disgust turns up, and, even quite suddenly, a baby who was eating soap and drinking bathwater will become prudish, and go off any kind of food that even looks like excretions, which were (till a few days previously) handled and pushed into the mouth.

Sometimes we see a return to the infant state in older children, and then we know that some difficulty has blocked the way to progress, and the child has a need to go back over the ground covered in infancy, in order to re-establish the rights of infants and the laws of natural development.

Mothers watch these things happening, and, as mothers, they do indeed play a part in it all; but they would rather watch a steady and natural developmental process than impose their own ideas of right and wrong.

One trouble that comes from trying to impose a pattern of right and wrong on an infant is that the infant's instincts come along and spoil it all. The moments of excited experience break down the baby's efforts to gain love through compliance. The result then is that he or she becomes upset, instead of strengthened, by the operation of the instincts.

The normal child has not too severely squashed the powerful instinctual feelings back, and is therefore subject to disturbances, and these look like symptoms to the ignorant observer. I have mentioned rage; temper tantrums and periods of absolute defiance are usual at two and three. Nightmares are frequently experienced by little children, and the piercing yells at midnight make the neighbours wonder what you are up to. But the truth is that the child has had a dream with some kind of sexuality in it.

Young children do not have to be ill to be frightened of dogs, doctors, and the dark, or to be imaginative about sounds and shadows, and vague shapes in the twilight; and they do not have to be ill to be liable to colic, or to sickness, or to going green when they are excited about something; they do not have to be ill to refuse to have anything to do with an adored father for a week or two, or to refuse to say 'ta' to an aunt; and they do not have to be ill to want to put the new sister in the dustbin, or to be rather cruel to the cat in a big effort to avoid hating the new baby.

And you know all about the way clean children become dirty, and dry ones wet, and how, in fact, in the period from two to five almost anything can happen. Put it all down to the workings of the instincts, and to the terrific feelings that belong to the instincts, and (since with all bodily happenings there are ideas) to the painful conflicts that result from all this in the child's imagination. Let me add that at this critical age the instincts are no longer just infantile in quality, and in describing them we do not say enough if we keep to the nursery terms, such as 'greediness' and 'messing'. When a healthy three-year-old child says 'I love you' there is meaning in it like that between men and women who love, and who are in love. It can, in fact, be sexual in the ordinary sense, involving the bodily sex parts, and including ideas that are like those of adolescents or adults in love. Tremendous forces are at work, yet all you need to do is to keep the home together, and to expect anything. Relief will come through the operation of time. When the child is five or six, things will then sober down a lot, and will stay sobered down till puberty, so you will have an easier few years, during which you can hand part of the responsibility and part of the task over to the schools, and to the trained teachers.

16

Growth and Development in Immaturity

Originally published in *The family and individual development* (pp. 21–29). London: Tavistock, 1965.

The reader should know that I am a product of the Freudian or psychoanalytic school. This does not mean that I take for granted everything Freud said or wrote, and in any case that would be absurd since Freud was developing, that is to say changing, his views (in an orderly manner, like any other scientific worker) all along the line right up to his death in 1939.

As a matter of fact, there are some things that Freud came to believe which seem to me and to many other analysts to be actually wrong, but it simply does not matter. The point is that Freud started off a scientific approach to the problem of human development; he broke through the reluctance to speak openly of sex and especially of infant and child sexuality, and he accepted the instincts as basic and worthy of study; he gave us a method for use and for development which we could learn, and whereby we could check the observations of others and contribute our own; he demonstrated the repressed unconscious and the operation of unconscious conflict; he insisted on the full recognition of psychic reality (what is real to the individual apart from what is actual); he boldly attempted to formulate theories of the mental processes, some of which have already become generally accepted.

Arising out of all this is something that is relevant here. Each individual starts and develops and becomes mature; there is no adult maturity apart from the previous development. This development is extremely complex, and it is continuous from birth or earlier right up to and through adulthood to old age. We cannot afford to leave anything out, not even the happenings of infancy, not even those of very early infancy.

Here we should pause to think about our aims in our work. We are concerned with the provision of the environment that is appropriate to the age of the infant, toddler, or child; the environment that will enable each individual gradually and in his own way to become a person who can take a place in the community without losing his or her own individuality. We do not want the children in our care to become persons who belong to an extreme category: either those who are indeed community-minded, but whose private lives are unsatisfactory so that they do not have a sense of the self going on; or those who maintain their own personal satisfactions only by neglecting their relation to society, or perhaps by being antisocial or insane. For we know that people who have to be classed in these two extremes are unhappy; they are suffering. Some of them achieve personal expression only in the act of suicide. Someone has failed them or something has gone wrong environmentally at one or more of the earlier stages, and at a late date it is hard to put things right.

But to return to the subject of young children. When we give children the right kind of good time there is really an aim in it all, namely, to make possible each child's ultimate growth to the adult state which collectively is called democracy. We know, however, how important it is not to put children in a position that is too advanced for them. Moreover, we know how futile it is to 'teach' democracy as distinct from enabling individuals to grow up, to mature, to become the stuff democracy is made of.[1]

I would mention here some of the early equivalents of what may later become, given favourable circumstances, the material for democracy. I leave out of account the management of older children, allowing them to take part in clubs and various institutions appropriate to their age. At an earlier stage, however, there is the germ of this, surely, in allowing children to take over community functions *temporarily*. We would not expect cubs or brownies to run their own groups, but we would expect there to be *moments* in which a cub or a brownie might wish to play at being in charge. And play is serious as well as enjoyable.

Sometimes an elder sister has to be a mother, with very great responsibilities, at an early age, and we can see how this task, well performed, drains away the girl's spontaneity and sense of her own self's rights; these things cannot be avoided. But ordinarily any child will like to be the responsible person *for limited periods of time*. This works best when it is the child's idea and not an idea imposed by ourselves. But gradually children become able to identify with us and so to accept our sensible impositions without too great a loss of their sense of self and the self's rights.

Is there not something of this in the evolution of children's drawings? First comes messing and then scribbling. Then the child means things in the scribbling, but we would not know what unless we were informed. The child sees anything and everything in the marks made. Perhaps the line goes over the edge and that is equivalent to bed-wetting, or to some actual messing (an upset teacup) that was nice for the child even if inconvenient for the adult. Then perhaps a rough circle turns up and the child says 'duck'. Now the child has begun to express more than the fun of instinctual experience. There is a new gain here, and for this the child is willing to forgo some of the pleasure of a more direct instinctual kind. Soon, all too soon, the child is putting legs and arms on the circle and eyes in the inside, and we say 'Humpty-Dumpty'. We all laugh, and already direct expression is a long way away and drawing has started. But once more there is a gain because of the constructive nature of what is being done, which is recognized by someone near and dear to the child, and also because a new form of communication has been discovered which is better than speech. In no time the child is drawing pictures. The size and shape of the page determine the placing of the objects depicted. There comes a balance of objects and of movements, and a subtle interrelationship of all the relative proportions. The child is now an artist for a brief spell. More important, the child has shown a developing capacity to retain spontaneity while respecting form and all the other controls. This is the democratic idea in miniature. It is but weakly established as yet because it depends on some person who is in relation to the child that is drawing. Later, this very personal tie is broken, and must be broken and diffused, and before the child is either eventually an artist, or more likely an ordinary citizen, he or she has to be able to supply *from within* this person in relation to whom, externally, the early artistry was so richly shown.

All this leads us back and back. In terms of environment, this earlier and earlier means more and more personal, and it means that the person who is personal with the child needs to be more and more reliable.

Gradually as we go still further back the person has to be able to be even more than reliable from the child's point of view. We know that with small children it is only love of the particular child that enables the person to be reliable enough. We love a child and maintain an uninterrupted relationship and half the battle is won. But let us go yet further back. Now even stronger words have to be used. I think that over the relatively short period of the first months the word 'devotion' takes us exactly where we need to go. I am not using words like 'clever', 'learned', 'well taught', although I do not despise them. Only a devoted mother (or mother-surrogate) can follow an infant's needs. As I see it, the infant at the start needs a degree of *active adaptation to needs* which cannot be provided unless a devoted person is doing everything. It is obvious that it is the infant's own mother to whom such devotion comes naturally, and even if it can be proved that infants do not know their mothers till they are some months old I still think we must assume that the mother knows her infant.

Education of Parents

I may be criticized here. The reader may say: 'But you are taking it for granted that mothers are normal and you are forgetting that many are neurotic and some are near-insane'. 'Many are getting a poor deal themselves, and they pass on their sexual frustrations to their infants by being irritable or in more direct ways'. 'It is absurd to talk about mothers acting naturally, or nurses or teachers or anyone. *They have all got to be taught*'.

My answer is not to disagree absolutely; but I would say that when people who care for infants and children are neurotic or near-insane (and many are), they cannot be taught. Our hope lies in those who are more or less normal. In our clinics we have to deal with the abnormalities, and we orientate towards abnormality. But in managing ordinary mothers and infants, and in teaching infants and young children, *we must resolutely keep orientated towards the normal or healthy*. And healthy mothers have much to teach us.

Are we quite sure that the doctors and nurses who so skilfully care for mothers in antenatal clinics, in maternity wards, and in welfare clinics really allow the ordinary healthy mother to function? Things have improved very much in the last few years. Now it is not so rare to see maternity hospitals with the babies in baskets beside their mothers. I need not draw a picture of the horrid alternative which is all too well known, of the infant in the infant ward, brought in at feed-time and pushed up against the breast of the bewildered and even frightened mother. Also, largely because of the work of Bowlby and Robertson,[2] there is now a greater tendency to allow parents to keep in touch with their infants and small children who unfortunately need to have a spell in hospital.

The fact is that doctors and nurses have to recognize that they are experts in one direction only. In regard to such a thing as the beginning of an emotional relationship between the mother and the baby (of which the establishment of breast-feeding is a part), the ordinary mother is not only the expert; she is actually the only one who can know how to act for that particular baby. There is a reason. It is because of her *devotion,* which is the only motivation that works.

When we attempt to carry over this consideration to such a complex thing as the nursery school, we can say, greatly simplifying, that in any nursery school there must be two kinds of children—and the same is true of all schools. There are those children whose parents have managed well and are managing well. These children will be the rewarding children, able to show and cope with all kinds of feelings. Then there are the children whose parents have not succeeded, and we must remember that the failure may not be their fault at all. It may be a doctor's fault, or a nurse's fault; or it may have come about through the operation of chance—for instance, a bad attack of whooping cough; or perhaps willing helpers got in the way. These children need, at nursery-school age, the active adaptation to needs that belongs truly to the earliest weeks and months. They may need it from persons who are not their actual parents. Active adaptation coming too late is called 'spoiling', and those who spoil a child are criticized. Moreover, since this active adaptation to needs comes too late the children cannot make proper use of it, or else they need it to a very great degree and over a long period. Thus the person who is able to supply it may find himself in a very difficult situation because the child may develop a dependence on him that he dare not break.

The thing is that all schools should be in triplicate:

(a) For the children of the first class that I have described, who can enrich themselves from what is offered to them and can contribute and gain by contributing.
(b) For the children who need from the teachers what home has failed to supply, that is psychotherapy rather than teaching.
(c) For the intermediates.

The Living Child

I would like now to turn this subject inside out, and to describe the infant and the child in terms of the development of the living child.

First I would simplify matters by separating out the *excited state* from the *unexcited state*. The *excited state* obviously implies the operation of instincts. As we know, every bodily functioning has its imaginative elaboration, and so the conflicts that develop in respect of ideas involve inhibitions and muddles in bodily happening; growth here implies not only going from stage to stage because of increasing age, but also the negotiation of each state as it is reached, without too much loss of the instinctual roots of feeling. It is just in these early stages of instinct development, however, that the serious repressions start that cripple the lives of many individuals. How necessary then, for the toddler, are a stability and a continuity of environment, in both its physical and its emotional aspects!

Although it is just here that the main forces of dynamic psychology are to be found I feel that I need not reiterate these points. Freud's work, which has chiefly dealt with these vital phenomena, is now fairly widely known, especially by those who study the psychology of children.

The various instinctual drives that almost rend the infant by their strength develop according to a natural progression. At first, naturally, it is the mouth and the whole intake mechanisms, including the grasping of the hands, that form the basis for the fantasy that exists at the height of excitement. Later the excretory phenomena provide material for excited fantasy, and what goes on inside too. In the course of time a genital type of excitement turns up and can be said to dominate the life of the little boy or girl in the two to five age group.

The natural progression of these various types of excited ideas and of excitement organizations is not usually clear and simple because at all stages conflicts arise, and the very best management cannot alter this fact. Good management is more of the nature of providing consistent conditions in which each infant can work out what is specific to that infant.

Naturally, the ideas that belong to excited times form the basis for play and for dreams. In play there is excitement of a special kind, and play is spoiled when direct instinctual need comes to the fore. Only gradually do infants come to the management of these matters. Indeed, all adults know how the pleasures of life can be spoiled by the intrusion of bodily excitement, and part of the technique of living is to find ways of avoiding bodily excitements that cannot come soon to climax. Naturally this is easier for those whose instinctual life is satisfactory than for those who cannot avoid having to tolerate a high degree of frustration in sexual relationships.

Fortunately, while children are gradually finding out these difficult things they can reach satisfactory climaxes in all sorts of ways that are characteristic for children. Food can do a lot, for instance. Also sleep resolves a great deal. Defecation and urination can be extremely satisfactory experiences, and so can a good fight or being smacked. Nevertheless, in every childhood there are manifold symptoms that quite clearly reflect the condition known as 'being all dressed up and nowhere to go'; excited, without the capacity for reaching a climax (bilious attacks, etc.). These things are not necessarily abnormal.

Many people now know a great deal about all these things, but they may not know about some of the more *indirect* results of instinctual experience. I refer how to the way the richness of the personality builds up through satisfactory and unsatisfactory experiences.

It is helpful to postulate here an early *ruthless* stage in order to draw attention to the fact that at first the excited and highly destructive ideas that go with instinctual experience are directed at the mother's breast without guilt. In health, however, the infant soon comes to put two and two together and to know that what is in fantasy so ruthlessly attacked is the same as that which is loved and needed. The ruthless stage gives way to a stage of *concern*.

The infant now has to deal with two sets of phenomena after a satisfactory excited experience. A good thing has been attacked and hurt and spoiled, and moreover the infant is richer for the experience; something good has been built up inside. The infant has to be able to stand feeling guilt. In the course of time a way out of the trouble appears, because the infant is able to find *ways of making reparation,* of mending, of giving in return, of putting back what has (in fantasy) been stolen. (Readers will recognize Melanie Klein in all this.)

We can see, then, that there is a specific need here which the environment must supply if the infant is to come through and grow (technically: to reach the 'depressive position' in emotional development). The infant has to be able to tolerate feeling guilt, and to alter this state of affairs by making reparation. If this is to happen, the mother (or someone in her place) has to stay there, alive and alert, over the guilt period. To put it crudely: an infant in an institution might be beautifully cared for by several nurses, but what if the guilt belonging to the morning's experiences comes up for repair in the evening when another nurse is there, and so the reparation misses fire. The mother caring for her own infant is more or less always there and recognizes the spontaneous constructive and reparative impulses. She can wait for them and she recognizes them when they come.

When all goes well it is not guilt that is experienced, but a sense of being responsible develops. The sense of guilt remains latent, to appear when reparation fails relative to destruction.

Much more could be said about all this guilt and reparation, and about the infant's anxieties in respect of the riches that are storing up inside. If we looked we should find frightening things in there too, inside the baby, arising out of the baby's angry impulses. But I now want to leave consideration of the excited states and of the consequences of excited experiences in order to get on to something else. Let me say in passing that difficulties in this field, associated with the repression of painful conflicts, lead on to the various neurotic manifestations and to mood disorders. If we study the material of the unexcited states, however, we shall be nearer to a study of psychosis. Disorders of what I describe under the heading of unexcited states will be found to be psychotic rather than neurotic in quality, the stuff insanity is made of. However, I am not dealing with disorders; instead I am briefly describing the tasks which the infant has to perform in making an ordinary healthy development.

Development Apart from Excitements

If we turn, then, rather artificially, to the *unexcited state,* what do we find? For one thing we find we are studying the ego in the self's journey towards autonomy. We are studying, for instance, the development in the infant of a sense of unity of personality, a capacity to feel (at any rate at times) *integrated.* Gradually, too, the infant begins to feel to be a dweller in what we so easily see as that infant's own body. All these things take time, and are greatly helped by sensible and consistent management of the body, bathing, exercising, and so on.

Then there is also the development of a capacity to *relate to* external reality. This task which every infant must achieve is complex and difficult, and very definitely needs the attention that a devoted mother is qualified to give. The *objectively* perceived world is *never* the same as what is conceived of, what is seen *subjectively.* This is a big trouble with all human beings, but by actively adapting at the start a mother superimposes external reality on what the infant conceives, of; she does this well enough, and often enough, so that the infant becomes contented to leave this problem to be taken up later as part of the game called philosophy.

One more thing: if the environment behaves well, the infant has a chance to maintain a sense of *continuity of being*; perhaps this may go right back to the first stirrings in the womb. When this exists the individual has a stability that can be gained in no other way.

If external reality has been introduced to the infant in small doses, accurately graded to the infant's or child's understanding, the child may grow up to be capable of making a scientific approach to phenomena, and may even perhaps carry a scientific method into the study of human affairs. If this happens, and if it is successful, then there is something owing to the devoted mother who laid the foundations, and then to both the fond parents, and then to a succession of minders and teachers, any of whom could have caused a muddle and could have made difficult the child's ultimate attainment of a scientific attitude. Most of us, alas, have to put at least some of human nature outside the realm of scientific inquiry.

Science and Human Nature

The main burden of this communication is that if what is true and good and natural in human nature and in the management of growing human beings is to be saved from being squashed out by science, it can only come about by an extension of scientific inquiry into the whole field of human nature. I think we are all travelling towards the same thing. To restate it: we want to make it possible for each individual to find and establish his or her own identity in such a solid way that eventually, in the course of time, and in that individual's own manner, there will be attained a capacity to become a member of society—an active, creative member, without loss of personal spontaneity and without loss of that sense of freedom which comes, in health, from within.

Clinical Coda

It may well be that the reader is left with a feeling of bewilderment. There is so much for the infant to go through, and the responsibility of the mothers and fathers and nurses and teachers who provide the environment suitable for the various stages is so great, how shall we ever manage? But it must be remembered that whenever we pause in our work and attempt to make some assessment of our aims, as we have done now, we have an artificial situation.

And so, let us return to the real thing, and conclude with the picture of a rather young baby boy. (It could as well be a girl.)

This baby has been through all the usual things, fist-sucking, finger-sucking, scratching the skin of his belly, pulling at his navel and his penis, and plucking at the wool of the cover. He is about eight months old and he has not yet quite taken up with the usual run of teddies and dolls. But he has found some soft object. He has adopted this object. Eventually there will be a special name for it. It will remain a necessary thing in the child's life for some years, and in the end will simply fade away like the old soldier. This object is halfway between everything. *We* know that it came from an aunt. From the infant's point of view however it is the perfect compromise. It is neither part of the self nor part of the world. Yet it is both. It was conceived of by the infant and yet he could not have produced it, it just came. Its coming showed him what to conceive of. It is at one and the same time subjective and objective. It is at the border between inside and outside. It is both dream and real.

We leave this baby with this object. In his relationship with it he is at peace, in the celtic twilight between a personal or psychic reality and reality that is actual and shared.

Notes

1. This theme is developed in 'Some Thoughts on the Meaning of the Word Democracy' [CW 3:5:17].
2. John Bowlby, *Maternal Care and Mental Health* (London: HMSO, 1951); abridged version, edited by Margery Fry, *Child Care and the Growth of Love* (Harmondsworth: Penguin Books, 1953). James Robertson, *Young Children in Hospital* (London: Tavistock Publications, 1958). See also two films by James Robertson, *A Two-year-old goes to Hospital and Going to Hospital with Mother* (Tavistock Child Development Research Unit, 2 Beaumont Street, London, W1).

Some Thoughts on the Meaning of the Word Democracy

Originally published in *Human Relations*, June 1950, 3(2). Also published in *The family and individual development* (pp. 155–169). London: Tavistock, 1965; and C. Winnicott, R. Shepherd, & M. Davis (Eds.), *Home is where we start from: Essays by a psychoanalyst* (pp. 239–259). Harmondsworth, UK: Penguin, 1986.

First of all let me say that I realize I am offering comments on a subject that is outside my own speciality. Sociologists and political scientists may at first resent this impertinence. Yet it seems to me to be valuable for workers to cross the boundaries from time to time, provided that they realize (as I do indeed) that their remarks must inevitably appear naive to those who know the relevant literature and who are accustomed to a professional language of which the intruder is ignorant.

This word *democracy* has great importance at the present time. It is used in all sorts of different senses; here are a few:

(i) A social system in which the people rule.
(ii) A social system in which the people choose the leader.
(iii) A social system in which people choose the government.
(iv) A social system in which the government allows the people freedom of:
    (a) thought and expression of opinion,
    (b) enterprise.
(v) A social system which, being on a run of good fortune, can afford to allow individuals freedom of action.

One can study:

(i) The etymology of the word.
(ii) The history of social institutions, Greek, Roman, etc.

(iii) The use made of the word by various countries and cultures at the present time, Great Britain, the United States, Russia, etc.
(iv) The abuse of the word by dictators and others; hoodwinking the people, etc.

In any discussion on a term, such as democracy, it is obviously of first importance that a definition should be reached, suitable for the particular type of discussion.

PSYCHOLOGY OF THE USE OF THE TERM

Is it possible to study the use of this term psychologically? We accept and are accustomed to psychological studies of other difficult terms such as 'normal mind', 'healthy personality', 'individual well-adjusted to society', and we expect such studies to prove valuable in so far as they give unconscious emotional factors their full import. One of the tasks of psychology is to study and present the latent ideas that exist in the use of such concepts, not confining attention to obvious or conscious meaning.

An attempt is made here to initiate a psychological study.

WORKING DEFINITION OF THE TERM

It does seem that an important latent meaning of this term can be found, namely, that a democratic society is 'mature', that is to say, that it has a quality that is allied to the quality of individual maturity which characterizes its healthy members.

Democracy is here defined, therefore, as 'society well-adjusted to its *healthy* individual members'. This definition is in accord with the view expressed by R. E. Money-Kyrle (Mental Health Congress, 1948 Bulletin).[i]

It is the way people use this term that is important to the psychologist. A psychological study is justified if there is implied in the term the element of *maturity*. The suggestion is that in all uses of the term there can be found to be implied the idea of maturity or relative maturity, though it is difficult, as all will admit, to define these terms adequately.

PSYCHIATRIC HEALTH

In psychiatric terms, the normal or healthy individual can be said to be one who is mature; according to his or her chronological age and social setting

---

[i] See Money-Kyrle, 'Some Aspects of State and Character in Germany' (1951).

there is an appropriate degree of emotional development. (In this argument physical maturity is assumed.)

Psychiatric health is therefore a term without fixed meaning. In the same way the term 'democratic' need not have a fixed meaning. Used by a community it may mean *the more rather than the less mature in society structure*. In this way one would expect the frozen meaning of the word to be different in Great Britain, the United States, and the Soviet Union, and yet to find that the term retains value because of its implying the recognition of maturity as health.

How can one study the emotional development of society? Such a study must be closely related to the study of the individual. The two studies must take place simultaneously.

Democratic Machinery

An attempt must be made to state the accepted qualities of democratic machinery. The machinery must exist for the *election* of leaders by free vote, true secret ballot. The machinery must exist for the people *to get rid of* leaders by secret ballot. The machinery must exist for the *illogical* election and removal of leaders.

The essence of democratic machinery is the free vote (secret ballot). The point of this is that it ensures the freedom of the people to express deep feelings, *apart from conscious thoughts*.[1]

In the exercise of the secret vote, the whole responsibility for action is taken by the individual, if he is healthy enough to take it. The vote expresses the outcome of the struggle within himself, the external scene having been internalized and so brought into association with the interplay of forces in his own personal inner world. That is to say, the decision as to which way to vote is the expression of a solution of a struggle within himself. The process seems to be somewhat as follows. The external scene, with its many social and political aspects, is made personal for him in the sense that he gradually identifies himself with all the parties to the struggle. This means that he perceives the external scene in terms of his own internal struggle, and he temporarily allows his internal struggle to be waged in terms of the external political scene. This to-and-fro process involves work and takes time, and it is part of democratic machinery to arrange for a period of preparation. A sudden election would produce an acute sense of frustration in the electorate. Each voter's inner world has to be turned into a political arena over a limited period.

If there is doubt about the secrecy of the ballot, the individual, however healthy, can only express by his vote his *reactions*.

IMPOSED DEMOCRATIC MACHINERY

It would be possible to take a community and to impose on it the machinery that belongs to democracy, but this would not be to create a democracy. Someone would be needed to continue to maintain the machinery (for secret ballot, etc.), and also to force the people to accept the results.

Innate Democratic Tendency

A democracy is an achievement, at a point of time, of a limited society, i.e. of a society that has some natural boundary. Of a true democracy (as the term is used today) one can say: *In this society at this time there is sufficient maturity in the emotional development of a sufficient proportion of the individuals that comprise it for there to exist an innate[2] tendency towards the creation and re-creation and maintenance of the democratic machinery.*

It would be important to know what proportion of mature individuals is necessary if there is to be an innate democratic tendency. In another way of expressing this, what proportion of antisocial individuals can a society contain without submergence of innate democratic tendency?

SUPPOSITION

If the second world war, and the evacuation scheme in particular, increased the proportion of antisocial children in Great Britain from X cent to, say, $5X$ per cent, this could easily have affected the education system, so that the educational orientation was towards the $5X$ per cent antisocials, crying out for dictatorship methods, and away from the $100-5X$ per cent children who were not antisocial.

A decade later this problem would be stated in this way, that, whereas society could cope with X per cent criminals by segregation of them in prisons, $5X$ per cent of them would tend to produce a general reorientation towards criminals.

IMMATURE IDENTIFICATION WITH SOCIETY

In a society at any one time, if there is X quantity of individuals who show their lack of sense of society by developing an antisocial tendency, there is Z quantity of individuals reacting to inner insecurity by the alternative tendency—identification with authority. This is unhealthy, immature, because it is not identification with authority that arises out of self-discovery. It is a sense of frame without sense of picture, a sense of form without retention of spontaneity. This is a pro-society tendency that is anti-individual. People who develop in this way can be called 'hidden antisocials'.

Hidden antisocials are not 'whole persons' any more than are manifest antisocials, since each needs to find and to control the conflicting force in the external world outside the self. By contrast, the healthy person, who is capable of becoming depressed, is able to find the whole conflict within the self as well as being able to see the whole conflict outside the self, in external (shared) reality. When healthy persons come together they each contribute a whole world, because each brings a whole person.

'Hidden antisocials' provide material for a type of leadership which is sociologically immature. Moreover, this element in a society greatly strengthens the danger that derives from its frank antisocial elements, especially since ordinary people so easily let those with an urge to lead get into key positions. Once in such positions, these immature leaders immediately gather to themselves the obvious antisocials, who welcome them (the immature anti-individual leaders) as their natural masters. (False resolution of splitting.)

THE INDETERMINATES

It is never as simple as this, because if there are $(X + Z)$ per cent antisocial individuals in a community, it is not true to say that $100 - (X + Z)$ per cent are 'social'. There are those in an indeterminate position. One could put it:

Antisocials X per cent
Indeterminates Y per cent
Pro-society but anti-individual Z per cent
Healthy individuals capable of social contribution $100 - (X + Y + Z)$ per cent
Total   100 per cent

The whole democratic burden falls on the $100 - (X + Y + Z)$ per cent of individuals who are maturing as individuals, and who are gradually becoming able to add a social sense to their well-grounded personal development.

What percentage does $100 - (X + Y + Z)$ per cent represent, for instance, in Great Britain today? Possibly it is quite small, say 30 per cent. Perhaps, if there are 30 per cent mature persons, as many as 20 per cent of the indeterminates will be sufficiently influenced to be counted as mature, thus bringing the total to 50 per cent. If, however, the mature percentage should drop to 20, it must be expected that there will be a bigger fall in the percentage of indeterminates able to act in a mature way. If 30 per cent maturity in a community collects 20 per cent indeterminates, i.e. a total of 50 per cent, perhaps 20 per cent maturity in a community collects only 10 per cent indeterminates, i.e. a total of 30 per cent.

Whereas a 50 per cent total might indicate sufficient innate democratic tendency for practical purposes, 30 per cent could not be counted sufficient to avoid submergence by the sum of the antisocials (hidden and manifest) and the indeterminates who would be drawn by weakness or fear into association with them.

There follows an anti-democratic tendency, a tendency towards dictatorship, characterized at first by a feverish bolstering up of the democratic facade (hoodwinking function of the term).

One sign of this tendency is the corrective institution, the localized dictatorship, the practising ground for the personally-immature leaders who are reversed antisocials (pro-social but anti-individual).

This, the corrective institution, has both the prison and the mental hospital of a healthy society perilously near to it, and for this reason the doctors of criminals and of the insane have to be constantly on guard lest they find themselves being used, without at first knowing it, as agents of the anti-democratic tendency. There must, in fact, always be a borderline in which there is no clear distinction between the corrective treatment of the political or ideational opponent and the therapy of the insane person. (Here lies the social danger of physical methods of therapy of the mental patient, as compared with true psychotherapy, or even the acceptance of a state of insanity. In psychotherapy the patient is a person on equal terms with the doctor, with a right to be ill, and also a right to claim health and full responsibility for personal political or ideational views.)

Creation of Innate Democratic Factor

If democracy is maturity, and maturity is health, and health is desirable, then we wish to see whether anything can be done to foster it. Certainly it will not help to impose democratic machinery on a country.

We must turn to the $100 - (X + Y + Z)$ group of individuals. All depends on them. Members of this group can instigate research.

We find that at any one time we can do nothing to increase the quantity of this innate democratic factor comparable in importance to what has already been done (or not done) by the parents and homes of these individuals when they were infants and children and adolescents.

We can, however, try to avoid compromising the future. We can try to avoid interfering with the homes that can cope, and are actually coping, with their own individual children and adolescents. These *ordinary good homes* provide the only setting in which the innate democratic factor can be created.[3] This is indeed a modest statement of positive contribution, but there is a surprising amount of complexity in its application.

FACTORS ADVERSE TO THE FUNCTIONING OF THE ORDINARY GOOD HOME

(i) It is very difficult for people to recognize that the essential of a democracy really does lie with the ordinary man and woman, and the ordinary, commonplace home.

(ii) Even if a wise government policy gives parents freedom to run their homes in their own way, it is not certain that officials putting official policies into practice will respect the parents' position.

(iii) Ordinary good parents do need help. They need all that science can offer in respect of physical health and the prevention and treatment of physical disease; also they want instruction in child care, and help when their children have psychological illnesses or present behaviour problems. But, if they seek such assistance, can they be sure they will not have their responsibilities lifted from them? If this happens they cease to be creators of the innate democratic factor.

(iv) Many parents are not ordinary good parents. They are psychiatric cases, or they are immature, or they are antisocial in a wide sense, and socialized only in a restricted sense; or they are unmarried, or in unstable relationship, or bickering, or separated from each other, and so on. These parents get attention from society, because of their defects. The thing is, can society see that the orientation towards these pathological features must not be allowed to affect society's orientation towards the ordinary healthy homes?

(v) In any case, the parents' attempt to provide a home for their children, in which the children can grow as individuals, and each *gradually add* a capacity to identify with the parents and then with wider groupings, starts at the beginning, when the mother comes to terms with her infant. Here the father is the protecting agent who frees the mother to devote herself to her baby.

The place of the home has long been recognized, and in recent years a great deal has been found out by psychologists as to the ways in which a stable home not only enables children to find themselves and to find each other, but also makes them begin to qualify for membership of society in a wider sense.

This matter of interference with the early infant-mother relationship, however, needs some special consideration. In our society there is increasing interference at this point, and there is extra danger from the fact that some psychologists actually claim that at the beginning it is only physical care that counts. This can only mean that in the unconscious fantasy of people in general the most awful ideas cluster round the infant-mother relationship. Anxiety in the unconscious is represented in practice by:

(a) Overemphasis by physicians and even by psychologists on *physical* processes and health.

(b) Various theories that breast-feeding is bad, that the baby must be trained as soon as born, that babies should not be handled by their mothers, etc.; and (in the negative) that breast-feeding *must* be established, that no training whatever should be given, that babies should never be allowed to cry, etc.

(c) Interference with the mother's access to her baby in the first days, and with her first presentation of external reality to the infant. This, after all, is the basis of the new individual's capacity eventually to become related to ever-widening external reality, and if the mother's tremendous contribution, *through her being devoted,* is spoilt or prevented, there is no hope that the individual will pass eventually into the $100 - (X + Y + Z)$ group that alone generates the innate democratic factor.

Development of Subsidiary Themes: Election of Persons

Another essential part of the democratic machinery is that it is a *person* who is elected. There is all the difference in the world between (i) the vote for a person, (ii) the vote for a party with a set tendency, and (iii) the support of a clear-cut principle by ballot.

(i) The election of a person implies that the electors believe in themselves as persons, and therefore believe in the person they nominate or vote for. The person elected has the opportunity to act as a person. As a whole (healthy) person he has the total conflict within, which enables him to get a view, albeit a personal one, of total external situations. He may, of course, belong to a party and be known to have a certain tendency. Nevertheless, he can adapt in a delicate way to changing conditions; if he actually changes his main tendency he can put himself up for re-election.

(ii) The election of a party or a group tendency is relatively less mature. It does not require of the electors a trust in a human being. For immature persons, nevertheless, it is the only logical procedure, precisely because an immature person cannot conceive of, or believe in, a truly mature individual. The result of the vote for a party or tendency, for a thing and not a person, is the establishment of a rigid outlook, ill-adapted for delicate reactions. This *thing* that is elected cannot be loved or hated, and it is suitable for individuals who have a poorly developed sense of self. It could be said that a system of voting is less democratic, because less mature (in terms of emotional development of the individual), when the accent is on the vote for the principle or party and not on the vote for the person.

(iii) Much further removed from anything associated with the word democracy is the ballot on a specific point. There is little of maturity about a referendum (although this can be made to fit in with a mature system on exceptional occasions). As an example of the way in which a referendum is un-useful can be cited the peace ballot, between the two world wars, in Great Britain. People were asked to answer a specific question ('Are you in favour of peace or war?'). A large number of people abstained from voting because they knew that the question was an unfair one. Of those who voted a big proportion put their crosses against the word peace, although in actual fact, when circumstances rearranged themselves, they were in favour of the war when it came, and took part in the fighting. The point is that in this type of questioning there is only room for the expression of the *conscious* wish. There is no relation between putting one's tick against the word 'peace' in such a ballot and voting for a person who is known to be eager for peace provided the failure to fight does not mean a lazy abandonment of aspirations and responsibilities and the betrayal of friends.

The same objection applies to much of the Gallup Poll and other questionnaires, even although a great deal of trouble is taken to avoid exactly this pitfall. In any case, a vote on a specific point is a very poor substitute indeed for the vote in favour of a person who, once elected, has a space of time in which he can use his own judgement. The referendum has nothing to do with democracy.

Support of Democratic Tendency: Summary

1. The most valuable support is given in a negative way by organized noninterference with the ordinary good mother-infant relationship, and with the ordinary good home.
2. For more intelligent support, even of this negative kind, much research is needed on the emotional development of the infant and the child of all ages, and also on the psychology of the nursing mother and of the father's function at various stages.
3. The existence of this study shows a belief in the value of education in democratic procedure, which of course can only be given in so far as there is understanding, and can only be usefully given to the emotionally mature or healthy individuals.
4. Another important negative contribution would be the avoidance of attempts to implant democratic machinery on total communities. The result can only be failure, and a setback to true democratic growth. The alternative and valuable action is to support the emotionally mature individuals, however few they may be, and to let time do the rest.

Person—Man or Woman?

The point that has to be considered is whether in the place of the word 'person' there can be put 'man' or 'woman'.

The fact is that the political heads of most countries are men, although women are increasingly used for responsible posts. It can perhaps be assumed that men and women have an equal capacity *qua* men and women; or, the other way round, it would not be possible to say that only men could be suitable for leadership on grounds of intellectual or emotional capacity for the highest political post. Nevertheless, this does not dispose of the problem. It is the psychologist's task to draw attention to the *unconscious* factors which are easily left out of account, even in serious discussions on this sort of subject. The thing that has to be considered is unconscious popular feeling in regard to the man or woman who is elected to the position of political chief. If there is a difference in the fantasy according to whether it be a man or a woman, this cannot be ignored, nor can it be brushed aside by the comment that fantasies ought not to count because they are 'only fantasies'.

In psycho-analytical and allied work it is found that all individuals (men and women) have in reserve a certain fear of *woman*.[4] Some individuals have this fear to a greater extent than others, but it can be said to be universal. This is quite different from saying that an individual fears a particular woman. This fear of *woman* is a powerful agent in society structure, and it is responsible for the fact that in very few societies does a woman hold the political reins. It is also responsible for the immense amount of cruelty to women, which can be found in customs that are accepted by almost all civilizations.

The root of this fear of *woman* is known. It is related to the fact that in the early history of every individual who develops well, and who is sane, and who has been able to find himself, there is a debt to a woman—the woman who was devoted to that individual as an infant, and whose devotion was absolutely essential for that individual's healthy development. The original dependence is not remembered, and therefore the debt is not acknowledged, except in so far as the fear of *woman* represents the first stage of this acknowledgement.

The foundation of the mental health of the individual is laid down at the very beginning when the mother is simply being devoted to her infant and when the infant is doubly dependent because totally unaware of dependence. There is no relation to the father which has such a quality, and for this reason a man who in a political sense is at the top can be appreciated by the group much more objectively than a woman can be if she is in a similar position.

Women often claim that if women were in charge of affairs there would be no wars. There are reasons why this may be doubted as a final statement of truth, but, even if the claim were justified, it would still not follow that men or women would ever tolerate the general principle of women generally at the highest points of political power. (The Crown, by being outside or beyond politics, is not affected by these considerations.)

As an offshoot of this consideration, one can consider the psychology of the dictator, who is at the opposite pole to anything that the word democracy can mean. *One of the roots of the need to be dictator can be a compulsion to deal with this fear of woman by encompassing her and acting for her.* The dictator's curious habit of demanding not only absolute obedience and absolute dependence but also 'love' can be derived from this source.

Moreover, the tendency of groups of people to accept or even seek *actual* domination is derived from a fear of domination by *fantasy woman*. This fear leads them to seek, and even welcome, domination by a known human being, especially one who has taken on himself the burden of personifying and therefore limiting the magical qualities of the all-powerful woman of fantasy, to whom is owed the great debt. The dictator can be overthrown, and must eventually die; but the woman figure of primitive unconscious fantasy has no limits to her existence or power.

Child-Parent Relationship

The democratic set-up includes the provision of a certain degree of stability for the elected rulers; as long as they can manage their job without alienating the support of their electors, they carry on. In this way the people arrange for a certain amount of stability which they could not maintain through direct voting on every point, even if that were possible. The psychological consideration here is that there is in the history of every individual the fact of the parent-child relationship. Although in the mature democratic way of political life the electors are presumably mature human beings, it cannot be assumed that there is no place for a residue of the parent-child relationship, with its obvious advantages. To some extent, in the democratic election mature people elect temporary parents, which means that they also acknowledge the fact that to some extent the electors remain children. Even the elected temporary parents, the rulers of the democratic political system, are children themselves outside their professional political work. If in driving their cars they exceed the speed limit they come under ordinary judicial censure because driving a car is not part of their job of ruling. As political leaders, and only as such, they are temporarily parents, and after being deposed at an election they revert to being children. It is as if it is convenient to play a game of parents and children because things work out better that way. In other words, because there are advantages in the parent-child relationship, some of this is retained; but, for this to be possible, a sufficient proportion of individuals need to be grown-up enough not to mind playing at being children.

In the same way, it is thought to be bad for these people who are playing at parents to have no parents themselves. In the game it is generally thought that there should be another house of representatives to which the rulers who are directly elected by the people should be responsible. In this country this function belongs to the House of Lords, which is to some extent composed of those who have a hereditary title, and to some extent of those who have won a position there by eminence in various branches of public work. Once again the 'parents' of the 'parents' are persons, and capable of making positive contributions as human beings. And it makes sense to love or to hate or to respect or to despise persons. There can be no substitute in a society for the human beings or being at the top, in so far as that society is to be rated according to its quality of emotional maturity.

And further, in a study of the social setting in Great Britain, we can see that the lords are children, relative to the Crown. Here in each case we come again to a person, who holds his or her position by heredity, and also by maintaining the love of the people by his or her personality and actions. It is certainly helpful when the reigning monarch quite easily and sincerely carries the matter a stage further and proclaims a belief in God. Here we reach the interrelated subjects of The Dying God and The Eternal Monarch.

Geographical Boundary of a Democracy

For the development of a democracy, in the sense of a mature society structure, it seems that it is necessary that there should be some natural geographical boundary for that society. Obviously, up to recently and even now, the fact that Great Britain is seabound (except for its relation to Eire) has been very much responsible for the maturity of our society structure. Switzerland has (less satisfactorily) mountain limits. America till recently had the advantage of a west which offered unlimited exploitation; this meant that the United States, while being united by positive ties, did not till recently need to start to feel to the full the internal struggles of a closed community, united in spite of hate as well as because of love.

A state that has no natural frontier cannot relax an active adaptation to neighbours. In one sense, fear *simplifies* the emotional situation, for many of the indeterminate Y and some of the less severe of the antisocial X become able to identify with the state on the basis of a cohesive reaction to an external persecution threat. This simplification is detrimental, however, to the development towards maturity, which is a difficult thing, involving full acknowledgement of essential conflict, and the non-employment of any way out or way round (defences).

In any case, the basis for a society is the whole human personality, and the personality has a limit. The diagram of a healthy person is a circle (sphere), so that whatever is not-self can be described as either inside or outside that person. It is not possible for persons to get further in society-building than they can get with their own personal development.

For these reasons we regard with suspicion the use of terms like 'world citizenship'. Perhaps only a few really great and fairly aged men and women ever get as far in their own development as to be justified in thinking in such wide terms.

If the whole world were our society, then it would need to be at times in a depressed mood (as a person at times inevitably has to be), and it would have to be able fully to acknowledge essential conflict within itself. The concept of a global society brings with it the idea of the world's suicide, as well as the idea of the world's happiness. For this reason we expect the militant protagonists of the world state to be individuals who are in a manic swing of a manic-depressive psychosis.

Education in Democratic Lore

Such democratic tendency as exists can be strengthened by a study of the psychology of social as well as of individual maturity. The results of such study must be given in understandable language to the existing democracies and to healthy individuals everywhere, so that they may become *intelligently self-conscious*. Unless they are self-conscious they cannot know what to attack and what to defend, nor can they recognize threats to democracy when these arise. 'The price of freedom is eternal vigilance'; vigilance by whom?—by two or three of the $100 - (X + Y + Z)$ per cent mature individuals. The others are busy just being ordinary good parents, handing on the job of growing up, and of being grown-up, to their children.

Democracy at War

The question must be asked, is there such a thing as democracy at war? The answer is certainly not a plain yes. In fact, there are some reasons why, in wartime, there should be an announcement of temporary suspension of democracy because of war.

It is clear that mature healthy individuals, collectively forming a democracy, should be able to go to war: (i) to make room to grow; (ii) to defend what is valued, already possessed, etc.; and (iii) to fight anti-democratic tendencies in so far as there are people to support such tendencies by fighting.

Nevertheless, it must be but seldom that things have worked out that way. According to the description given above, a community is never composed of 100 per cent of healthy, mature individuals.

As soon as war approaches, there is a rearrangement of groups, so that by the time war is being fought it is not the healthy who are doing all the fighting. Taking our four groups:

(a) Many of the antisocials, along with mild paranoiacs, feel better because of actual war, and they welcome the real persecution threat. They find a pro-social tendency by active fighting.
(b) Of the indeterminates, many step over into what is the thing to do, perhaps using the grim reality of war to grow up as they would not otherwise have done.
(c) Of the hidden antisocials, probably some find opportunity for the urge to dominate in the various key positions which war creates.
(d) The mature, healthy individuals do not necessarily show up as well as the others. They are not so certain as the others are that the enemy is bad. They have doubts. Also they have a bigger positive stake in the world's culture, and in beauty and in friendship, and they cannot easily believe war is necessary. Compared with the near-paranoiacs they are slow in getting the gun in hand and in pulling the trigger. In fact, they miss the bus to the front line, even if when they get there they are the reliable factor and the ones best able to adapt to adversity.

Moreover, some of the healthy of peace-time become antisocial in war (conscientious objectors), not from cowardice but from a genuine personal doubt, just as the antisocials of peace-time tend to find themselves in brave action in war.

For these and other reasons, when a democratic society is fighting, it is the whole group that fights, and it would be difficult to find an instance of a war conducted by just those of a community who provide the innate democratic factor in peace.

It may be that, when a war has disturbed a democracy, it is best to say that at that moment democracy is at an end, and those who like that way of life will have to start again and fight inside the group for the re-establishment of democratic machinery, after the end of the external conflict.

This is a large subject, and it deserves the attention of large-minded people.

Summary

1. The use of the word democracy can be studied psychologically on the basis of its implication of maturity.
2. Neither democracy nor maturity can be implanted on a society.
3. Democracy is an achievement of a limited society at any one time.
4. The innate democratic factor in a community derives from the working of the ordinary good home.

5. The main activity for promotion of democratic tendency is a negative one: avoidance of interference with the ordinary good home. Study of psychology and education according to what is known provide additional help.
6. There is special significance in the devotion of the ordinary good mother to her infant, the capacity for eventual emotional maturity being founded as a result of the devotion. Mass interference at this point, in a society, would quickly and effectually lessen the democratic potential of that society, just as it would diminish the richness of its culture.

Notes

1. In this respect proportional representation is anti-democratic, even when secret, because it interferes with free expression of *feelings,* and it is only suitable for specialized conditions in which clever and educated people wish for a test of *conscious* opinions.
2. By 'innate' I intend to convey the following: the natural tendencies in human nature (hereditary) bud and flower into the democratic way of life (social maturity), but this only happens through the healthy emotional development of individuals; only a proportion of individuals in a social group will have had the luck to develop to maturity and therefore it is only through them that the innate (inherited) tendency of the group towards social maturity can be implemented.
3. The ordinary good home is something that defies statistical investigation. It has no news value, is not spectacular, and does not produce the men and women whose names are publicly known. My assumption, based on 20,000 case histories taken personally over a period of twenty-five years, is that in the community in which I work the ordinary good home is common, even usual.
4. It would be out of place to discuss this here in detail, but the idea can be reached best if approached gradually:
    (i) Fear of the parents of very early childhood.
    (ii) Fear of a combined figure, a woman with male potency included in her powers (witch).
    (iii) Fear of the mother who had absolute power at the beginning of the infant's existence to provide, or to fail to provide, the essentials for the early establishment of the self as an individual.

This is further discussed in 'The Mother's Contribution to Society' [CW 5:3:30], and in the Introduction to *The Child, the Family, and the Outside World* [CW 7:1:17].

18

'Yes, But How Do We Know It's True?'

Originally published in R. Shepherd, J. Johns, & H. Taylor Robinson (Eds.), *Thinking about children* (pp. 13–18). London: Karnac, 1996.

A talk to students of psychology and social work at the London School of Economics, 1950.

Students who are for the first time meeting instruction of a psychological nature rather regularly pass through two stages. In the first stage, they learn what is being taught about psychology just as they learn the other things. In the second stage, they begin to wonder—yes but is it true, is it real, how do we know? In the second stage, the psychological teaching begins to separate out from the other as something that can't just be learnt. It has to be felt as real, or else it is irritating and even maddening.

It is not difficult to see that there must be a difference between the effects of one kind of teaching and another. For instance, you are being instructed in administration. You read the Child Care and Protection Act, and trace the social development that led up to the Curtis Report.[i] Or you find out about the workings of Juvenile Courts, the use made of probation officers, and so on. You form your own ideas from reading and from actual visits to the Courts.

Contrast this with what happens when you learn psychology. The old academic psychology has died a natural death, and this is a loss to you because you could have learnt it just as you learned about Acts of Parliament and about the procedure of courts, without trouble but without value. Psychology is now a matter of *feelings*, of *live people*, of *emotions* and *instincts*, and also it deals with the unconscious, and conflicts in the unconscious that cause symptoms because they are not available to consciousness.

---

[i] Home Office Report of the Care of Children Committee. London: HMSO, 1946.

Do you see? Whereas most types of teaching take you out of yourself, psychology, the psychology that matters, tends to throw you back into yourself. For we are all human beings ourselves, and if we learn about another we learn about ourselves. We can try to be objective and we can make every effort to learn about people without developing morbid introspection, but this requires effort, and you notice this effort, and you feel disturbed; this psychology is not going to behave itself properly as the other subjects in the curriculum do.

Indeed, psychology is not going to help eventually in the same way as the other subjects help, and the result of what you learn will always be the recognition that the care of human beings is more complex than you thought. You can be taught how to proceed in a Juvenile Court case, but you cannot be taught how to cope with a child who is unhappy in a foster-home. In the latter case, you can only be given more and more insight into the factors involved, so that in coping with the trouble you can do what you feel like doing with more and more understanding of the reasons.

Here I have introduced a new idea, and I want to follow it up.

When you learn ordinary things you make no contribution from your own person, you just learn what is taught. The past tense of 'je suis' is 'j'étais'; the way to address a magistrate is 'yer 'onor' (or whatever it is), and that's that. When you learn psychology, however, you never learn anything cut and dried. There is no instruction that can be carried out as such. In the end it will always be you acting as you feel. The only thing is that you can be enriched by knowing of other situations similar to the one you find yourself in, and also you can be enabled to have the power to see more and more clearly what you are doing and why.

Let me give a homely illustration. A friend of yours goes into a mild depression. She rings you up and you agree to go round to her flat, but you don't know what to do. You first take a book on psychiatry and look up 'depression', and after a brief glance at the clinical description you rush on to the paragraph on treatment. You get no help. You are bewildered. 'Keep the patient from suicide' is not applicable, because your friend is not so ill as all that.

Psychology has so far not helped you much.

Let us say, however, that your friend had the good sense to have 'flu or sciatica. She is alone in her flat and you are feeling unwell yourself, and so you fly round and you do all the necessaries. You know exactly what to do. You serve an appropriate meal, you make the bed comfortable, slipping in a hot-water bottle, you go around and get the rations, and when you leave you put some water or milk within easy reach, and tell your friend exactly at what time tomorrow she may expect you.

To do this, you certainly did not have to consult a psychiatry textbook.

The fact is that you knew exactly what to do for a friend with a mild depression. It was easy because in this case the patient had a physical complaint that made it all seem sensible. (She probably had a depression too; most people are ready with a depression if only they can find someone to cherish them, and why waste the opportunity provided by the 'flu, and your response?)

Psychology does not try to teach you what to do when your friend needs your help. It can do a lot, however, towards enabling you to be more sure of yourself, to understand what is going on, to grow on experiences, to see where mistakes might have been made, to prevent distress and disasters.

Take another example. It is possible to talk to mothers about the management of their children and to give instructions based on our knowledge. In the matter of physical health and the prevention of disease, there is plenty of room for instruction, and this corresponds with what I have referred to as your gaining instruction in such things as the Children's Act.[ii] When it comes to telling mothers about mothering, however, psychological instruction can easily be harmful. Mothers either turn a deaf ear or else they get muddled, and feel hopeless, and the extreme is expressed in the cartoon of the parent smacking her child's bottom with one hand and holding in the other a book on child psychology which she is feverishly reading with the aid of strong glasses.

To talk to mothers usefully, I think it is necessary to discover and strengthen what comes naturally to them. This will be enough for many, perhaps for the majority. Some will want to go further and learn more about what they do and why they do it. Mothers who have actually done their job well can stand very deep instruction indeed, because they are not afraid to discover what tremendous forces were at work, and what a lot depended on just that being done just that way, just then. They know they did not do what they did by chance, or by cleverness, but by deeply rooted intuitive or instinctive feeling, strengthened by the self-confidence that belongs to health.

The reason why I am going into all this about mothering is that I think it is relevant.

The trouble is that you are being taught dynamic *psychology at a time when you are not in fact dealing with children*, or with people for that matter. For the time being, although you are experienced men and women, you are *in statu pupillari*, you are divorced from just those things that make you feel confident in your power to draw on intuition.

Perhaps you have been teachers, or you have actually been parents, or you have had charge of people in an office or a factory. Every day you found

---

[ii] The Children's Act, 1948. London: HMSO, 1948.

yourselves surprising yourselves, acting or not acting in a way that exactly fitted the situation, as much as Hamlet's speech 'To be or not to be' fits into the exposition of the theme of the play exactly. When you were so placed you could have stood a great deal of digging down into the psychology of your fellow human beings and of yourselves.

Here, in the temporary state of being learners, you can easily develop that lack of self-confidence that makes dynamic psychology seem dangerous. Telling an expectant mother that 'her baby can never make a satisfactory contact with the world unless she knows how to introduce external reality to her infant in small doses' may alarm her, and even make her have a miscarriage, for she becomes alarmed at her own lack of conscious knowledge. Yet, if left to it, she will do just this thing perfectly, simply because of her devotion to her baby.

Similarly, if I tell you that a baby's whole future depends on your knowing that a certain foster-mother has an unconscious revenge feeling against her own mother that renders her unfit for the job of fostering, you may recoil. How can you ever know these things? If, however, you were on the job, you would be finding yourselves suspicious here, and doubtful there, and you would be asking to have a chance to discuss the hidden aspects of the case.

And now, what about the teaching that tremendous forces are at work in the infant from the word 'go!'; that the foundations of the mental health of the adult are laid down in infancy and childhood, that the little boy of 2, 3, 4 years has instincts that make him in his dreams just like an adult, so that he is (in that sense) a sexual rival of his father; that infants who are bandied about from one minder to another do not develop a capacity to believe in the effectiveness of their own love impulses—what about all this kind of thing that you will meet during the year's course? You see, if you believe all these things, you are believing that these things were true of you, and yet you obviously can't get at these same things by remembering. Also, if these things are true things, you and I and all who have come through in a satisfactory way at all owe a debt to someone. Someone saw us through the early stages. In fact we couldn't have done without the care we received at the start. We were dependent, and as we think further and further back so we must admit we were more and more dependent, and at the time of birth and for a few months the degree of this dependence is alarming to contemplate. It must remain alarming to everyone always.

No wonder it is difficult to learn about psychology.

What is the answer? One thing is to go slow.

Another is to get relief from the fact that some of what is taught is bound to be wrong, although psychology can teach a good deal about human nature that is true as far as it goes. Also, whenever you can, travel from experiences you have had, from things you have done, towards the insight that psychology may be able to provide; the reverse direction from psychology to experience is no good at all.

Lastly, here is a half-way house. You can lodge there while you are growing. I refer to intelligence tests. These valuable tests have one foot in the academic psychology of the past, and therefore they are restful. Fortunately, they also have a foot in the dynamic psychology of the present, and therefore, if you go in for I.Q. estimations thoroughly, you will eventually find yourselves in the deep waters of feeling and unconscious conflicts. However, testing for I.Q. provides a very neutral territory and can be recommended interim.

PART 6

1951

1

Review: *The Child and the Magistrate*
BY J. A. F. WATSON (LONDON: JONATHAN CAPE, 1950)

Review originally published in *British Medical* 6 January 1951, 1(4696), 22.

Although Mr Watson is not a doctor, his book can be safely recommended to any medical man who is clinically minded. This second edition of his well-known book, largely rewritten and brought up to date, must be studied as a textbook by every magistrate of a juvenile court, but it is written in such a way that anyone who has to do with children can thoroughly enjoy it from beginning to end. Those of us who do not exclude psychological cases from our out-patient clinics will recognize on every page the children with whom we are concerned, and it is very important for us to be able to see these same children through the eye, the human and kindly eye, of this magistrate.

If the book gives one qualms at all, it is by making one realize what a great deal depends, in the management of the delinquent who has arrived at the stage of court proceedings, on the clinical sense and the human understanding of the magistrates, and there cannot be many in whom are combined (as they are in Mr Watson and his colleague Mr Basil Henriques) a love of children with a knowledge of the law and of court procedure. Sentimentality will not do. The complexities of the Education Act, 1944, the Children Act of 1948, the Criminal Justice Act of 1948, and the Justices of the Peace Act of 1949 have to be known to the magistrate as anatomy and physiology have to be known to the doctor. Moreover, magistrates need to keep in mind that it is 'the public interest which, as a court of justice, must always be their paramount consideration'.

I think that general practitioners as well as psychiatrists should know what to expect of the juvenile court, and there can be no better way of getting this knowledge than through the enjoyment of this book. Incidentally, there are plenty of amusing tit-bits to help the reader along.

There is one thing which will come as new to many readers. There is a gap in management left by the serious attempt which is being made to eliminate corporal punishment. This gap is to be filled by attendance centres, provision for which is laid down in the Criminal Justice Act of 1948. However, only one exists as yet. Mr Watson has great hopes from this new provision, but one feels that their success will depend not only on the way they are run but on their being used by the magistrates for the right kind of case—that is to say, for the child who is able to make use of a limited corrective.

Letter to W. R. Bion

Wilfred R. Bion (1897–1979) was a British psychoanalyst, President of the British Psychoanalytical Society (1962–65), and a follower and developer of the ideas of Melanie Klein.

22 January 1951

Dear Bion,

I read your paper immediately you gave it to me, but I had to keep it till now before I could read it again.[i] I've just re-read it backwards.

I think I understand what you are saying but I do find it very difficult. This is due to me mostly. Whatever else I have got from the paper I get from it an insight into your doing analysis, and I feel very confident about the future of your analytic work. There is something essentially individual about whatever you do and write, and eventually your contribution to the Society will be a big one. It is for us to gradually find out how to understand what you say.

Every good wish,
Yours,
D. W. Winnicott

---

[i] Bion had read 'The Imaginary Twin', his first paper to the British Psychoanalytical Society, the previous November.

3

Letter to James Strachey

Originally published in Rodman, F. R. (Ed.), *The spontaneous gesture. Selected letters of D. W. Winnicott* (Letter 18, p. 24). Cambridge, MA: Harvard University Press, 1987.

James Strachey (1887–1967) was Winnicott's training analyst and the translator and general editor of *The Standard Edition of the Complete Psychological Works of Sigmund Freud*.

1 May 1951

Dear Strachey,

You may have seen from the notices sent round that I am due to give a paper on 30th May on what I am calling 'Transition Objects'. Actually I am trying to get some of this written out clearly before Whitsun so that it can be circulated. The full paper would be rather a long one.

    I am writing to you because I am wondering whether you would agree to read through what I have roughly made of this paper already and let me come and discuss it with you. I am particularly keen to pick up the ordinary psychoanalytic theory in the theoretical section of the paper enough to make what I think is my own contribution acceptable.

    You will be relieved to hear that I have done quite a bit of psychoanalytic reading, thanks to having been ill twice; however, it is still true to say that if I were to take a year off and do nothing but read, I would be in a better position for writing papers.

I will be ringing you up about this, but to make a rough suggestion, I would very much like to be able to see you, perhaps Tuesday 8th May any time between 7 P.M. and midnight; if you prefer a morning time, I could probably manage the morning of 8th between 11 and 2. I know that you will tell me if you would rather not burden yourself with this.

Yours very sincerely,
D. W. Winnicott

4

The Foundation of Mental Health

Originally published as an editorial leader article in *British Medical Journal*, 16 June 1951, *1*(4719), 1373–1374. Also published in C. Winnicott, R. Shepherd, & M. Davis (Eds.), *Deprivation and delinquency* (pp. 168–171). London: Tavistock, 1984.

Mental hygiene, although an extension of ordinary public-health work, goes further in that it alters the kind of people that compose the world. It is significant that the report[1] of the second session of W.H.O.'s Expert Committee on Mental Health concerns itself mainly with the management of infancy and childhood, thus taking for granted something which might not have been accepted by doctors 50 years ago—namely, that the basis of adult mental health is laid down in infancy and childhood, and of course in adolescence. The introduction to the report begins with the statement: 'The most important single long-term principle for the future work of W.H.O. in the fostering of mental health, as opposed to the treatment of psychiatric disorders, is the encouragement of the incorporation into public-health work of the responsibility for promoting the mental as well as physical health of the community'. The report then discusses the maternity services, the management of the infant and the pre-school child, the dependence of the pre-school child on the mother, school health in its wider aspects, and the emotional problems arising from physical handicap and from the isolation of children suffering from infectious diseases such as leprosy and tuberculosis. The committee recognizes that the mental health worker in training has more to do than to learn. The student is faced with 'an emotional problem because of the nature of the subject matter quite apart from any intellectual difficulty in understanding the facts. Its initial emotional impact is far greater than that of the dissecting room or the operating theatre'.

Along with the publication of this report there comes a W.H.O. monograph on 'Maternal Care and Mental Health', written by Dr John Bowlby, consultant in mental health to W.H.O., as a contribution to the United

Nations programme for the welfare of homeless children.[2] Dr Bowlby, in his work at the Tavistock Clinic, has already shown that he appreciates the need for presenting psychological concepts in a form which appeals to the scientific worker trained to make the statistical approach, and it can be said at once that he has been successful in writing a remarkably interesting and valuable report. Compared with the amount of individual psychotherapy that is being done all over the world the investigations giving clear-cut results are few and far between: perhaps there are aspects of psychology which cannot yield results for the statistician. The success of this monograph is due in part to the choice of subject—the effect of the separation from their homes, and specifically from their own mothers, on the emotional development of infants and children, who, as Dr Bowlby writes, 'are not slates from which the past can be rubbed by a duster or a sponge, but human beings who carry their previous experiences with them and whose behaviour in the present is profoundly affected by what has gone before'. Quoting convincing figures, he is able to show how separation can augment the tendency to the development of a psychopathic personality. Bowlby found that almost all workers in this field had arrived at the same conclusion: 'What is believed to be essential for mental health is that the infant and the young child should experience a warm, intimate, and continuous relationship with the mother (or permanent mother-substitute) in which both find satisfaction and enjoyment'. This is not new: it is what mothers and fathers feel, and it is what those who work with children have found. But what is new in this report is the attempt to translate the idea into figures.

There are three main sources of information: studies by direct observation of infants and small children; studies based on the investigation of early histories of those who are ill; and follow-up studies of groups of deprived children in various categories. Perhaps the main result of these inquiries, especially when they have been confirmed and amplified, will be to serve as a lesson for the medical profession, including the administrators. It must always be difficult for those who are making physical health their speciality to keep the greater importance of mental health in mind. Emotional development can so easily be disturbed: the child in hospital who has forgotten its mother and who has reached the stage of making friends with anyone who comes along may be delightful to have in the ward, but it is a fact that a child, and especially a small child, cannot forget a parent without damage to the personality. Happily in children's wards and children's hospitals there is now a tendency to allow daily visiting. Admittedly this presents great difficulties to the nurses, but even the small amount of carefully controlled work which Bowlby is able to report on this limited aspect of the subject shows how worthwhile the extra trouble is.

Naturally the effect on the child of separation from its mother will depend on the degree of deprivation and also on the age of the child. The care of infants brought up in an institution from their earliest days was obviously due for reform, and in this country public opinion was firmly behind the Curtis Committee and the Children Act which followed in 1948. It is now becoming generally accepted that no child should be removed from the mother's care if this can be avoided—and this simple statement must not be obscured by the subsidiary fact that a minority of parents are themselves ill (in a psychiatric sense) and therefore bad for their children.

It would be a large task to teach the parents of the world how to be good parents, especially as most of them already know much better than we can ever tell them. It is appropriate therefore that W.H.O. should start at the other end in its consideration of mental hygiene, at the end at which teaching can have effect. The two important conclusions are that the impersonal upbringing of children tends to produce unsatisfactory personalities and even active antisocial characters and, secondly, that when there is anything like a good relationship between the developing infant or child and the parent the continuity of this relationship must be respected and must never be broken without good cause. Bowlby likens the acceptance of these facts to the acceptance of certain facts on the physical side of paediatrics, such as the importance of vitamins in the prevention of scurvy and rickets. Acceptance of the principle to which Bowlby's statistics point could lead to a reduction of antisocial tendencies and the suffering that lies behind them, exactly as vitamin D has lessened the incidence of rickets. Such a result would be a great achievement of preventive medicine, even without taking into account the deeper aspects of emotional development, such as richness of personality, strength of character, and the capacity for full, free, and mature self-expression.

Notes

1. *World Health Organisation Technical Report Series*, No. 31, 1951, Geneva.
2. *Maternal Care and Mental Health*, Geneva, 1951.

5

Visiting Children in Hospital

Originally published in *Child-Family Digest*, October 1952; and *New Era in Home and School*, 1952, 33. Also published in *The child and the family: First relationships* (pp. 121–126). London: Tavistock, 1957; and *The child, the family, and the outside world* (pp. 221–226). Harmondsworth, UK: Penguin, 1964. Broadcast in two parts, 16 and 23 May 1951. Benzie, I. (Producer) *Woman's Hour*. Light Programme. London: British Broadcasting Corporation (see the broadcast list [CW 12:3:2]).

[Added 1964:] *In the past decade great changes have come about in hospital practice. In many hospitals parents visit freely and they are where necessary admitted with their children. The results are generally recognized as good for the children, good for the parents, and even helpful to the hospital staff in a big proportion of cases. Nevertheless I have kept this chapter as it was written in 1951 because of the fact that the changes have not by any means reached all the hospitals, and also because there are inherent difficulties in the modern method, and these difficulties should be recognized.*

Every child has a line of life that starts at any rate from birth, and it is our job to see that it does not get broken. There is a continuous process of development within, which can make steady progress only if the care of the infant or small child is steady too. As soon as the infant as a person has begun to make relationships with people, these relationships are very intense and cannot be tampered with without danger. There is no need for me to labour this point since mothers naturally hate to let their children go away until the children are ready for the experience, and of course they are eager to go and see them if they have to be away from home.

At the present time there is a wave of enthusiasm for ward visiting. The trouble with waves of enthusiasm is that they may override real difficulties and sooner or later there comes a reaction. The only sensible thing is to get people to understand the reasons for and against visiting. And there are some really big difficulties from the nursing point of view.

Why, in fact, does a nursing sister do this work? Perhaps at first nursing was just one of many ways of earning a living; but eventually as a nurse she got caught up in the work and became keen on it, and took tremendous trouble to learn all the very complicated techniques; eventually she became a sister. As a sister she works long hours, and this will always be the case because there will never be enough good nursing sisters, and the work is difficult to share out. The nursing sister has absolute responsibility for twenty to thirty children who are not her own. Many of these children are very ill and require skilled handling. And she is responsible for all that is done for them, even for what the junior nurses do when she is not looking. She becomes terribly keen to get the children well, and this may mean following very definite lines laid down by the doctor. In addition to all this she has to be ready to deal with doctors and medical students, and these are human beings too.

When there is no visiting, the Sister takes the child into her care and the very best that is in her is roused. She would much rather be on duty than off duty very often, because she is always wondering what is happening in her ward. Some of the children get very dependent on her and cannot bear her to go off duty without saying good-bye. And they want to know exactly when she is coming back. The whole thing appeals to the best in human nature.

Now what happens when we have visiting? Immediately there is a difference, or at any rate there can be. From now on the responsibility for the child is never wholly with the Sister. This can work wonderfully well, and the Sister may be glad to share responsibility; but if she is very busy, and especially if there are some rather trying cases in the ward, and some rather trying mothers visiting it, it is much simpler to do the whole thing oneself than to share.

You would be surprised if I were to start to tell you things that happen during visiting. After the parents have gone the children are quite often sick, and what they bring up tells tales. Perhaps it does not matter much, this little episode of sickness after visiting, but it may reveal that children have been given ice cream or carrots, and that the child on a diet has had sweets, this completely upsetting the whole investigation on which his future treatment is to be based.

The fact is that in the visiting-hour the Sister has to let go of the control of the situation, and I think she sometimes really has no idea what goes on during that time. And there is no way round this. And, quite apart from food indiscretions, there is the menace of infection.

Another difficulty, as a very good Sister of a ward in a hospital has told me, is that since they have been allowed to visit daily, mothers think that their children are always crying in hospital, which of course is just not true. It is true that if you visit your child, your visits will often cause distress. You keep up the child's memory of you every time you go to the ward. You revive the wish to be home, so it must be that often you will leave the child crying. But this kind of distress, we think, is not nearly as harmful to the child as the distress that has gone over into indifference. If you have to leave the child so long that you are forgotten, the child will recover after a day or two and stop being distressed, and will adopt the nurses and the other children, and will develop a new life. In this case you have been forgotten and you will have to be remembered again afterwards.

It would not be so bad if the mothers were contented to go in and see their children for a few minutes and then go out again; but mothers do not feel like this, naturally. As will be expected, they go into the ward and use the whole time that is allowed. Some seem to be almost 'making love' to their child; they bring presents of all kinds, and especially food, and they demand affectionate response; and then they take quite a long time going, standing waving at the door till the child is absolutely exhausted by the effort of saying good-bye. And the mothers are quite liable to go to the Sister on the way out, and say something about the child's not being warmly enough clad or not having enough to eat for dinner or something like that. Only a few mothers take the moment of leaving as the right opportunity to thank the Sister for what she is doing, which is really quite a big thing. It is very difficult to admit that someone is looking after your own child as well as you could yourself.

So you see that if the Sister were asked, just after the patents have gone: 'Sister, what would you do about visiting if you were a dictator?' she might very likely say, 'I would abolish it'. But still she may agree, at a more favourable moment, that visiting is a natural and a good thing. The doctors and nurses can see it is worth while to allow it if they can stand it, and if the parents can be asked to cooperate.

I was saying that we find that anything that breaks up the child's life into fragments is harmful. Mothers know this, and they welcome daily visiting which makes it possible for them to keep in touch with their children during those unfortunate times when there is a need for hospital care.

It seems to me that when children *feel* ill the whole problem is much easier; everyone understands what to do. Words seem so useless when one is talking to a small child, and they are unnecessary when a child feels very ill. The child just feels that something will be arranged that will help, and if this involves a stay in hospital this is accepted, even if tearfully. But when a child has to be put into hospital at a time when there is no feeling of being unwell, it is altogether different. I remember a child who was playing in the street when suddenly the ambulance came up, and she was whisked away to a fever hospital, although she was feeling well, because the day before it had been discovered at the hospital (through a throat examination) that she was a diphtheria carrier. You can imagine how awful this was for the child, who could not even be allowed to go in and say good-bye to her family. When we cannot explain ourselves we must expect a certain amount of loss of faith; actually, the particular child I am thinking about never really recovered from the experience. Perhaps, if visiting had been allowed, the outcome would have been more happy. If for nothing else it seems to me that the parents should be able to visit such a child so as to be able to take his anger while it is at white heat.

I have spoken of a need for hospital care as being *unfortunate,* but it can work out the other way. When your child is old enough, a hospital experience, or a stay away from home with an aunt, may be very valuable, enabling the home to be looked at from outside. I remember a boy of twelve who said, after he had been away at a convalescent home for a month, 'You know, I don't think I really am my mother's darling. She always gives me everything I want, but she doesn't really love me, somehow'. He was quite right too; his mother was trying hard, but she had big difficulties of her own which got in the way in her dealings with her children, and it was quite healthy for this particular boy to be able to see his mother from a distance. He went back ready to tackle the home situation in a new way.

Because of their own difficulties some parents are not ideal. How does this affect hospital visiting? Well, if when parents visit they bicker in front of the child it is naturally a very painful thing at the time, and the child worries about it afterwards. Such a thing can seriously affect the child's return to bodily health. And some people just cannot keep promises; they say they will come, or they will bring some special toy or book, but they do not. And then, again, there is the problem of parents who, although they give presents and make clothes and do all sorts of things which of course are very important, just cannot give a hug at the right moment. Such parents may find it easier to love their child in the difficult conditions of a hospital ward. They come early and stay as long as possible, and bring more and more presents. After they have gone the child can hardly breathe. A girl once implored me (it was round about Christmas time), 'Take all those presents off the cot!' She was so weighed down by the burden of the expression of love which had taken this indirect form and had nothing to do with her mood.

It seems to me that the children of overbearing, unreliable, and highly excitable parents can get a great deal of relief for a while from being in hospital *unvisited*. The Sister of the ward has some children like this in her care, and we can see her point of view when she feels at times that *all* children are better unvisited. Also she is looking after the children whose parents live too far away to visit, and, most difficult of all, children who have no parents at all. Naturally, the visiting-hour does not help the Sister in the management of *these* children, who make special demands on her and the nurses because of their poor belief in human beings. For children with no good home a stay in hospital may provide the first good experience. Some of them do not even believe in human beings enough to be sad; they must make friends with anyone who turns up, and when they are alone they rock backwards and forwards, or bang their heads on the pillow, or on the sides of the cot. You have no reason to let your child suffer on account of there being these deprived children in the ward, but at the same time you should know that the Sister's management of these less fortunate children can be made more difficult by the fact that other children are being visited by their own parents.

When all goes well, it may very likely be that the main effect of a stay in hospital is that afterwards the children have a new game; there was 'Fathers and Mothers', and then of course 'Schools', and now it is 'Doctors and Nurses'. Sometimes the victim is the baby, and sometimes it is a doll, a dog, or a cat.

The main thing I want to say is that the introduction of frequent visiting of children in hospital is an important step forward, and is in fact a reform long overdue. I welcome the new tendency as something which lessens distress and which, in the case of children of the toddler age, can easily make all the difference between good and thoroughly bad when a child must spend a certain length of time in hospital. I have drawn attention to the difficulties, which can be very real, because of the fact that I think that hospital visiting is so important.

Nowadays when we go into a children's ward we see a little child standing up in a cot, eager to find someone to talk to, and we may easily be greeted with these words, 'My mummy comes to see me!' This proud boast is a new phenomenon. And I can tell you about a little boy of three who was crying and the nurses were trying hard to find out how to make him happy. Cuddling was no good; he did not want it. At last they found that a certain chair had to be placed beside his cot. This calmed him down but it was some time before he could explain, 'That's for daddy to sit on when he comes to see me tomorrow'.

So you see, there must be something in this visiting business more than just preventing damage; but it is a good idea for parents to try to understand the difficulties so that the doctors and nurses will be able to keep up something which they know is good, but which they also know can spoil the quality of the very responsible work which they are doing for you.

6

Transitional Objects and Transitional Phenomena

Notes for the first presentation of this paper, as distributed to members of the British Psychoanalytical Society prior to the meeting in which it was given, 30 May 1951.

The paper was revised for its first publication [CW 4:2:21] in the *International Journal of Psychoanalysis*, 1953, 34, 89–97, and became available to a wider readership after its republication, with minor alterations, [CW 5:4:24] in *Collected papers: Through paediatrics to psycho-analysis* (1958). This second publication in 1958 included formatting alterations such as the adding of capitals to the term Not-Me, italicizing certain key ideas, for instance 'The intermediate area to which I am referring is the area allowed to the infant between primary creativity and objective perception based on reality-testing', and some further changes to paragraph headings, references and footnotes.

Winnicott prepared a third version [CW 9:3:5] as the first chapter of his book *Playing and reality* (1971), His archives show that he planned a further book of papers on transitional objects and transitional phenomena [CW 12:1:5].

In order to provide the opportunity for scholarly comparison, these notes, circulated for its original presentation, and all three published versions; have been included in the *Collected Works*. For more on this paper, see also the General Introduction to the Collected Works (in Volume 1) and the Introductions to Volume 5 and Volume 9.

Part I. Statement of main ideas.
Part II. Clinical descriptions.
Part III. Theoretical study.
Part IV. Quotation of relevant passages in psychoanalytic and other literature.

Part I. Statement of Main Idea

I wish to draw the attention of the Society to a well known clinical phenomenon, to ask whether this phenomenon deserves a name, and if so to ask whether the name I have given it is suitable. I also wish to invite discussion as to the significance of the phenomenon in the theory and the practice of psychoanalysis.

Clinical Description. What I am studying is the first 'not-me' possession of the infant, and the wide variations in the infant's relationship to this possession. I find that in the infant's behaviour there can be seen a sequence of objects and of relationship-patterns (and of diffuse phenomena), and that health and ill-health can be detected by the study of this particular sequence in the same way as it can be detected by study of any other sequence in infant development.

Definition. I am using these terms, transitional object and transitional phenomena, to describe certain features of child behaviour which seem to belong to a transition which the infant is making in several different ways from one kind of experience to another: from auto-erotism to allo-erotism, from the use of part of the self to the use of external objects, from the pleasure principle to the reality principle, from an excited type of relationship to an affectionate one, from imagination in its primary creative form to reality acceptance, from subjectivity to objective perception. A transitional object is an hallucination taken for granted because of the immaturity of the infant.

Attempt to State a Normal Sequence. After birth infants employ all sorts of mouth techniques. I must pass over these.

Ordinarily the baby uses a fist and shoves it almost down the throat. First the fist, then a thumb or perhaps two or three fingers. Almost immediately the infant's own personal pattern is showing pretty strongly. No one who respects infants would want to try to alter this pattern which is simply part of the infant's profile, and it is noticed and loved by the parents along with the other characteristics of the offspring.

The fist and the thumb are part of the infant from our point of view, and in health it must be very early that an infant, at certain moments, feels virtue flow from the ego reservoir into the fist, thumb, fingers, etc., as well as into the mouth, lips, gums, salivary glands, throat. In other words, from the infant's point of view as well as from ours the fist and the digits are part of the self.

It is possible to see that the phenomena we are studying occur at certain times:

(1) when loneliness begins to be felt
(2) when hunger threatens
(3) when between waking and sleeping

There is one thing common to these three states, namely *anxiety*, and it must be presumed that in the early stages anxiety constantly threatens, and that there is natural provision for defence against anxiety.

There is plenty of reference in psychoanalytic literature to the progress from 'hand to mouth' to 'hand to genital'. There appears to be less written about progress to the handling of truly external objects. However, there comes sooner or later a tendency on the part of the infant to weave other-than-me objects into the personal pattern.

In the case of some infants the thumb is placed in the mouth while fingers are made to caress the face by pronation and supination movements of the forearm. The mouth is then active in relation to the thumb, but not in relation to the fingers. The fingers caressing the upper lip or some other part may become more important than the thumb engaging the mouth.

In common experience one of the following occurs, complicating an auto-erotic experience such as thumb-sucking:

(1) with the other hand the baby takes a part of a sheet, or blanket, into the mouth along with the fingers:
(2) somehow or other the bit of cloth is held but not actually sucked. The objects used naturally include napkins and (later) handkerchiefs.
(3) the baby starts from early months to pluck wool and to collect it and to use it for the caressing part of the activity. Less commonly, the wool is swallowed, even causing trouble.
(4) mouthing, accompanied by sounds of mum mum, babbling, anal noises, and the first musical notes and so on.

Out of all this if we study any one infant there may emerge something or some phenomenon—perhaps a bundle of wool or the corner of a blanket or eiderdown, or a word or tune or a mannerism, which becomes vitally important to the infant for use in defence against anxiety, especially of depressive type. Perhaps some soft object has been offered and accepted by the infant, and this then becomes what I am calling a Transitional Object. This object goes on being important. The parents get to know its value and carry it round when travelling. Indeed by washing it the mother may destroy its value (but it would not be wise to assume that the smelliness of the object indicates no more than its value as faeces-substitute).

I suggest that the transition is usually ready to be made at about (4) – 6 – 8 – 12 months. Purposely I leave room for wide variations. What is the nature of the transition I shall discuss later.

Patterns set in infancy may persist into later life so that the original soft object continues to be absolutely necessary at bed-time or at time of loneliness or when a depressed mood threatens. Quite normally patterns that started at a very early date may reappear at a later age under such condition. In health there is, however, a gradual extension of range of interest, even when anxiety threatens.

This first object is used in conjunction with special techniques derived from very early infancy and which can include the more direct auto-erotic activities. Gradually teddies and dolls and hard toys are acquired. Boys tend to go over to use hard objects, whereas girls tend to proceed right ahead to the acquisition of a family. It is important to note, however, that there is no noticeable difference between boy and girl infants in their use of the original not-me object, which I am calling the transitional object.

The name given by the infant to these earliest objects is often significant.

I should mention that sometimes there is no transitional object except the mother herself. At the other end of the scale, an infant may be so disturbed in emotional development that the transitions cannot be made in an orderly way.

SUMMARY OF SPECIAL QUALITIES IN THE RELATIONSHIP

(1) The infant assumes rights over the object and we agree to this assumption.
(2) It is affectionately cuddled as well as excitedly loved and mutilated.
(3) It must never change, unless changed by the infant (one eye pulled off, etc.)
(4) Yet it must seem to give warmth, or to move, or to have texture, or to do something to show it has vitality of its own.
(5) It comes from without from our point of view, but not necessarily so from the point of view of the baby.
(6) Its fate is to be gradually allowed to be decathected, so that in the end it becomes not so much forgotten as relegated to limbo. By this I mean that in health the transition object does not 'go inside' nor does the feeling about it necessarily undergo repression. It is not forgotten and it is not mourned. It just loses meaning, but this is simply because the transition phenomena have become diffused, spread out over the whole intermediate territory between 'inner psychic reality' and 'the external world as perceived by two persons in common'.

The subject widens out into that of play and of artistic creativity, and appreciation, and of religious feeling, and of dreaming, and also of fetishism, lying and stealing, loss of affectionate feeling, drug addiction, the talisman of obsessional rituals.

Abnormalities. The main abnormality, I suggest, arises out of *discontinuity of experience* relative to transitional objects and phenomena. As a result there is either no transitional object or else an exaggeration of the dependence on the original transitional object with limitation of spread of interests. I attempt to explain this in Part III, but at this point I wish to refer to one clinical type, the anti-social child, typically a thief.

Psychology of Stealing. The thief is trying, (amongst other things) to fill the gap in experience of transitional objects. While he has hope he steals. He seeks the affectionate relationship which belongs to transitional phenomena. In the lying that goes with stealing is hidden the claim that a story can he both fantasy and fact.

The aetiology of thieving cannot, in fact, be fully worked out except on a basis of the thief's attempt to recover lost transitional phenomena. It must be remembered that the delinquent is not depressed or mad *when delinquent*, though depression or madness may in some cases be the *alternatives* to anti-social behaviour.

Part II. Clinical

There is an infinite variety of clinical material and only enough is given to remind members of the Society of similar material in their own experiences with children or with histories taken from parents.

BAAs and EEs. Mrs X, who has had four children (now healthy adults) has given me an alternative title for my paper, one which arises out of her own experiences, and which has the advantage of not committing me in advance to a new term. She calls it 'my paper on BAAs and EEs'. I give her story.

Her first boy, A, has had to fight his way towards maturity. The fact is that the mother learned how to be a mother in her management of A when he was an infant and she was able to avoid certain mistakes with the other children because of this. There were also external reasons why she was anxious at the time of her rather lonely management of A when he was born. She took her job very seriously and she breast-fed him for 7 months. She is sure that in his case this was too long and he was very difficult to wean. He never sucked his thumb or his fingers and when she weaned him 'he had nothing to fall back on'. He had never had the bottle or a dummy or any other form of feeding. He had a very strong and early attachment to her herself as a person and it was her actual person that he needed.

From 12 months he adopted a rabbit which he would cuddle and his affectionate regard for the rabbit eventually transferred to real rabbits. This particular rabbit lasted till he was 5 or 6 years old. It could be described as a *comforter* (but it never had the true quality of a transitional object). In the case of this particular boy the sort of anxieties which were brought to a head by the weaning at 7 months produced asthma and only gradually did he conquer this. It was important for him that he found employment in the colonies. His attachment to his mother is still very powerful although he and all these four children come within the wide definition of the term normal, or healthy.

The second boy, B, has developed in quite a straightforward way right through. He now has three healthy children of his own. This boy was fed at the breast for 4 months and then weaned without difficulty. (The mother had learned from her first child that it was a good idea to give one bottle feed while breast feeding and by this means she produced easier weaning in the case of the 2nd, 3rd and 4th children.) He sucked his thumb in the early weeks and this made weaning easier for him than for his older brother. Soon after weaning at 5–6 months he adopted the end of the blanket where the stitching finished. He was pleased if a little bit of the wool stuck out at the corner and with this he would tickle his nose. This very early became his 'BAA'; he invented this word for it himself as soon as he could use organised sounds. From about the time when he was about a year old he was able to substitute for the end of the blanket a soft green jersey with a red tie. This was not a 'comforter' as in the case of the depressive older brother but a 'soother'. It was a sedative which *always worked*. When he was a little boy it was always certain that if anyone gave him his BAA he would immediately suck it and lose anxiety, and in fact go to sleep within a few minutes if it were at all the time for sleep. The thumb-sucking continued at the same time until he was 3 or 4 years old and he remembers thumb-sucking and a hard place which resulted from it. He is now interested (as a father) in the thumb-sucking of his children and their use of BAAs.

The next two children were twins. They were extremely different from one another. The girl, C, was born first and she was a placid fat ball. On the other hand, the boy, D, was long and skinny and sensitive from the moment of birth. These characteristics persisted. C, the girl, was not a thumb- or finger-sucker. The mother decided that in order to be fair to twins one would have to use a dummy and she quickly discovered that the girl could use a dummy and that the boy could not. C therefore had a dummy which enabled her to wait for her feeds. She was weaned at 3 months easily. The dummy was used by C till 12 months and would always keep her quiet for 5 minutes, which was vitally important because of the extreme sensitivity of the twin brother, whose feeding or sleep would be disturbed by the twin's crying. At 12 months she adopted a woolly donkey which was given her, without giving it a name.

D never sucked his fingers or thumb. As I have said, he refused a dummy and so the mother did not persist in offering it to him. He adopted a corner of the eiderdown from 6 months and this was vitally important to him until he was two. He very early named it 'EE'. Even after two he liked to have it. It was *protective* for him, something that he needed because of being always on the verge of anxiety (paranoid type). Of the four children he was the one who was more difficult to manage in later childhood, and he could have developed along psychopath lines with careless management. Nevertheless he came through well. He was the one who had the most intimate relationship with the father but it could be said that this relationship had its dangers and was solved by his finding a life in the colonies; whereas his older brother solved his relation to his *mother* that way, this boy solved his relation to his *father* by going abroad. Eventually he was killed after gaining distinction in fighting in the Far East.

This family naturally watches with interest what there is of 'BAAs' and 'EEs' in the grandchildren, children of B. The eldest girl, E, early adopted a 'BAA' which she only used at night-time. It was a blanket or a piece of soft cotton material. Naturally in this case the name was implanted and at first only used by the parents. The father was expecting his child to have a BAA as he had had. The next child, a girl, F, sucked her thumb and this continues at the age of 4 at nighttime or if she is bored. She had no BAA. The third child, a boy, G, uses three fingers when bored and no BAA. In this generation there is a great difference in management in that the mother has always used other techniques along with breast-feeding. She has given orange juice by spoon and by cup. The anxieties associated with weaning are thereby much reduced. The three children are developing normally.

I also have notes about a cousin of these children, E. He was an afterthought. It was at first wondered how he would manage in a family where the other children were so much older. He has done well, however. He sucked his thumb from early times and also had what he called a Mimi. Soon he had a selection of Mimis and he had his own reasons for choosing a long or short or flat one, etc. This became quite a cult and lasted till he was 3. Without his Mimi he was unhappy. He is now 11.

The story of those four healthy children brings out the following points, arranged for comparison:

	Thumb	Transitional Object	Development	Type
A.	o	Mother	Rabbit (comforter)	Mother-fixated
B.	+	BAA	Jersey (soother)	Free
C.	–	Dummy	Donkey	Late maturity
D.	o	EE	(protective)	Latent psychopath
E.	+	Mimi	Cult (company)	Developing well

In consultation with a parent it is often valuable to get information about these phenomena in respect of all the children of the family. This starts the mother off on a comparison of her children one with another and brings to light early roots of personality characteristics.

Jennifer and Judith. Judith, aet 11½, normal sister, sucked her thumb satisfactorily and was a contented child. She quite early adopted the habit of having a piece of satin, the important thing about which was its smoothness. This she placed on her face whilst sucking her thumb.

Jennifer, aet 10, was never normal. Four days before her birth the house was badly bombed; as a result the mother was in a very bad state from which she has not yet properly recovered; this affected the breast feeding, so that Jennifer was never contented and breast feeding was abandoned at 2 months. It was not till 6 months that a feed was found which suited her. There was also the complication of much hospitalisation due to (possibly) infective gastro enteritis. This child that was never contented was nevertheless very lively, very friendly, and more popular than the normal sister, and thought to be markedly happy. *She did not suck her thumb: the mother often wished she would. She would adopt teddies and gollywogs but they were never important to her. She just liked them.* (i.e. no organised transitional phenomena). Very early she started nightmares which continued until she was 8. During her infancy there were frequent air raids. When she could say what the nightmares were about she explained that the wall was coming in on her slowly and the ceiling coming down, etc., etc.

It may happen that one has to see a child without the mother. It is surprising what information can sometimes be obtained from a child in regard to transition objects; for instance, *Angus* (11 yrs. 9 mths): he told me that his brother has 'tons of teddies and things' and before that he had little bears. This made it possible for Angus to talk about his own history in this respect. He never had teddies. There was a bell rope which hung down and of which he would go on hitting a tag end and so go off to sleep. Probably in the end it fell and that was the end of it. There was, however, something earlier. He was very shy about this. It was a purple rabbit with red eyes. 'I wasn't fond of it. I used to throw it around'. 'Jeremy has it now. I gave it to him. I gave it to Jeremy because it was naughty. It would fall off the chest of drawers. It still visits me. I like it to visit me'. He surprised himself when he drew the purple rabbit.

> *Paul*: A detail in a carefully taken history may be very informative, for instance, Paul. The first thing he cuddled was a gauze cot sheet. This was important to him till he was 5. At that time the mother reasoned with him and got him to give it up, whereupon he substituted nail-biting. He had many teddies and then Dinky Cars which he still uses (aet 12 years).

> *Barbara*: (now 3½ years) The mother's description of Barbara's early development indicates abnormality. Here again the mother could very easily see the contrast between the boy and the girl in terms of the study of those early phenomena.

In regard to early object relations, the *brother* put everything to his mouth and quickly adopted a teddy and other objects for going to bed with. *This child*, however, 'never had any hand to mouth instinct'. She had no cuddly object. Recently she has started sucking her clothes. If put to bed with dolls she threw them all out before going to sleep. She gets under her blanket and pulls it over her head. It is not really possible to say what she would adopt if mopey because she does not get into that kind of mood. The brother, being normal, gets tired and mopey and needs consolation. From 12–18 months she had one toy she liked. This was a rag-bag and she repeatedly sorted out the objects in it according to texture, accurately.

It would be impracticable to give more case material in this shortened version of the paper.

Part III. Theoretical

Auto-erotism and allo-erotism. In the early stages of the development of psychoanalytic theory there is postulated a stage of auto-erotism; this gradually develops into a capacity for allo-erotic experience. The child at the beginning is concerned with *zones* at which experiences lead to lessening of instinct tension. At the beginning the child is therefore thought to be concerned with the pleasure-pain principle, with gratification of instincts and of course with reactions to frustration increasing instinct tension and interfering with orgasm or with gratification of a more diffuse kind. These things dominate the infant's waking life. At first the picture of the infant depicted by this method was as follows; either the infant is asleep or else awake. If awake, the infant is excited and very quickly in pain unless gratified. Crying, which in itself does no good, produces the mother. The mother provides the feed and the infant sinks back happily to renewed sleep. This is an allo-erotic experience. Gradually the infant is awake for longer periods and has to stand instinct tension which cannot be immediately gratified, and by the sucking of the fist the need for the mother's activities is lessened and the infant is beginning to know how to wait. In the course of time the thumb and the fingers are substituted. The infant's use of the fist and thumb and fingers constitutes an auto-erotic experience. Then the infant finds other parts of the body. Notably the boy child finds the male genital and discovers a new zone for auto-erotic experience. What the girl child discovers is not made clear in this part of the theory. There are other explorations going on at the same time such as the discovery of the tongue which can be sucked.

In this part of the theory the idea of object relationship is not stressed.

It must be remembered that in psychoanalytic theory it is implied all the time that the body functions are enriched by an imaginative elaboration, and only a few analysts care to put a date to the beginning of such enrichment of body function.

Transitional objects can be used in the service of erotic experience at almost any zone.

The pleasure-pain principle. The theory is then extended to cover developments in respect of object-relationships. At first the breast is not felt by the infant as an other-than-me object. Gradually the infant comes to recognise the not-me nature of the breast. (Obviously the essential condition in all this is that the mother is able to act well.) The concept of *omnipotence* is introduced here. The baby has magical control over the object and the concept of the pleasure-pain principle is an attempt at giving the statement of the situation as perceived at the time by analysts. The idea of the reality principle is introduced to describe the infant's gradual acceptance of the not-me quality of objects, and next that there is no magical control over objects. Fist-sucking and thumb-sucking etc. come in as methods by which the infant has *a measure of control* (assuming the arms are allowed to be free), so that magical control is converted into muscular and sensory control. By gaining gratification without dependence on other people the baby is able to command the instinct situation to some extent.

The transitional object here is something rather like the thumb or finger in that it helps in the transition from omnipotence to reality-acceptance. Nevertheless it can be out of reach and therefore a distressing reminder of the infant's dependence on others.

At this point a number of valuable concepts become relevant, notably those of *displacement*, of *symbol formation* and of *part objects*. The transitional object can stand for the mother's breast or the mother or for the child's genital or faeces or anything else. There can be a displacement on to the cuddling of a transitional object from oral and anal erotism. Moreover the transitional object can stand for a part or a whole person.

There is nothing so far in the statement of the child's emotional development about the infant's creativity. This received attention from Freud under the term 'primary identification'. By everything the infant does and feels the infant is creating. I shall deal with this idea later.

Introjection and projection. The concept of introjection and projection was added to make possible a statement of what was understood of the gradual enrichment of the individual from external reality and along with it the gradual enrichment of external reality for the infant.

There will be many who will feel that there is no need to go further than this in an attempt to include in psycho-analytic theory that which I am describing as the transitional object. These objects are used in the imaginative elaboration of auto- and allo-erotic functioning, and are part of the machinery for the lessening of instinct tension and for a lessening of the amount of frustration which compels reaction. I am suggesting however that there is value in the close observation of infants in every respect and that here is an example of something which can be observed easily in the case of every child and which may lead us to make welcome developments in psychoanalytic theory.

Note in passing. For healthy development an infant must have a 'good enough' mother, i.e. one who actively adapts to the needs of the infant. This active adaptation cannot be done except through the fact of the mother's love, and it depends very little if at all on cleverness.

Instinct tension and the quiet states. Psychoanalytic theory has always paid full attention to instinct tensions, and much of the early work was concerned with the elaboration of this theme. Anxiety is related to instinct tension, and to the reactions to frustration. Also an attempt has been made to explore the periods between instinct tension along lines of instinct inhibited in aim, and of displacement of feeling.

There is much work to be done on these quiet states and probably it is being done by the study of ego-development.

Belonging to these quiet states is the affectionate type of relationship, that which we can easily take too much for granted in the normal; in the case of the anti-social person all observers are struck by the importance of the lack of the capacity for affectionate response or even for the affectionate impulse. Bowlby has forcibly drawn our attention to this point.

In my opinion the infant's relationship to the transitional object is evidence of the early development of that infant's capacity for the affectionate type of feeling. The word cuddle implies all this, and I suggest that some of the meaning of the cuddling of an early toy has a positive quality, a half-way state between love with instinct tension and indifference. Behind cuddling there is also a greater or less degree of depressive anxiety.

The depressive position. The contribution of Klein to psycho-analysis includes the concept which she calls the depressive position in normal development. Two main features can be drawn from this wide concept; let me take one first. This is the developing concern in the healthy infant for the object loved; primitive love impulse is crude and originally ruthless, and in any case there is the aggression reactive to inevitable frustrations. At the depressive position the infant has come by a very complex route to innate guilt feelings which simply belong to the maintenance of the capacity to love in spite of recognition of the nature of the loved object and the nature of the primitive love impulse (cannibalism). This guilt is intolerable to the human infant, and cannot be felt as such except in so far as reparation can be made, and for this purpose consistent environment is again necessary and the care of a person who can tolerate aggression, thereby introducing a time factor and the opportunity for reparation. In this respect the transition object is quite clearly used as a substitute for the mother and the mother's breast. It is notoriously badly used, but it survives. It has the advantage that it can be really damaged. It is not vindictive. It is not actually the mother or her breast. At the same time it has the disadvantage that it does not give out warmth or breathe, properties of the mother which are vitally important. It can smell, however. It is a kind of objectified hallucination.

The other main feature of the Klein concept is the complex alteration of the internal situation in the infant following instinctual experience and following the process of introjection and projection. *Forces* which are felt to be good and bad by the infant are set up as a result of instinctual experiences and strive with each other in the internal world except in so far as this inner world is projected. It is a valuable simplification at times to talk of internal *objects* which are felt to be good and bad by the infant and which threaten each other or defend each other and which can be dead or alive. The word object is useful because it begs the question as to whether one refers to part or whole objects. The relationship between the transition object and internal objects has to be considered.

In my opinion it would not be useful to say that the transitional object is an *internal* object because it obviously is *external*, and even felt to be such by the infant. Nevertheless it would be wrong simply to say that in a certain case the transitional object represents the actual mother (or her breast). I suggest that only in so far as there are good *internal* objects which have liveliness and value can the infant employ the transitional object, which is intermediate between internal and external.

In a certain case, therefore, the transitional object may stand for the internal mother who represents the external mother. A depression implying a lack of liveliness of the internal mother would destroy the infant's ability to use a transitional object even if the external mother were alive and present and loving. Contrariwise if an infant's mother is absent the transitional object can take her place provided there is a live internal good mother. It is only by a theory at least as complex as this that the facts can be explained.

ILLUSION-DISILLUSIONMENT

Positive value of illusion. I now come to the contribution which I feel I can make to this subject which is for discussion:

This part is reserved for the actual reading of the paper.

Part IV. Quotations

(My own comments in brackets.)

M. Wulff, M.D. (Tel Aviv, Palestine). 'Fetishism and Object Choice in Early Childhood'. *Psychoanalytic Quarterly* 1946 Vol. 15, p. 450. The author is clearly concerned with the same problem (but he relates these too closely in my opinion to that of Fetishism).

Freud. 'Interpretation of Dreams' p. 189. Reference to a forgotten toy, a china yellow lion, that appeared in a dream.

Freud. 'Collected Papers' Vol. 3 pp 63/4. Case of Dora. Sucking left thumb while tugging with right hand at lobe of brother's ear. Another case (1st half of second year) sucking at breast while pulling rhythmically at lobe of nurse's ear.

Freud. 'Three Essays on the Theory of Sexuality' 1915. p. 75 .... infantile sexual life essentially auto-erotic component instincts relatively independent of one another in search for pleasure. (Emphasis on zones of erotogenicity)

(In this paper the term 'affectionate current' of sexual life at puberty).

p. 78 convergence of affectionate current and sensual current in health.

Freud. 'Introductory Lectures on Psychoanalysis (1916–1917)' p. 263 reference to sucking for enjoyment, use of comforter; statement of sexual nature of pleasure derived from sucking for its own sake.

p. 264 object replaced by part of infant's own body (thumb, tongue). Independence of outer world, and excitation spread to thumb, tongue and genitalia.

p. 265 extension of these ideas to consideration of excretory functions. (accent on gratification)

p. 275 'Objects are not wanting to the component-instincts in this period, but these objects are not necessarily all comprised in one object'.

p. 276 Development of theme of the *object*. Sequence A allo-erotic B auto-erotic C allo-erotic (at oral zone, other zones B and C only). (At the present day this seems rather obscure)

p. 311. Discussion of phantasy-making. (N.B. In this paragraph Freud describes what I suggest is the essential need for transitional phenomena, namely 'renunciation has always been very hard to man; he cannot accomplish it without some kind of compensation. Accordingly he has evolved for himself a mental activity . . .'.)

(There follows a description of the artist which always seems to me to be a bit of an anti-climax).

Abraham. 'Collected Papers on Psychoanalysis'. The first Pregenital Stage of the Libido (1916) p. 267. A case description:

Thumb-sucking 'cured'; replaced by adoption of corner of pillow. Later: drug addiction, compulsive masturbation, etc. Return of thumb-sucking in transference situation.

(Positive value of latter occurrence not noted by Abraham)

p. 396. Migration of pleasure in sucking. First statement in psychoanalytic literature (?) of faeces as having a pre-history resulting from previous incorporation. (Transitional object can be substitute for good anal possession, or internal object).

A. Retention of good stuff—possession.
B. Retention of bad stuff—fear of persecution.

Basis laid for subsequent development of psychoanalytic theory of persecution ideas.

Also normal anal functioning is dependent on previous oral functioning, i.e. oral or acquisitive aims not displaced to anal erotic experience (in health).

Freud. The Ego and the Id. p. 35. 'at the very beginning, in the primitive oral phase of the individual's existence, object-cathexis and identification are hardly to be distinguished from each other'. (and p. 39)

Isaacs, Susan. Childhood and After, p. 14. 'or, to put it differently it is very truly a part of the child's own psyche which is differentiated to act as if it were external to the id impulses. One suspects that Freud's "primary identification" may perhaps play a greater part in the total drama than was originally thought'.

Freud. Group Psychology and the Analysis of the Ego. Discussion of identification theme. p. 65. 'What we have learned from these three sources may be summarised as follows. First, identification is the original form of emotional tie with an object; secondly, in a regressive way it becomes a substitute for a libidinal object tie, as it were by means of the introjection of the object into the ego; and thirdly, it may arise with every new perception of a common quality shared with some other person who is not an object of the sexual instinct. The more important this common quality is, the more successful may this partial identification become, and it may thus represent the beginning of a new tie'.

Riviere, Joan. *International Journal of Psychoanalysis*, Vol.17 1936, p. 399. 'I said this world was without objectivity; but from the very beginning there exists a core and a foundation in *experience* for objectivity ... the psyche responds to the reality of its experiences by interpreting them—or rather *mis*-interpreting them—in a subjective manner ... phantasy life is never "pure phantasy". It consists of true perceptions and of false interpretations, all phantasies are thus *mixtures* of external and internal reality'.

(This word 'mixture' contains the idea that I am trying to convey by the terms transitional objects and phenomena.)

Klein, Melanie. see in 'The Psychoanalysis of Children' and in subsequent papers the child Rita's use of her doll in her obsessional rituals. (It would be interesting to know the early history of this doll, or more especially of its precursor).

Freud, Anna. The Ego and the Mechanisms of Defence. p. 97. 'The defensive method of denial by word and act is subject to the same restrictions in time as I have discussed in the previous chapter in connection with denial in phantasy. It can be employed only so long as it can exist side by side with the capacity for reality-testing without disturbing it'.

p. 98. 'The single possible exception in neurosis is the "talisman" of obsessional neurotics, but I should not care to commit myself to an opinion as to whether the possession to which such patients cling so convulsively represents a protection against prohibited impulses from within or against dangerous forces from without, *or whether perhaps it combines both types of defence*'. (my italics)

Hoffer, Willi. The Psychoanalytic Study of the Child. Vol. III–IV p. 51. Observation of Bertie, 16 weeks, who combines sucking ring-finger with other employment of 3 fingers. 'The position of his fingers while finger-sucking might therefore also be interpreted as a voluntary reproduction of an epidermic stimulation which he felt when sucking at the breast'. Also refers to Gesell and Ilg.

Spitz, René, A. 'Autoerotism'. pp. 108–9. Reference to the 'libidinal object' (perhaps a good alternative term for my transitional object?) Important reference to 'the consistent retardation of the majority of rocking infants in the sectors of 'things' and libidinal objects is a measurable proof of these infants' disturbance in the field of object relations in general. For we find it permissable to assume from unpublished observations of K. M. Wulf that libidinal object relations have to be firmly established to enable infants to form relations with inanimate objects'.

Freud. Fliess Letters, 1895, p. 402 and 413.[i] It has been pointed out to me that Freud wrote that it is only by outside help that certain early functioning can proceed satisfactorily; the scream of the infant does not produce a clearing up of the inner tension by direct means: nevertheless through the reactions of the mother to the screaming satisfaction and relief of tension may be achieved. One can say of this that Freud is not bringing into the picture the mother who (through identification with the infant) knows the infant's needs without having to wait for the screaming. Freud then refers to the original helplessness which he relates to the development of the moral sense. In this is implied everything that one could now say in a broader way about the relation of maternal care to mental health. A reference to the same point occurs in 'Interpretation of Dreams' p. 521.

Illingworth, R. S. *British Medical Journal*. 'Sleep Disturbances in Young Children'. 7th April 1951.

Spitz, René A. The Psychoanalytic Study of the Child, Vol. V. Relevancy of Direct Infant Observation.

Fairbairn, W. R. D. International Journal of Psychoanalysis, Vol. 25. 1944. p. 70. Endopsychic structure considered in terms of object relationships.

(Object relationships stressed, though perhaps without due recognition of developments that had already taken place in psychoanalytic theory).
Milner, Marion. (Joanna Field) On Not Being Able to Paint.
Klein, Melanie. The Psycho-genesis of the Manic-Depressive States (and other papers).

---

[i] In *Aus den Anfängen der Psychoanalyse*. These references can be found in English in Freud's *Project for a Scientific Psychology*. For 'p. 402', see Part 1: Section 11: The Experience of Satisfaction (p. 318). For 'p. 413', see Part 1: Section 16: Cognitive and Reproductive Thought (p. 329).

7

Review: *The Inner World of Man: With Psychological Drawings and Paintings*
BY FRANCES G. WICKES (LONDON: METHUEN, 1950)

Review originally published in *The Lancet*, 14 July 1951, 258(6672), 66.

Although this book was published in New York in 1939, this is its first appearance in England. It began as a record of the rich inner world of fantasy revealed by dream analysis according to the methods of Jung. As it became evident to the author that the psychological theory which explained the findings needed to be itself explained or expounded for the majority of readers, the arrangement and proportions of the book changed, and it is now an exposition of analytical psychology illustrated by case-histories, drawings, dreams, and visions. The first nine chapters, which deal with the ego, the persona, the shadow, the anima, the animus, and other familiar material of Jungian analytical psychology, are followed by six chapters replete with clinical records, images from the inner life, and the interpretation put upon them. Vivid and poetical though these often are, it is hard to gather from them the nature of the therapeutic process they mediate, upon which Mrs Wickes lays strong emphasis. The language, like the thought, is closer to religion than to psychology or medicine.

8

Letter to *The Lancet*

LEUCOTOMY IN PSYCHOSOMATIC DISORDERS

Originally published in *The Lancet*, 258 (6677) 314–315.

18 August 1951

SIR: In your issue of July 21 Dr Sargant set out his views in an article under this heading. May I have space to proclaim my absolute belief that the human being has the right to suffer, and even to commit suicide, *intact*—that is to say, with the brain, the somatic basis for his psyche, inviolate.

Is there anywhere that the simple ethics of leucotomy (and all the magic box of the physical treatments) can be objectively presented and discussed? I think that except for the correspondence columns of medical journals there is no forum. No scientific psychiatric group will allow the ethics of leucotomy as matter for scientific discussion. The philosophical societies are too aloof, and moreover scared of madness. The B.B.C. has lent itself to propaganda for the physical treatments, and the religious bodies and the theologians are afraid that the argument will lead to an examination of the basis for the human soul: does it exist even in an anencephalic monster through investment from God, or does it depend on the existence in each individual of a brain?

All that can be said (until a series of serious discussions are organised by a responsible body) is that most doctors feel that the physical treatments of mental disorder are running a bit wild, that leucotomy is of doubtful taste; further, that when Dr Sargant claims the right to cut the brain about in 'dermatitis, effort syndrome, nervous vomiting, anorexia nervosa, and the like' a titter can be heard, as well as a sigh, from those who can remember the long series of such thought-systems about these groups of symptoms.

Is the neurologist coming to psychiatry already warped? There is a great deal to be said for an approach to psychology through general practice or paediatrics, in each of which specialties human nature is given its proper dignity.

London, W.1.   D. W. WINNICOTT

9

Letter to the *British Medical Journal*
ETHICS OF PREFRONTAL LEUCOTOMY

Originally published in the *British Medical Journal*, 2 (4729), 496,

25 August 1951

SIR: I write to welcome Mr Joseph Schorstein's letter (July 28, p. 239) in which he refers to the article by Dr G. D. F. Steele (July 14, p. 84). This article on the treatment of a case of persistent anxiety and tachycardia by leucotomy omits all reference to the deeper issues and contains the following statement: 'One year after the operation she remained well; her mental equilibrium has been restored at the price of the familiar personality changes associated with leucotomy. These have not seriously impaired her *functional efficiency* [my italics]. Both the patient and her husband believe the operation well justified'.

One can only hope with Mr Schorstein that this case may have 'the welcome result of shocking medical opinion into reconsidering the whole problem in its basic aspects'. The leucotomy enthusiasts have abandoned their initial claim that they cut the brain about only in the hopeless mental hospital case. Gradually the indications for this treatment have encroached on the psychoneuroses. According to Dr William Sargant obsessional neurosis often calls for this treatment, and in the *Lancet* (July 21, p. 87) he advocates leucotomy for 'dermatitis, effort syndrome, nervous vomiting, anorexia nervosa, and the like'. Further, a new psychology is developing, as represented by his article 'The Mechanism of Conversion' (August 11, p. 311), and we may expect a rapid growth of this theorizing which conveniently by-passes the psychology of the dynamic unconscious. Nevertheless very few find it good to protest, and it is for this reason that I write in support of Dr Schorstein.

The fundamental principle for which I think we must fight is that the human being has the right to suffer, and even to commit suicide, with the brain, the somatic basis for the psyche, inviolate.—I am, etc.,

London, W.1.   D. W. WINNICOTT

Review: *Jealousy in Children*
BY EDMUND ZIMAN, M.D. (LONDON: VICTOR GOLLANCZ, 1951)

Review originally published in the *British Medical Journal*, 1 September 1951, 2(4730), 532.

This book is mostly descriptive. The author writes to inform parents about their children so that they may manage them along sensible lines. Instead of talking about emotional development as a whole, he has chosen this one theme, jealousy, and has built a book around it. He has plenty of case material, given in a simple way which parents can understand and which will enlarge their experience, and he is all the time sympathetic with parents and children.

 The author has derived more than theoretical formulations from psychoanalysis. He has an appreciation of dynamic psychology, and thinks of the individual in terms of the continuity of emotional development. Nevertheless this book remains descriptive and suitable for parents. It therefore contains nothing that an informed psycho-analyst does not know about jealousy, and it avoids its deeper significances. Psychiatrists will read the book only in order to form an opinion on its suitability for being recommended to parents. I think they will want to recommend it.

Letter to *The Times*

NURSERY SCHOOLS: A DEFINITION OF FUNCTIONS

Originally published in *The Times*, Issue 52101, p. 7.

8 September 1951

Sir: I would like to write as one who has been concerned both as clinician and as a teacher of psychology to nursery school teachers with the problems discussed in the correspondence opened by Lady Astor on August 18.

It is generally known that nursery schools and day nurseries are widely different from each other. In out-patient pediatric work one constantly experiences a need for increased day nursery accommodation. A mother with a family burden that is just too big can keep the home going with the help of a nursery, and without such help the home breaks up; or perhaps a mother must work for economic or temperamental reasons, and the nursery makes all the difference between success or failure in the home, and so on. In each case recommended there has been a careful weighing-up of alternatives, keeping in mind the basic principle that the right place for a small child is that child's own home, and nearly always the matter is urgent once the decision is made, so that a waiting list is useless.

Behind the day nursery is urgent need, so that considerations of quality are secondary. Behind the nursery school, on the other hand, is not need so much as value. Here the idea is to enrich the lives of children who have good homes of their own. The mothers have made a good start and they begin to be able to make use of help; also they lack certain facilities: an only child needs gradually to mix in with other children, a child in a flat needs to make a noise, a child in small apartments needs room to run round. The nursery school justifies its existence only by being well equipped and by having an enlightened staff trained to meet the individual needs, physical, emotional, and educational of growing small children. A good nursery school is an extension of the child's own home, and it naturally becomes a place where parents meet and gather ideas.

In Mr C. H. Dobinson's letter of September 3 certain fears are usefully expressed, such as the idea that the aim and effect of nursery schools might be to make children clean, cooperative, and obedient, with serious loss of individuality. The nursery school is referred to as an 'organized group'. In this country, however, the nursery school tradition is of the very opposite kind, so much so that it is generally accepted that the tendency towards enabling children to be individuals first, which characterizes modern education as a whole, derives very largely from the pioneer work in the nursery schools. The names of Margaret McMillan and Susan Isaacs immediately occur to one's mind. Day nurseries deserve support because they meet urgent needs, and the nursery school movement deserves support because it gives us something very good.

Yours faithfully,
D. W. Winnicott

Paddington Green Children's Hospital, W.2, Sept. 4.

Review: *The Psychoanalytic Study of the Child, Volumes 3–4 and Volume 5*
EDITED BY ANNA FREUD, WILLIE HOFFER, AND EDWARD GLOVER (LONDON: IMAGO PUBLISHING COMPANY, 1949)

Review originally published in *British Medical Journal*, 13 October 1951, 2(4736), 894.

Delay in reviewing the combined Vols. III–IV has put the reviewer in the humiliating position of being overtaken by Vol. V. His difficulties are thereby increased, since the trouble with these volumes is the quantity of the material they contain. They are indeed a kind of journal appearing in book form, and it is to be hoped that they will continue to appear yearly.

To read all that these two volumes contain would be a big experience for anyone to whom the subject has meaning, and the task of sorting out the very good from the mediocre a heavy one. In any case this task belongs to the more specialist journals. Here it is perhaps sufficient to remind those who are interested in child psychiatry and in the roots of mental health and mental disorder that these volumes contain important contributions to every aspect of dynamic psychology and its practice. Most happily, it can be reported that there is less 'in-breeding' in the articles and references than in the first two volumes. Hitherto the contributions have come largely from one half of the psycho-analytic grouping—that which seems to the other half to edge away from the child's ideas of the inside of the psychosoma—but there is good reason why there should exist a place for publication of all kinds of sincere work.

The really valuable articles are too numerous in these volumes even to be listed here, but they include (Vol. III–IV) Anna Freud's contribution to a symposium on aggression, and an article by the late August Aichhorn, pioneer in the study and management of delinquents, on female juvenile delinquents. There is also an article in each volume by René A. Spitz, who is widely known through his observations, which appeared in Vol. II, on infants deprived of natural human relationships. These volumes provide, incidentally, a valuable link between psycho-analysis in the U.S.A. and psycho-analysis in Great Britain and Holland, and indicate the extent of the circle of friendships that has near its centre the personality of Miss Anna Freud.

13

Letter to Edward Glover

Originally published in Rodman, F. R. (Ed.), *The spontaneous gesture. Selected letters of D. W. Winnicott* (Letter 19, pp. 24–25). Cambridge, MA: Harvard University Press, 1987.

Edward Glover (1888–1972) was a psychoanalyst and, with Ernest Jones, a founding member of the British Psychoanalytical Society. Glover resigned from the British Psychoanalytic Society in 1944.

23 October 1951

Dear Glover,

Your letter does not need an answer,[i] but I feel like writing nevertheless as we are colleagues and both human beings.

The point you make gets to the centre of our scientific differences, I think, because you genuinely hold the view that D. W. W.'s ideas (or M. K.'s) are not derived from objective perception of children's ideas, whereas I genuinely believe that they are. At this point I think we can comfortably leave the solution to future observers.

I am sure that your scepticism has a valuable effect, making me a more careful observer, and I expect that my observations have some effect or other on you although I cannot for the moment say exactly what. In any case the review was signed so that everyone is free to feel as you felt when reading the review, that I was talking about 'edging away from D. W. W.'s ideas of the child's ideas of the psyche-soma'.

With good wishes,
Yours,
D. W. Winnicott.

---

[i] Glover had written to Winnicott to comment on Winnicott's review of *The Psychoanalytic Study of the Child, Vol. II* [CW 3:3:9], of which Glover was one of the series editors.

14

Notes on the General Implications of Leucotomy

Originally published in C. Winnicott, R. Shepherd, & M. Davis (Eds.), *Psychoanalytic explorations* (pp. 548–552, part of the chapter 'Physical therapy of mental disorder: Leucotomy'). Cambridge, MA: Harvard University Press, 1989.

These notes were used to open a discussion on leucotomy held at the London School of Economics on 13 November 1951.

Preliminary Survey

1. The fact of mental illness
2. The actual problems of management
3. The revolution in mental-hospital nursing
4. The value of the physical treatments
5. The gradual evolution of professional opinion about the various treatments

Statement of present position of the physical treatments in psychiatry.

Personal Standpoint

Consider a series of types of physical treatments: at one end, physical care, permission to regress

then: added narcotics
then: drugs aiding reliving of forgotten situations
then: insulin shock (skilled team work)
then: electric convulsion therapy [E.C.T.] (relatively unskilled)
then: leucotomy
then: euthanasia

Philosophical Considerations

1. E.C.T.—being unskilled has an effect on the practitioner's theories of human personality growth and abnormality.
2. Leucotomy alters the seat of the self, puts a premium on relief of suffering and creates teams of skilled neurosurgeons who constitute a type of vested interest, which can affect scientific evaluation. Theory of insanity as an organisation of the self appropriate to the circumstances.

Influence of Emotions on Judgement

Separation off one from another of two themes (inter-related of course): (a) Efficacy of (say) leucotomy compared with that of (say) psychoanalysis. This involves discussion of meaning of word 'efficacy' in this setting. And (b) Philosophical considerations, ethics of interference with brain functioning, ethics of therapy involving irreversible changes.

Observation In psychiatric papers at the present time (a) is being fully discussed without reference to (b).

Relative Importance of Various Body Organs for the Existence of an Individual Psyche

Obviously the healthy psyche needs a healthy and intact body. Nevertheless, it is possible to examine the relative values of various parts of the body to the psyche.

MUTILATION OF BRAIN VIS-À-VIS CASTRATION:

Anxiety about brain mutilation, anxiety about castration (conscious, unconscious)
Brain mutilation as *symbolical* of castration
False implication: that brain mutilation is *only* symbolical of castration, i.e. not in itself deserving fear, avoidance, condemnation, etc.

ILLUSTRATIONS (FOR SIMPLICITY, CONSIDERING ONLY MALES):

a. *Mutilation of main motor nerves to upper limbs.* Result, helplessness. It might be done (let us suppose) as a cure for masturbation, or stealing, or aggressive acts toward people. *This is unthinkable, we know no surgeon would perform this operation in this country.*

Yet it would leave the psyche intact. A biographer could write 'he bore the insult with dignity'. Perhaps the victim might have said 'Forgive them, for they know not what they do!' Circumcision is often performed to cure or prevent enuresis, masturbation, sexual aberrations—showing that surgery can easily become the handmaid of superstition and unconscious hate.

b. *Castration, i.e. removal of testicles.* Here we know about the results. To some extent the psyche is affected, in that the instinctual drives are modified. The effect on the psyche is more direct therefore than the removal of other (so called) internal glands, i.e. glands producing hormones.

At the present day castration would never be performed as a treatment of behaviour disorder, nor at the request of the individual (though it is part of the masochistic organisation for exactly this request to be made). The operation leaves the psyche to some extent intact, but the change is irreversible unless a testicular extract could be prepared exactly to replace the internal hormones lost, in which case the psyche would be again intact, though the individual would have to adjust to being unable to procreate. Surgeons sometimes tie the two ducts that carry spermatozoa from testicles, so that the patient need not fear he will impregnate the woman with whom he compulsively cohabits. This is not necessarily irreversible. (Cf. women after removal of [a] womb, [b] ovaries, adding ovarian extracts replacing hormones.)

c. *Subsidiary considerations.* Removal of both kidneys can be said to leave the psyche intact, except that gradually uraemia develops, and there is an increasing toxic distortion of the personality up to death. Removal of a limb naturally affects the individual, the cause of the removal of the limb being important. But the psyche is intact. Blindness, deafness, etc., all affect the individual, but leave the psyche intact; it is the person himself or herself who adjusts or fails to adjust to the mutilation.

As far as can be told there is not usually any injury to the brain tissue as a result of electrically induced fits, though it is very difficult to prove this. Few of us would voluntarily undergo a course of ten fits. (We can ignore the accidents that belong to this form of treatment as to any other—overdosage, fracture of the spine, etc.—as they do not affect the main problem.)

d. *Surgical treatment of the brain* has now to be considered. Brain tumour can often be removed, the operation being one of the most remarkable in surgery. It may in some cases be completely successful. In other cases more or less brain substance is involved, so that after the operation the patient is not able to make a complete return to normal. Something of the personality has gone or altered. This is unavoidable. The same can be said of other operations on the brain tissue for *surgical cure of brain abnormalities*.

It is not this group of phenomena that is under discussion. Consideration of these phenomena is important, however, as it brings forward the axiom that *the brain tissue* by and large *is the somatic (or physical) prerequisite for the existence of the psyche*. Some parts of a brain are more important than others in this respect (the motor and sensory centres are less, for instance), but there is no other organ that has comparable importance for the psyche's existence.

Question: Is this self-evident, or is it something that needs to be established?

Main Theme

What is being discussed is *the mutilation of normal, healthy brain tissue for the treatment of disorders of the psyche,* i.e. to alter an individual's behaviour, to lessen suffering, to make nursing easier, to restore *functional efficiency*. Here something is being done which attacks the psyche itself, by disturbing its physical basis.

Of a person so treated we can no longer say: 'he bore the mutilation with fortitude', because the meaning of the word 'he' has altered. We cannot say 'she suffers less now than before', because 'she' is not the same as before. All we could say would be: 'whereas the total he or she suffered (or misbehaved), the new sub-total he or she suffers (or misbehaves) less'.

I have said that it is unthinkable that (a) or (b) would be performed by a surgeon today in this country. Yet this infinitely more terrible operation has been done on thousands of people in the last ten years, and the advocates of this treatment are claiming a wider and wider field for their activities. At first it was only the hopeless mental hospital case that was leucotomised. Then gradually, obsessional neurotics were so treated, and melancholics whose own suffering could not be tolerated by the doctors in charge of them. Now the treatment is advocated for all sorts of psycho-somatic disorders. Soon the only symptom not qualifying a person for this treatment will be the obsession towards treatment by leucotomy, a contagious disorder to be found chiefly (alas!) in psychiatrists.

Effect on the General Public

This is a subject for research by the social psychologist. Does the fact that leucotomy is practised make one more afraid of madness, or less? Can it be that the apathy of the public to this problem, which is like that of euthanasia if it were being daily practised, is due to fear?

Fear Associated with the Leucotomy Problem

1. Conscious fear that some dependent who is insane will be sent home from the mental hospital.
2. Fear that if one becomes a voluntary boarder in a mental hospital one will be irreversibly mutilated.
3. Fear of the wish to be mutilated (masochistic, unconscious guilt, etc.); cf. fear of suicide.
4. Fear of the idea of a malevolent doctor; this fear always lurks behind the usual belief in one's doctor when one is ill. A malevolent doctor is unthinkable when one is ill.
5. The question of the soul and its relation to the psyche-soma. Does a newly conceived baby start at par in respect of soul, or at some degree above par? Very deep religious convictions are involved in this problem, and most people like to take it for granted that the soul is implanted, in the same way that God is not conceived of but perceived.

The Crude Issue

To put the matter crudely, either I or the psychiatrist in question is mad.

In the former case Dr X will sign me up (i.e. certify) and order my leucotomy (with the very best of intentions) and there will no longer be a D. W. W.; the resulting yes-man will be a sub-total D. W. W., no doubt much happier and free from missionary zeal and social sense, and released for the pleasures that belong to lack of true aim.

In the latter case, the psychiatrist is mad and I psycho-analyse him. He, of course, does not want to be psycho-analysed, so he remains unanalysed, and I remain a frustrated analyst. But he retains his psyche intact. This is the difference between the two awful alternatives.

You can see why for me it is a very serious matter, this which is the world's choice. For society of today must decide, not the psychiatrists who are cluttered up with immediate clinical problems. Who is to be considered mad? But whereas I am fighting for the very existence of my psyche my adversary knows that his psyche will be left to him intact and he knows that when he resists psycho-analytic treatment it will at least be himself resisting. I envy him.

15

Review: *On Not Being Able to Paint*
BY MARION MILNER (LONDON: HEINEMANN, 1950)

Review originally published in *British Journal of Medical Psychology*, March 1951, 24(1), 75–76, as 'Critical notice'. Also published in C. Winnicott, R. Shepherd, & M. Davis (Eds.), *Psycho-analytic explorations* (pp. 390–392). Cambridge, MA: Harvard University Press, 1989.

Let no one think that this book is just about painting or not painting. Yet it had to have its title because in that way the writing of the book started. The real purpose of the book only becomes clear to the author in the course of her experience of writing, in fact the book is itself an example of its main theme. This theme, which gradually becomes clear to the reader, is foreshadowed in an early quotation: 'Concepts can never be presented to me merely, they must be knitted into the structure of my being, and this can only be done through my own activity' (M. P. Follett, *Creative Experience*).

The central concept which is presented to the reader and apprehended by the writer through the writing of the book has to do with the subjective way of experiencing and the role of this in creative process. Thus the book is in one sense a plea for the recognition of subjectivity as having its own place and way of functioning, just as legitimate and as necessary as objectivity, but different. As applied to education, it is pointed out that subjectivity must be understood by teachers, otherwise the objectivity aimed at must be in danger of fatal distortion. Painting comes in as a jumping-off place; it was the surprise of discovering the power to make 'free' drawings that concentrated the writer's attention on this problem of subjectivity or subjective action.

The concept of the role of subjectivity which emerges has two main aspects, one to do with illusion, the other with spontaneity. Both are connected with what the writer calls the interplay of differences, out of which creativity proceeds, but if interplay is to be allowed in oneself one must be prepared for mental pain. Such an interplay needs various descriptions according to the level being considered. At a comparatively late stage of emotional development, what is familiar in psycho-analytic literature about unconscious conflict between love and hate in interpersonal relationships is relevant, and indeed this paved the way for all other statements. Such conflict involves the problem of the preservation of the loved object from hate and from erotic attacks (whether in fact or in fantasy) and creation is seen in this setting as an act of reparation. If one considers earlier stages in emotional development of the individual, one must use other language, such as the statement that magical creativity is an alternative to magical annihilation.

If I understand the author aright she wishes to make a yet more fundamental statement about creativity. She wishes to say that it results from what is for her (and perhaps for everyone) the primary human predicament. This predicament arises out of the non-identity of what is conceived of and what is to be perceived. To the objective mind of another person seeing from outside, that which is outside an individual is never identical with what is inside that individual. But there can be, and must be, for health (so the writer implies), a meeting place, an overlap, a stage of illusion, intoxication, transfiguration. In the arts this meeting place is pre-eminently found through the medium, that bit of the external world which takes the form of the inner conception. In painting, writing, music, etc., an individual may find islands of peace and so get momentary relief from the primary predicament of healthy human beings.

Psycho-analysts are accustomed to thinking of the arts as wish-fulfilling escapes from the knowledge of this discrepancy between inner and outer, wish and reality. It may come as a bit of a shock to some of them to find a psycho-analyst drawing the conclusion, after careful study, that this wish-fulfilling illusion may be the essential basis for all true objectivity. If these moments of fusion of subject and object, inner and outer, are indeed more than islands of peace, then this fact has very great importance for education. For what is illusion when seen from outside is not best described as illusion when seen from inside; for that fusion which occurs when the object is felt to be one with the dream, as in falling in love with someone or something, is, when seen from inside, a psychic reality for which the word illusion is inappropriate. For this is the process by which the inner becomes actualised in external form and as such becomes the basis, not only of internal perception, but also of all true perception of environment. Thus perception itself is seen as a creative process. In practice psycho-analysts, just like other people, love the arts and value the work of those who traffic in illusion. This book is showing psychoanalysts a way in which they may bring their theory into line not only with their psychotherapy but also with their daily lives.

Moreover the author is reminding psycho-analysts and all teachers that teaching is not enough; each student must create what is there to be taught, and so arrive at each stage of learning in his own way. If he temporarily forgets to acknowledge debts this is easily forgiven, since in place of paying debts he re-discovers with freshness and originality and also with pleasure, and both the student and the subject grow in the experience.

The second thread of the book, the role of spontaneity in creativeness, is also something that analysts tend to allow for more in their practice than in their theory. They are well used to theorising about the effects of too rigid control of spontaneity, imposed in the interests of social living and propriety. What they, and also other teachers, are less used to considering is the stultifying effect on the creative spirit of too great insistence not just on propriety but on objectivity. This insistence on objectivity concerns not only perception but also action, and creativity can be destroyed by too great insistence that in acting one must know beforehand what one is doing.

Review: *Problems of Infancy and Childhood*

TRANSACTIONS OF THE THIRD CONFERENCE, MARCH 7–8, 1949, NEW YORK, N.Y. (NEW YORK: JOSIAH MACY, JR. FOUNDATION. 1949)

> Review originally published in *British Journal of Medical Psychology*, June 1951, 24(2).

For me these verbatim accounts of discussions between pediatricians, psycho-analysts, psychiatrists, psychiatric social workers, obstetricians, and various other workers in the infant and child field (twenty-five of them in this instance) are always welcome.

Here is the third instalment, and may there be a steady stream from the same source.

In this volume are recorded informal discussions around three subjects: 'Anxieties of Mothers as Verbalized to Physicians', 'The Psychological Situation of Mother and Child upon Return from Hospital', and 'Observations on the Emotional Reactions of Children to Tonsillectomy and Adenoidectomy'. I feel that the reviewer's job here is not to pick out significant details but to recommend strongly that the discussions shall be read. This is the very opposite of eclectic exposition, and the main feature is that everyone's point of view is expressed and respected.

The best thing would be if some of us over here could start up discussion groups as widely representative as these that are faithfully reproduced in these reports. The Medical Director of the Foundation is Dr Frank Fremont-Smith and the Chairman at the discussions is Dr Leo H. Bartemeier, psychiatrist of Detroit.

17

Review: *Papers on Psycho-Analysis*
BY ERNEST JONES, FIFTH EDITION (LONDON: BAILLIÈRE, TINDALL AND COX, 1948)

Review originally published in *British Journal of Medical Psychology*, June 1951, 24(2).

A fifth edition does not always call for a new appraisal. In this case, however, in each new edition much has been discarded and much has been added. A possessor of the five editions has access to eighty-nine lectures and papers on psycho-analysis, surely a comment in itself of the author's capacity for work. The first edition published thirty-eight years ago had to meet a public very different from that which welcomes this latest and last edition, and naturally the author's main concerns were also different in 1912 from what they are in 1950. One thing remains, a love of Freud and a loyalty to him, combined with an easy freedom seriously to question the validity of Freud's findings where occasion arises.

In the full and useful index the author has allowed himself one irregularity. Against the name Freud the reader will find not page numbers, but the two words 'every page'. This is nearly true.

The reviewer has read nearly all the eighty-nine and certainly the twenty-seven papers that comprise this volume, and he is deeply impressed with the author's prowess as a writer of scientific papers. Each essay is a masterpiece in itself. There is no need to stress the wide 'scatter' of Jones's interests because this is well known, but this is perhaps a good moment to pay tribute to some other features. In each chapter one meets a clear development of the theme, an understandable setting out of the main points and a statement of the author's conclusion. There is personal conviction combined with modesty, as befits scientific work, with evidence all through of the author's very wide reading in three languages. (Once there comes through evidence of the author's fourth language, Welsh.) Jones seems to be always pleased when he can quote another author and so pin down priority in respect of an idea, and in this he resembles Freud.

It would be useful perhaps to make special reference to three papers. Chapter III on the Theory of Symbolism is a long essay and is a real *tour de force*. It necessarily makes difficult reading, but the subject is covered well. A great deal of loose and valueless talk about symbolism could be avoided if this study could be taken as the accepted jumping-off ground for new exploration. Jones gives a short summary at the end, but to quote from it would be to detract from the value of the paper, which is the comprehensive discussion of symbolism, metaphor and simile. Nevertheless, the following is indicative of the main trend: '... in the psycho-analytical sense the symbol is a substitute for the primary idea compulsorily formed as a compromise between the tendency of the unconscious complex and the inhibiting factors ...'.

The second outstanding chapter is no. V; 'Psycho-analysis and the Instincts'. This lecture leads up to a presentation of Freud's difficult Death Instinct Theory, which Freud himself had doubts about, and about which Jones still keeps an open mind. The evolution of the idea in Freud's mind is traced in a masterly way, and the reader is left at any rate with an understanding of the problem which Freud attempted to solve in this way and which is perhaps (or perhaps not) being solved in other ways by modern psycho-analytic research.

The third outstanding contribution is Jones's frank discussion of Freud's theories of early sexual development in the female, comparing these theories with those of Horney, Deutsch, Klein, Riviere, and others. The importance of penis envy is not denied at all, and yet the possibility of a fundamental female sexuality developing without the idea of castration as a primary element in the emotional development of girls is kept open. Here again Jones's contribution gives a good solid basis for the founding of urgently needed development in psycho-analytical theory in this direction.

Perhaps Jones would have chosen other chapters as his favourites. That on Fear, Guilt and Hate, for instance, is outstanding, and I understand that he does actually like this chapter best. One can easily agree that it was a brave thing to do to lecture on Jealousy in France, but one hopes that Jones's wide reading of the French writers impressed the French audience and helped them to accept his insistence on the unconscious factors in the motivation of pathological jealousy, indeed of jealousy itself.

In short, in these eighty-nine papers Jones has given invaluable help to any student of the psychology that has grown out of Freud's work.

18

Review: *Infant Feeding and Feeding Difficulties*
BY PHILIP EVANS AND RONALD MACKEITH (LONDON: J. AND A. CHURCHILL, 1951)

> Review originally published in *British Journal of Medical Psychology*, December 1951, 24(4), 304–305.

This book must stand or fall on the success or failure of its presentation of modern scientific pediatrics, with the accent on the physical side. In my opinion the authors have given those who work with infants and their mothers an accurate, up-to-date and easily read exposition of available knowledge and opinion. From this basis one can examine the psychological tendency.

There is a general acceptance of the importance of infant feeding as the start of a relationship between persons. This is very welcome and it makes the book into one that can be studied by the student of the psychology of infant feeding since it nowhere irritates by implied jeering at the psychologist or even by denial of emotional factors. In fact, it contributes on the psychological side both by direct reference and also by the quotations at the chapter heads. In this way three types of human experience are represented in this book, each of which contributes to the other two.

To illustrate my point I take chapter XII. This begins 'Levez vers le ciel vos faces radieuses; l'univers esculent est ouvert devant vous'. If I understand what is meant here aright, this quotation gives the reader the idea that the early feeding experience is related to the whole problem of the introduction of external reality to the individual, and the creation of the world by each individual afresh. A chapter on this would be out of place in this book, but because of the triple approach of the two authors (and how well they have worked together!) the deeper psychological implications of the developing infant-mother experience has tribute paid to it without offence being given to those who dislike logical psychology.

Assuming the soundness of the physical facts about infants and mothers, what I value most in this book is the choice of quotations from a wide field of cultural experience.

> A child born yesterday
> A thing on mother's milk and kisses fed.
>
> SHELLEY

Till quite recently pediatrics forgot the kisses, and these authors quietly make amends.

It does seem strange that the good work of Bakwin and Spitz on infant depression is respectable for quotation, whereas other and much older work pointing to the laying down of the mental health of the individual in the early months of that individual's life fails to impress people. One can only be glad that these authors have found a way of presenting clinical material which catches the pediatric eye. The danger is that the pediatrician will think this matter of infantile depression is quite a simple one. What is needed is a first-class pediatrician who recognizes that the psychology of infantile emotional development is at least as complex as the physiology of which he is an eager and humble student.

The paragraph on adopted infants raises a whole host of problems that cannot be dealt with usefully in a book of this nature. I would like to pull out of this paragraph one sentence: 'As an infant's interest is self-centred it does not come to know its mother as opposed to any other loving mother-substitute until it is five or six months old; there is from the point of view of the child's emotional development no urgency for some months for it to come into the care of the person who is to have permanent charge'.

This idea is being taught even by some of the psycho-analysts, and it is to say the least inadequate. Perhaps it is really very bad teaching. When those who spread this teaching see this sort of quotation might they not decide to go slow for a while, until more is known? *Festina lente* is put at the head of the chapter on Prematurity (chapter XV). Is not this teaching premature too?

It is true that changes occur somewhere about the fifth to sixth month, which make clear to observers that a capacity for a relationship as between *whole human beings* has developed. Also it is true that in the early stages *techniques* are appreciated more easily than the shape of the mother's nose. These two observations simply need co-ordinating.

It is at any rate possible that an infant can be muddled by loss of a breast, or technique, or smell (or whatnot) even in the first weeks and even the first days. Certainly a baby can be so confused at adoption at nine weeks that already a paranoid 'constitution' results, and the adopting parents find they have taken over an ill baby.

I would personally ask: let those who teach about the emotional development of infants at any rate keep an open mind during the next few years, and not yet give out the edict that before five months nothing much can happen adversely except physical damage.

But the book is a good one, and I like to think the medical students and nurses and health visitors for whom it is written will meet the facts of physical infant care in this form, a form that is friendly to psychology.

CHRONOLOGY

	Biography	Significant Publications
1896	Donald Woods Winnicott born in Plymouth, Devon, England. Youngest son, with two older sisters, of Elizabeth Martha Woods Winnicott and John Frederick Winnicott, a merchant who was twice mayor of Plymouth.	
1910	Enters The Leys School, a boarding school in Cambridge.	
1914	Studies Natural Science at Jesus College, Cambridge University, in preparation to read medicine.	
1917	Enters St Bartholomew's Hospital Medical School, London. Enlists in the Royal Navy, serving during the war on H.M.S. Lucifer as Surgeon-Probationer.	
1920	Graduates from Barts and continues to work there as House Physician.	
1923	Appointed Assistant Physician at Paddington Green Children's Hospital, eventually becoming Physician-in-Charge. Appointed Assistant Physician at the Queen's Hospital for Children. Marries Alice Taylor. Begins his analysis with James Strachey.	
1924	Opens his own practice in Belgravia, London.	
1925	His mother, Elizabeth, dies of cardiac disease. Becomes a Fellow of the Royal Society of Medicine.	
1927	Begins his psychoanalytic training at the Institute of Psychoanalysis, London, supervised by Ella Freeman Sharpe and Nina Searl.	
1928	Appointed Physician in charge of a newly formed Rheumatism Clinic at the Queen's Hospital.	
1931		*Clinical Notes on Disorders of Childhood* [CW 1:3:1–20]
1933	Finishes his ten-year analysis with James Strachey.	
1934	Qualifies as an adult psychoanalyst and becomes an associate member of the British Psychoanalytical Society (BPAS). Resigns from the Queen's Hospital but continues to run the rheumatism clinic. Continues training as a child analyst under the supervision of Melanie Klein, Melitta Schmideberg, and Nina Searl.	
1935	Qualifies as the first male child psychoanalyst at the BPAS. Melanie Klein asks him to analyse her son Eric. Gives his membership paper, 'The Manic Defence', to the BPAS.	'The Manic Defence' [CW 1:4:6]

	Biography	Significant Publications
1936	Begins his second analysis, with Joan Riviere, lasting until 1941. Becomes a full member of the BPAS.	'Appetite and Emotional Disorder' [CW 1:4:11]
1939	Gives his first broadcasts on BBC Radio. Freud dies in London.	'Aggression' [CW 2:1:8] Letter to the *British Medical Journal*, 'The Evacuation of Small Children', with E. Miller and J. Bowlby [CW 2:1:6]
1940		'Children and Their Mothers' [CW 2:2:2]
1941	Appointed as psychiatric consultant to the scheme for evacuated children in Oxfordshire and meets Clare Britton, social worker in charge of the scheme.	'The Observation of Infants in a Set Situation' [CW 2:3:6]
1941–3	Named as one of five Kleinian training analysts and participates in the 'Controversial Discussions' in the BPAS. Becomes Director of the Child Department of the BPAS, holding the post until 1960.	'Resolution K: On Scientific Aims in Psychoanalysis' [CW 2:4:1] 'Child department consultations' [CW 2:4:2]
Mid-1940s	No longer regarded as a Kleinian. Broadcasts 'Getting to Know Your Baby' and other programmes on BBC radio, for 'the ordinary devoted mother'.	
1944	Becomes a Fellow of the Royal College of Physicians.	
1945		*Getting to Know Your Baby* 'Primitive Emotional Development' [CW 2:7:8]
1947		'Hate in the Countertransference' [CW 3:2:1] 'Residential Management as Treatment for Difficult Children' [CW 3:2:3]
1948	Chairman of the Medical Section of the British Psychological Society. His father, Sir John Frederick Winnicott, dies. Suffers his first coronary. Paddington Green Hospital is absorbed into St Mary's Hospital.	'Paediatrics and Psychiatry' [CW 3:3:2] 'Children's Hostels in War and Peace' [CW 3:1:1] 'Reparation in Respect of Mother's Organized Defence Against Depression' [CW 3:3:1]
1949	Leaves his first wife, Alice. Suffers his second coronary.	*The Ordinary Devoted Mother and Her Baby* 'Mind and Its Relation to the Psyche-Soma' [CW 3:4:20] 'Birth Memories, Birth Trauma, and Anxiety' [CW 3:4:8]
1950	Suffers a third coronary after a patient commits suicide. Named Scientific Secretary of the BPAS.	'Some Thoughts on the Meaning of the Word Democracy' [CW 3:5:17] 'Aggression in Relation to Emotional Development' [CW 3:5:2]

	Biography	Significant Publications
1951	Divorces Alice. Marries Clare Britton. Becomes Training Secretary of the BPAS. Begins analysis of Masud Khan in October, continuing until April 1954.	'Transitional Objects and Transitional Phenomena' [CW 3:6:6; CW 4:2:21; CW 5:4:24; CW 9:3:5]
1952	President of the Paediatric Section of the Royal Society of Medicine. Broadcasts the series 'The Ordinary Devoted Mother and Her Baby' on BBC radio. Suffers his fourth coronary.	'Psychoses and Child Care' [CW 4:1:5] 'Anxiety Associated with Insecurity' [CW 4:1:11]
1953	Clare Winnicott begins analysis with Melanie Klein.	'Symptom Tolerance in Paediatrics' [CW 4:2:4] 'The Mother's Contribution to Society' [CW 5:3:30]
1954	Suffers his fifth coronary	'Withdrawal and Regression' [CW 4:3:29] 'The Depressive Position in Normal Emotional Development' [CW 4:3:5] 'Metapsychological and Clinical Aspects of Regression Within the Psycho-Analytical Set-up' [CW 4:3:6]
1955	Gives the first of many annual courses of lectures at the Child Development Department, Institute of Education, University of London.	'Clinical Varieties of Transference' [CW 5:1:11]
1956	Elected President of the BPAS for the first time, on a three-year term.	'Primary Maternal Preoccupation' [CW 5:2:16] 'The Antisocial Tendency' [CW 5:2:8] 'Paediatrics and Childhood Neurosis' [CW 5:2:11]
1957		*The Child and the Family* *The Child and the Outside World* 'On the Contribution of Direct Child Observation to Psychoanalysis' [CW 5:3:21]
1958		*Collected Papers: Through Paediatrics to Psychoanalysis* 'The Capacity to Be Alone' [CW 5:3:20] 'Child Analysis in the Latency Period' [CW 5:4:13]
1959	Spends August in Finland giving courses and lectures as part of a World Health Organisation conference.	'Classification: Is There a Psycho-analytic Contribution to Psychiatric Classification?' [CW 5:5:5]

	Biography	Significant Publications
1960	Broadcasts the series 'The Ordinary Devoted Mother and Her Children' on BBC radio. Melanie Klein dies. Steps down as Director of the Child Department of the BPAS, but remains Consultant Physician.	'The Effect of Psychosis on Family Life' [CW 6:1:6] 'The Theory of the Parent–Infant Relationship' [CW 6:1:21] 'Ego Distortion in Terms of True and False Self' [CW 6:1:22] 'String: A Technique of Communication' [CW 6:1:20] 'Counter-transference' [CW 5:5:20]
1961	Retires from St Mary's Hospital after forty years.	'Varieties of Psychotherapy' [CW 6:2:5]
1962	Undertakes a lecture tour in the United States in October, speaking in Los Angeles, San Francisco, Topeka, Boston, and New York.	'The Aims of Psycho-analytical Treatment' [CW 6:3:2] 'A Personal View of the Kleinian Contribution' [CW 6:3:8] 'Ego Integration in Child Development' [CW 6:3:19] 'Providing for the Child in Health and Crisis' [CW 6:3:10]
1962–8	Analyses Harry Guntrip 'on demand', continuing for over 150 sessions.	
1963	Undertakes a lecture tour in the United States in October, visiting Atlanta, Philadelphia, and Baltimore.	'The Development of the Capacity for Concern' [CW 6:3:11] 'Fear of Breakdown' [CW 6:4:21] 'From Dependence Towards Independence in the Development of the Individual' [CW 6:4:11] 'Morals and Education' [CW 6:3:18] 'Communicating and Not Communicating Leading to a Study of Certain Opposites' [CW 6:4:8] 'Training for Child Psychiatry' [CW 6:3:5] 'Psychotherapy of Character Disorders' [CW 6:4:9] 'The Mentally Ill in Your Caseload' [CW 6:4:5] 'Psychiatric Disorder in Terms of Infantile Maturational Processes' [CW 6:4:12] 'Dependence in Infant-Care, in Child-Care, and in the Psycho-analytic Setting' [CW 6:3:9] 'Adolescence: Struggling Through the Doldrums' [CW 6:2:4] 'The Value of Depression' [CW 6:4:10]

	Biography	Significant Publications
1964		*The Child, the Family and the Outside World* 'The Concept of the False Self' [CW 7:1:1] 'The Relationship of a Mother to Her Baby at the Beginning' [CW 6:1:8]
1965	Elected President of the BPAS for a second three-year term	*The Family and Individual Development* *The Maturational Processes and the Facilitating Environment* 'The Value of the Therapeutic Consultation' [CW 7:2:22] 'A Clinical Study of the Effect of a Failure of the Average Expectable Environment on a Child's Mental Functioning' [CW 10:1:4]
1966		'The Absence of a Sense of Guilt' [CW 7:3:32] 'The Ordinary Devoted Mother' [CW 7:3:3] 'The Child in the Family Group' [CW 7:3:17] 'On the Split-Off Male and Female to be Found in Men and Women' [CW 7:3:2]
1967	President of the Association for Child Psychology and Psychiatry. Chair of the International Psychoanalytic Association's Sponsoring Committee for the Finnish Psychoanalytic Society, which gains status as a provisional society. Lectures in Boston, USA.	'The Location of Cultural Experience' [CW 7:3:31] 'Mirror-Role of Mother and Family in Child Development' [CW 8:1:38] 'The Concept of a Healthy Individual' [CW 8:1:4]
1968	Wins the *James Spence* Gold Medal for Paediatrics. Appointed Honorary Member of the Royal Medico-Psychological Association. Undertakes a lecture tour in the United States, speaking in New York, but suffers a serious coronary after reading 'The Use of an Object' to the New York Psychoanalytic Society.	'The Squiggle Game' [CW 8:2:47] 'Breast-Feeding as Communication' [CW 8:2:26] 'Communication Between Infant and Mother, and Mother and Infant, Compared and Contrasted' [CW 8:2:2] 'The Use of an Object and Relating Through Identifications' [CW 8:2:28] 'Sum, I Am' [CW 8:2:10]
1969		'The Use of an Object in the Context of *Moses and Monotheism*' [CW 9:1:4] 'Mother's Madness Appearing in the Clinical Material as an Ego-Alien Factor' [CW 9:1:29]
1970	Prepares to give keynote paper to the IPA Congress in Vienna in July.	'Dependence in Child-Care' [CW 9:2:15] 'On the Basis for Self in Body' [CW 9:2:12] 'Residential Care as Therapy' [CW 9:2:9]

	Biography	Significant Publications
1971	Dies of a coronary in January.	*Playing and Reality* *Therapeutic Consultations in Child Psychiatry* [CW 10] 'Dreaming, Fantasying and Living: A Case-History Describing a Primary Dissociation' [CW 9:3:6] 'Playing: A Theoretical Statement' [CW 8:2:15] 'Playing: Creative Activity and the Search for the Self' [CW 8:1:27] 'Creativity and Its Origins' [CW 9:3:7] 'The Place Where We Live' [CW 8:2:1] 'Interrelating Apart from Instinctual Drive and in Terms of Cross-Identifications' [CW 9:3:8] 'Contemporary Concepts of Adolescent Development and Their Implications for Higher Education' [CW 9:3:9]
1977		*The Piggle: An Account of the Psychoanalytic Treatment of a Little Girl* (Ed. I. Ramzy) [CW 11:2:1–17]
1981	The Squiggle Foundation established.	
1984	Clare Winnicott dies. The Winnicott Trust founded.	*Deprivation and Delinquency* (Eds. C. Winnicott, R. Shepherd, M. Davis)
1986		*Home Is Where We Start From* (Eds. C. Winnicott, R. Shepherd, M. Davis) *Holding and Interpretation: Fragment of an Analysis*
1987		*Babies and Their Mothers* (Eds. C. Winnicott, R. Shepherd, M. Davis) *The Spontaneous Gesture: Selected Letters of D. W. Winnicott* (Ed. F. R. Rodman)
1988		*Human Nature* [CW 11:1]
1989		*Psychoanalytic Explorations* (Eds. C. Winnicott, R. Shepherd, M. Davis)
1993		*Talking to Parents* (Eds. C. Bollas, R. Shepherd, M. Davis)
1996		*Thinking About Children* (Eds. R. Shepherd, J. Johns, H. Taylor Robinson)
2002		*Winnicott on the Child*
2017		*The Collected Works of D. W. Winnicott* (Eds. L. Caldwell, H. Taylor Robinson)

REFERENCES

Volume 3

Abraham, K. (1916). The first pregenital stage of the libido. In *Collected papers on psycho-analysis* (pp. 248–279). London: Hogarth.

Aichhorn, A. (1949). Some remarks on the psychic structure and social care of a certain type of female juvenile delinquents. *Psychoanalytic Study of the Child*, 3–4, 439–448.

Astor, Lady Nancy. (1951, 18 August). Letter: Fewer nursery schools: Need for objective survey. *The Times*, Issue 52083.

Bion, W. R. (1950). The imaginary twin. In *Second thoughts*. London: Karnac.

Bowlby, J. (1951). *Maternal care and mental health*. Geneva: World Health Organization.

Bowlby, J., & Fry, M. (Eds.). (1953). *Child care and the growth of love*. Abridged version. Harmondsworth: Penguin.

Bowley, A. H. (1947). *The psychology of the unwanted child*. Edinburgh: E. and S. Livingstone.

Bradley, C. (1941). *Schizophrenia in childhood*. New York: Macmillan.

Bradley, C. (1942). Biography of a schizophrenic child. *The Nervous Child*, 1(2–3), 141.

Brierley, M. (1951). *Trends in psycho-analysis*. London: Hogarth.

Britton, C., & Winnicott, D. (1944). The problem of homeless children. [CW 2:6:14]

Britton, C., & Winnicott, D. (1957). Residential management as treatment for difficult children: The evolution of a wartime hostels scheme. *Human Relations*, 1(1), 87–97. [CW 3:2:3]

Bruch, H., & Cottington, F. (1942). Diary of a psychotic child. *The Nervous Child*, 1 (2–3), 232.

Casteret, N. (1947). *My caves*. London: Dent.

Cottington, F. (1942). Treatment of schizophrenia in childhood. *The Nervous Child*, 1 (2– 3), 172.

Creak, E. M., & Shorting, B. J. (1944). Child psychiatry. *Journal of Mental Science*, 90, 365–381.

Curtis, M. (chair). (1946). *Report of the Care of Children Committee* (The Curtis Report), Command 6922. London: HMSO.

Davies, W. H. (1914). Infancy. In *The bird of paradise, and other poems*. London: Methuen.

Despert, J. L. (1942). Prophylactic aspect of schizophrenia in childhood. *The Nervous Child*, 1(2–3), 189.

Dobinson, C. H. (1951, 3 September). Nursery schools. Letter. *The Times*, Issue 52096.

Evans, P. R., & MacKeith, R. (1951). *Infant feeding and feeding difficulties*. London: Churchill.

Fain, M., & Marty, P. (1955). La motricité dans la relation d'objet. *Revue française de psychanalyse*. Tome XIX, Nos. 1–2. Paris: Presses Universitaires de France.

Fairbairn, W. R. D. (1944). Endopsychic structure considered in terms of object-relationships. *International Journal of Psychoanalysis*, 25, 70–93.

Follett, M. P. (1924). *Creative experience*. New York: Longmans, Green, & Co.

Freud, A. (1937). *The ego and the mechanisms of defence*. London: Hogarth. [Original work published 1936.]
Freud, A. (1947). Aggression in relation to emotional development: Normal and pathological. *The Psychoanalytic Study of the Child, 3–4*, 37.
Freud, A. (1947). Emotional and instinctive development. In R. W. B. Ellis (Ed.), *Child health and development* (ch. 10). London: Churchill.
Freud, A., Hoffer W., Glover, E., et al. (Eds.). (1946). *The Psychoanalytic Study of the Child, 2*.
Freud, A., Hoffer, W., & Glover, E. (Eds.). (1949). *The Psychoanalytic Study of the Child, 3–4*.
Freud, A., Hoffer, W., & Glover, E. (Eds.). (1949). *The Psychoanalytic Study of the Child, 5*.
Freud, S. (1895/1950). *Aus den Anfängen der Psychoanalyse*. London: Imago.
Freud, S. (1895). Project for a scientific psychology. *Complete psychological works of Sigmund Freud, 1*. London: Hogarth.
Freud, S. (1900). *The interpretation of dreams*. A. A. Brill (Trans.). London: George Allen & Co.
Freud, S. (1905). Dora: Fragments of an analysis of a case of hysteria. In J. Strachey (Ed.), *Complete psychological works of Sigmund Freud, 7*. London: Hogarth.
Freud, S. (1909). Notes upon a case of obsessional neurosis. In J. Strachey (Ed.), *Complete psychological works of Sigmund Freud, 10*. London: Hogarth.
Freud, S. (1915). Instincts and their vicissitudes. In J. Strachey (Ed.), *Complete psychological works of Sigmund Freud, 14*. London: Hogarth.
Freud, S. (1915). *Three essays on the theory of sexuality*, 3rd ed. Leipzig/Vienna: Deuticke.
Freud, S. (1916–1917). Introductory lectures on psychoanalysis. In J. Strachey (Ed.), *Complete psychological works of Sigmund Freud, 15–16*. London: Hogarth.
Freud, S. (1920). Beyond the pleasure principle. In J. Strachey (Ed.), *Complete psychological works of Sigmund Freud, 18*. London: Hogarth.
Freud, S. (1921). *Group psychology and the analysis of the ego*. London/Vienna: International Psycho-Analytical Press.
Freud, S. (1923). *The ego and the id*. London: Hogarth.
Freud, S. (1926). *Inhibitions, symptoms and anxiety*. London: Hogarth.
Friedlander, K. (1947). *The psycho-analytical approach to juvenile delinquency: Theory, case-studies, treatment*. London: K. Paul, Trench, Trübner.
Glover, E. (1945). An examination of the Klein system of child psychiatry. *The Psychoanalytic Study of the Child, 1*, 75–118.
Glover, E. (1949). The position of psycho-analysis in Great Britain. In *On the early development of mind* (ch. 23). London: Imago.
Goodenough, Sir W. (1944). *Report of inter-departmental committee on medical schools*. Ministry of Health. London: HMSO.
Greenacre, P. (1941). The predisposition to anxiety. *Psychoanalytic Quarterly, 10*, 66–94.
Greenacre, P. (1941). The predisposition to anxiety, part II. *Psychoanalytic Quarterly, 10*, 610–638.
Greenacre, P. (1945). The biological economy of birth. In *Trauma, growth and personality*. London: Hogarth.
Harms, E. (1947). *Handbook of child guidance*. New York: Child Care Publications.
Hartmann, H. (1952). The mutual influences in the development of ego and id. *The Psychoanalytic Study of the Child, 7*, 9–30.

Heimann, P., Klein, M., & Money-Kyrle, R. (1977). *New directions in psycho-analysis.* London: Karnac.

Hill, A. (1948). *Art versus illness*, 2nd ed. London: George Allen & Unwin.

Hoffer, W. (1949). Mouth, hand and ego-integration. *The Psychoanalytic Study of the Child*, 3–4, 49–56.

Illingworth, R. S. (1951). Sleep disturbances in young children. *British Medical Journal*, 1(4709), 722–728.

Isaacs, S. (1929). *The nursery years.* London: Routledge.

Isaacs, S. (1930). *The intellectual growth in young children.* London: Routledge.

Isaacs, S. (1932). *The children we teach: Seven to eleven years.* London: University of London, Institute of Education.

Isaacs, S. (1933). *Social development in young children.* London: Routledge.

Isaacs, S. (1948). *Childhood & after: Some essays and clinical studies.* London: Routledge & Kegan Paul.

Jones, E. (1946). A valedictory address. *International Journal of Psycho-Analysis*, 27, 7–11.

Jones, E. (1948). *Papers on psycho-analysis*, 5th ed. London: Baillière, Tindall and Cox.

Kanner, L. (1943). Autistic disturbances of affective contact. *The Nervous Child*, 2, 217–250.

Klein, M. (1932). *The psycho-analysis of children.* London: Hogarth.

Klein, M. (1935). A contribution to the psychogenesis of the manic-depressive states. *International Journal of Psycho-Analysis*, 16, 145.

Klein, M. (1946). Notes on some schizoid mechanisms. *International Journal of Psycho-Analysis*, 27, 99.

Klein, M. (1948). *Contributions to psycho-analysis, 1921–1945.* London: Hogarth.

Little, H. M. (1947). The psychotic child. *Pennsylvania Medical Journal*, 51, 174.

MacAlpine, I. (1952). Psychosomatic symptom formation. *Lancet*, 259 (6702), 278–282.

Malleson, J. (1948, 18 December). Letter: Taking children's temperatures. *British Medical Journal*, 2(4589), 1078.

Middlemore, M. P. (1941). *The nursing couple.* London: Hamish Hamilton Medical Books.

Milner, M. (1950). *On not being able to paint.* Madison, CT: International Universities Press.

Moncrieff, A., & Hussey, B. J. (1948). Temperature recording in sick children. *British Medical Journal*, 2(4587), 972–973. [see CW 3:4:2]

Money-Kyrle, R. (1951). *Psychoanalysis and politics.* London: Duckworth.

Money-Kyrle, R. (1951). Some aspects of state and character in Germany. In G. Wilbur & W. Munsterberger (Eds.), *Psychoanalysis and culture* (pp. 280–292). New York: International Universities Press.

Pennington, Sarah. (1784). *An unfortunate mother's advice to her absent daughters in a letter to Miss Pennington.* London: printed for J. Walter. [see CW 3:4:11]

Rank, O. (1929). *The trauma of birth.* London: Kegan Paul, Trench, Trubner.

Rapoport, J. (1942). Therapeutic process in case of childhood schizophrenia. *The Nervous Child*, 1(2–3), 188.

Read, G. D. (1942). *Revelation of childbirth: The principles and practice of natural childbirth.* London: Heinemann.

Riviere, J. (1936). On the genesis of psychic conflict in earliest infancy. *International Journal of Psychoanalysis*, 17, 395–422.

Robertson, J. (1953). *A two-year-old goes to hospital* [Motion picture]. London: Concord Video and Film Council.

Robertson, J. (1958). *Going to hospital with mother* [Motion picture]. London: Tavistock Child Development Research Unit.

Robertson, J. (1958). *Young children in hospital*. London: Tavistock.

Sandy, J. R. (1948, 31 January). Letter: Mr Bevan and the B.M.A. *The Times*, Issue 50983.

Sargant, W. (1951). Leucotomy in psychosomatic disorders. *Lancet*, 258(6673), 87.

Sargant, W. (1951). The mechanism of 'conversion'. *British Medical Journal*, 2(4727), 311–316.

Sargant, W., & Stewart, C. M. (1947). Chronic neurosis treated with leucotomy. *British Medical Journal*, 2(4534), 866–869.

Schorstein, J. (1951, 28 July). Letter: Prefrontal leucotomy. *British Medical Journal*, 2(4725), 239.

Scott, W. C. M. (1949). The 'body scheme' in psychotherapy. *British Journal of Medical Psychology*, 22, 139–150.

Sechehaye, M. A. (1951). *Symbolic realization*. New York: International Universities Press.

Senn, M. J. (Ed.) (1949). *Problems of infancy and childhood. Transactions of the Third Conference*. New York: Josiah Macy, Jr. Foundation.

Shakespeare, W. *Hamlet*.

Shakespeare, W. *Romeo and Juliet*.

Shelley, P. B. (1824). Hymn to Mercury. In *Posthumous poems*. London: John and Henry L. Hunt.

Spitz, R. A. (1949). Autoerotism. *The Psychoanalytic Study of the Child*, 3–4, 85–120.

Spitz, R. A. (1950). Relevancy of direct infant observation. *The Psychoanalytic Study of the Child*, 5, 66–73.

Spitz, R. A., & Wolf, K. M. (1949). Anaclitic depression. *The Psychoanalytic Study of the Child*, 2, 313–342.

Steele, G. D. F. (1951). Persistent anxiety and tachycardia successfully treated by prefrontal leucotomy. *British Medical Journal*, 2(4723), 84.

Stein, L. (1949). *The infancy of speech and the speech of infancy*. London: Methuen.

Stungo, E. (1946, 15 June). Letter: Psychology in the child's education. *British Medical Journal*, 1(4458), 930.

The Children's Act. (1948). London: HMSO.

Watson, J. A. F. (1950). *The child and the magistrate*. London: Jonathan Cape.

Weiss, E. (1953). *Ego psychology and the psychoses*. London: Imago.

Whitehead, A. N. (1933). *Adventures of ideas*. Harmondsworth: Penguin.

Wickes, F. (1950). *The inner world of man: With psychological drawings and paintings*. London: Methuen.

World Health Organization Expert Committee on Mental Health. (1951). *Report on the second session, Geneva, 11–16 September 1950*. Technical Report Series, No. 31. Geneva: World Health Organisation.

Winnicott, D. W. (1943, 21 August). Letter: Responsibility and freedom. *British Medical Journal*. [CW 2:5:7]

Winnicott, D. W. (1943, 25 December). Letter: Shock treatment of mental disorder. *British Medical Journal*. [CW 2:5:10]

Winnicott, D. W. (1945). Primitive emotional development. [CW 2:7:8]

Winnicott, D. W. (1954). Mind and its relation to the psyche-soma [1949]. [CW 3:4:20]

Winnicott, D. W. (1947). Physical therapy of mental disorder. [CW 3:2:2]

Winnicott, D. W. (1948). Pediatrics and psychiatry. [CW 3:3:2]

Winnicott, D. W. (1948). Review: *The psychoanalytic study of the child, Vol. II*. [CW 3:3:9]
Winnicott, D. W. (1949). Hate in the countertransference [1947]. [CW 3:2:1]
Winnicott, D. W. (1949). Leucotomy. [CW 3:4:21]
Winnicott, D. W. (1949, 23 August). Letter: Punishment and crime: A psychologist's view. *The Times*. [CW 3:4:16]
Winnicott, D. W. (1950). Childhood psychosis. [CW 3:5:5]
Winnicott, D. W. (1950). Some thoughts on the meaning of the word democracy. [CW 3:5:17]
Winnicott, D. W. (1951). Book review: *The psychoanalytic study of the child, Vols. III–IV, & Vol. V*. [CW 3:6:12]
Winnicott, D. W. (1953). Psychoses and child care [1952]. [CW 4:1:5]
Winnicott, D. W. (1955). Metapsychological and clinical aspects of regression within the psychoanalytical set-up [1954]. [CW 4:3:6]
Winnicott, D. W. (1946). Some psychological aspects of juvenile delinquency. [CW 3:1:7]
Winnicott, D. W. (1957). The mother's contribution to society. [CW 5:3:30]
Winnicott, D. W. (1958). Aggression in relation to emotional development [1950]. [CW 3:5:2]
Winnicott, D. W. (1958). Appetite and emotional disorder [1936]. [CW 1:4:11]
Winnicott, D. W. (1958). Birth memories, birth trauma, and anxiety [1949]. [CW 3:4:8]
Winnicott, D. W. (1958). Primary maternal preoccupation [1956]. [CW 5:2:16]
Winnicott, D. W. (1958). Transitional objects and transitional phenomena. [CW 5:4:24]
Winnicott, D. W. (1964). Introduction to *The child, the family, and the outside world*. [CW 7:1:17]
Winnicott, D. W. (2017) The infancy of Juliet [1949]. [CW 3:4:4]
Winnicott, D. W. (2017). Report on Q camps [1941]. [CW 2:3:1]
Wolff, W. (1947). *The personality of the preschool child: The child's search for his self*. London: William Heinemann Medical Books.
Wordsworth, W. (1807). Ode: Intimations of mortality. *Poems, in Two Volumes*. London: Longman, Hurst, Rees and Orme.
Wulff, M. (1946). Fetishism and object choice in early childhood. *Psychoanalytic Quarterly*, 15, 450.
Ziman, E. (1951). *Jealousy in children: A guide for parents*. London: Victor Gollancz.

CONTRIBUTORS

Lesley Caldwell, General Editor
Lesley Caldwell is a member of the British Psychoanalytic Association in private practice in London. She is an Honorary Professor in the Psychoanalysis Unit and Honorary Senior Research Associate in the Italian Department at University College, London. As Chair of the Squiggle Foundation (2000–03) and editor of the Winnicott Studies Monograph Series (2000–08), she published four edited collections on D. W. Winnicott. She has been an editor for the Winnicott Trust since 2002 and was the Chair of Trustees from 2008 to 2012. With Angela Joyce, she published *Reading Winnicott* (2011). She has a continuing interest in psychoanalysis and the arts and has also written on film and the city of Rome.

Helen Taylor Robinson, General Editor
Helen Taylor Robinson is Fellow of the Institute of Psychoanalysis, British Psychoanalytical Society, London, and was a clinical psychoanalyst with adults and children until her retirement. She was an Editor and Trustee of the Winnicott Trust for seventeen years and co-edited *Thinking About Children* with Jennifer Johns and Ray Shepherd. Her special interest is in the relationship of psychoanalysis to the arts, literature, and cinema. She has been Honorary Senior Lecturer at the Psychoanalysis Unit of University College, London. She has contributed to books and journals in the field of psychoanalysis and to the European Psychoanalysis and Film Festival.

Vincenzo Bonaminio
Vincenzo Bonaminio, PhD, is training and supervising analyst of the Italian Psychoanalytic Society (SPI) and works in Rome in private practice with adults, adolescents, and children. He is Adjunct Professor at the Department of Child Psychiatry, La Sapienza, University of Rome, where he teaches child psychotherapy, works clinically with children, and coordinates a research group on brief psychoanalytic psychotherapy with latency children. He is Director of the D. W. Winnicott Institute for the Psychoanalytic Treatment of Children, Adolescents and Parental Couples attached to the University and is Director of Winnicott-Centro, Rome. He is Honorary Visiting Professor at UCL, London. He is co-editor of *Richard e Piggle*, the *Italian Journal for the Psychoanalytic Study of the Child and the Adolescent*, and co-editor of the series Psicoanalisi Contemporanea.

He has published extensively and was the Winner of the Frances Tustin Trust Memorial Prize in 2001.

Paolo Fabozzi
Paolo Fabozzi, PhD, is a full member of the Società Psicoanalitica Italiana (SPI), a component Society of the International Psychoanalytical Association (IPA), and also a child analyst. He is in private practice with adult patients and with adolescents. He is an adjunct professor in the Department of Dynamic and Clinical Psychology, La Sapienza, University of Rome, and has published widely.

CREDITS

Sources for the *Collected Works* include the published volumes of Winnicott's work, together with additional material from the Winnicott Archives, held at the Wellcome Library, London, and the Oskar Diethelm Library, Cornell Medical Center, New York; the Archives of the Institute of Psychoanalysis, London; the National Archives, Kew, UK; the British Library; the University of London Library at Senate House; the Bodleian Library, Oxford; and the archives of individual past editors of the Winnicott Trust. The *Collected Works* is as comprehensive as current sources allow; the online edition will enable the addition of any further material, should it become available. The Winnicott Archives at Wellcome and Cornell contain considerable material that cannot legally be accessed for reasons of confidentiality. Unless otherwise noted, all works appear courtesy of the Winnicott Trust.

Part 1

Chapter 1. 'Children's Hostels in War and Peace'. Published by arrangement with Routledge, an imprint of the Taylor & Francis Group and courtesy of John Wiley and Sons, Inc.

Chapter 2. 'Educational Diagnosis'. Published by arrangement with Routledge, an imprint of the Taylor & Francis Group and courtesy of The Froebel Trust.

Chapter 7. 'Some Psychological Aspects of Juvenile Delinquency'. Published by arrangement with Routledge, an imprint of the Taylor & Francis Group.

Part 2

Chapter 1. 'Hate in the Countertransference'. Published by arrangement with Routledge, an imprint of the Taylor & Francis Group and courtesy of John Wiley and Sons, Inc. Copyright Institute of Psychoanalysis.

Chapter 2. 'Physical Therapy of Mental Disorder'. Reprinted courtesy of BMJ Publishing Group.

Chapter 3. 'Residential Management as Treatment for Difficult Children'. Reproduced with permission of Sage Publications Ltd., London, Los Angeles, New Delhi, Singapore, and Washington, DC, from D. W. Winnicott, 'Residential Management as Treatment for Difficult Children', Human Relations, Copyright D. W. Winnicott, 1947.

Chapter 4.	'Further Thoughts on Babies as Persons'. Published by arrangement with Routledge, an imprint of the Taylor & Francis Group.
Chapter 5.	'The Child and Sex'. Routledge: Reprinted from *The Practitioner* by Permission of Practitioner Medical Publishing Ltd.

Part 3

Chapter 1.	'Reparation in Respect of Mother's Organized Defence Against Depression'. Published by arrangement with Routledge, an imprint of the Taylor & Francis Group.
Chapter 2.	'Paediatrics and Psychiatry'. Published by arrangement with Routledge, an imprint of the Taylor & Francis Group and courtesy of John Wiley and Sons, Inc.
Chapter 6.	'Review: *The Psychology of the Unwanted Child*' by A. Bowley. Reprinted courtesy of BMJ Publishing Group.
Chapter 7.	'Review: *Parents' Questions*' by Child Study Association of America. Reprinted courtesy of BMJ Publishing Group.
Chapter 8.	'Disorders of Childhood'. Reprinted courtesy of the Royal Society for Public Health.
Chapter 9.	'Review: *The Psychoanalytic Study of the Child, Vol. II*'. Reprinted courtesy of BMJ Publishing Group.
Chapter 10.	'Review: *The Personality of the Pre-School Child*' by W. Wolff. Reprinted courtesy of BMJ Publishing Group.
Chapter 12.	'Primary Introduction to External Reality'. Reprinted courtesy of Perseus Books Group.
Chapter 13.	'Environmental Needs'. Reprinted courtesy of Perseus Books Group.

Part 4

Chapter 8.	'Birth Memories, Birth Trauma, and Anxiety'. Published by arrangement with Routledge, an imprint of the Taylor & Francis Group.
Chapter 15.	'Review: *Handbook of Child Guidance*' edited by E. Harms. Reprinted courtesy of the BMJ Publishing Group.
Chapter 20.	'Mind and Its Relation to the Psyche-Soma'. Published by arrangement with Routledge, an imprint of the Taylor & Francis Group and courtesy of John Wiley and Sons, Inc.
Chapter 22.	'Review: *Art Versus Illness*' by Adrian Hill. Reprinted courtesy of John Wiley and Sons, Inc.
Chapter 23.	'A Man Looks at Motherhood'. Published by arrangement with Routledge, an imprint of the Taylor & Francis Group.
Chapter 24.	'The Baby as a Going Concern'. Published by arrangement with Routledge, an imprint of the Taylor & Francis Group.

Chapter 25.	'Where the Food Goes'. Published by arrangement with Routledge, an imprint of the Taylor & Francis Group.
Chapter 26.	'The End of the Digestive Process'. Published by arrangement with Routledge, an imprint of the Taylor & Francis Group.
Chapter 27.	'The Baby as a Person'. Published by arrangement with Routledge, an imprint of the Taylor & Francis Group.
Chapter 28.	'Close-up of Mother Feeding Baby'. Published by arrangement with Routledge, an imprint of the Taylor & Francis Group.
Chapter 29.	'The World in Small Doses'. Published by arrangement with Routledge, an imprint of the Taylor & Francis Group.
Chapter 30.	'The Innate Morality of the Baby'. Published by arrangement with Routledge, an imprint of the Taylor & Francis Group.
Chapter 31.	'Weaning'. Published by arrangement with Routledge, an imprint of the Taylor & Francis Group.
Chapter 32.	'Young Children and Other People'. Published by arrangement with Routledge, an imprint of the Taylor & Francis Group.
Chapter 33.	'Stealing and Telling Lies'. Published by arrangement with Routledge, an imprint of the Taylor & Francis Group.
Chapter 34.	'The Impulse to Steal'. Published by arrangement with Routledge, an imprint of the Taylor & Francis Group.

Part 5

Chapter 2.	'Aggression in Relation to Emotional Development'. Published by arrangement with Routledge, an imprint of the Taylor & Francis Group.
Chapter 5.	'Childhood Psychosis'. Reprinted courtesy of BMJ Publishing Group.
Chapter 8.	'Review: *Infancy of Speech and Speech of Infancy*' by Leopold Stein. Reprinted courtesy of John Wiley and Sons, Inc.
Chapter 10.	'The Deprived Child and How He Can Be Compensated for Loss of Family Life'. Published by arrangement with Routledge, an imprint of the Taylor & Francis Group.
Chapter 14.	'Knowing and Learning'. Published by arrangement with Routledge, an imprint of the Taylor & Francis Group.
Chapter 15.	'Instincts and Normal Difficulties'. Published by arrangement with Routledge, an imprint of the Taylor & Francis Group.
Chapter 16.	'Growth and Development in Immaturity'. Published by arrangement with Routledge, an imprint of the Taylor & Francis Group.
Chapter 17.	'Some Thoughts on the Meaning of the Word Democracy'. Published by arrangement with Routledge, an imprint of the Taylor & Francis Group and with permission of Sage Publications Ltd., London, Los Angeles, New Delhi, Singapore

	and Washington, DC, from D. W. Winnicott, 'Some Thoughts on the Meaning of the Word Democracy', *Human Relations*, Copyright D. W. Winnicott, 1950.
Chapter 18.	'Yes, But How Do We Know It's True?' Reprinted courtesy of Perseus Books Group.

Part 6

Chapter 1.	'Review: *The Child and the Magistrate*' by J. A. F. Watson. Reprinted courtesy of the BMJ Publishing Group.
Chapter 4.	'The Foundation of Mental Health'. Published by arrangement with Routledge, an imprint of the Taylor & Francis Group and courtesy of the BMJ Publishing Group.
Chapter 5.	'Visiting Children in Hospital'. Published by arrangement with Routledge, an imprint of the Taylor & Francis Group.
Chapter 7.	'Review: *The Inner World of Man: With Psychological Drawings and Paintings*' by F. Wickes. Reprinted from *The Lancet*, 258 (6672), D. W. Winnicott, *Review of The Inner World of Man*, 66. Copyright 1951, with permission from Elsevier.
Chapter 10.	'Review: *Jealousy in Children*' by E. Ziman. Reprinted courtesy of the BMJ Publishing Group.
Chapter 12.	'Review: *The Psychoanalytic Study of the Child, Vol. III & IV, Vol. V*'. Reprinted courtesy of the BMJ Publishing Group.
Chapter 15.	'Review: *On Not Being Able to Paint*' by Marion Milner. Reprinted courtesy of John Wiley and Sons, Inc.
Chapter 16.	'Review: *Problems of Infancy and Childhood*' by Ernest Jones. Reprinted courtesy of John Wiley and Sons, Inc.
Chapter 17.	'Review: *Papers on Psychoanalysis*' by Ernest Jones. Reprinted courtesy of the BMJ Publishing Group.
Chapter 18.	'Review: *Infant Feeding and Feeding Difficulties*' by Evans & MacKeith. Reprinted courtesy of John Wiley and Sons, Inc.

Additionally, some chapters in this volume were previously published in the following books:

The Child and the Family, 1957. Originally published by Tavistock Publications Ltd. Copyright 1957, D. W. Winnicott.

The Child and the Outside World, 1957. Originally published by Tavistock Publications Ltd. Copyright 1957, D. W. Winnicott.

Through Paediatrics to Psychoanalysis. First published 1958 by Tavistock Publications Ltd. First published 2001 by Routledge. Routledge is an imprint of the Taylor & Francis Group, an Informa Business. Copyright Tavistock, 1958.

The Family and Individual Development. First published 1965 by Tavistock Publications Ltd. First published 1989 by Routledge. Routledge Classics 2006. Routledge is an imprint of the Taylor & Francis Group, an Informa Business. Copyright 1965, D. W. Winnicott. Introduction to Routledge Classics edition: Copyright 2006, Martha Nussbaum.

Deprivation and Delinquency. First published 1984 by Tavistock Publications Ltd. First published 1990 by Routledge. Routledge Classics 2012. Routledge is an imprint of the Taylor & Francis Group, an Informa Business. Copyright 1984, Clare Winnicott. Foreword to Routledge Classics edition, Copyright 2012, Jan Abram.

INDEX

Page numbers in **bold** indicate reprinted letters and texts. Page numbers in *italics* indicate illustrations. In the index, DWW stands for Donald Woods Winnicott.

Abraham, K., 'The first Pregenital Stage of the Libido' (1916), 459–460
Adler, Alfred, 54
adolescents
  Romeo and Juliet, 185–193
  'Sex Education in Schools' (1949), **323–326**
  sexual activity and risk of pregnancy, 324–325
adoption
  emotional development of child affected by, 370
  of illegitimate children of adolescent mothers, 325
aggression. *See also* rage; hate and hatred
  'Aggression' (Royal Society of Medicine paper, 1948), 148, 333
  'Aggression in Relation to Emotional Development' (1950), 9, 148*n*iii, **333–347**
  Aggression in the Relationship Between Mature Persons (1947), 339*n*iii
  anger and frustration, 336
  concern and guilt, stage of, 335–336
  correlation between DWW's concepts of transitional objects and space and, 9–10
  early roots of, 335, 340–343
  external world and, 344–347
  identification with the aggressor, 347*n*6
  inner world, growth of, 336–339
  at intermediate stage of emotional development, 335–340
  letter to Anna Freud on (1948), 147–148
  in maturity, 339*n*iii
  mother-child relationship and, 5, 165–166, 311–312
  new semantics introduced by DWW, 4–5
  organisation of, 334
  social value of, 339
agoraphobia and DWW's concept of potential space, 12
Aichhorn, August, 473
Alexander, Franz, 147*n*i
allo-erotism, auto-erotism, and transitional objects, 448, 455, 456, 459, 461

anal erotism, 108, 110, 181
anger
  aggression and, 336
  primitive love impulse and, 394
angst, 208
antisocial behaviour
  deprivation of home life leading to, 439
  deprived children and, 371
  of evacuated children in WWII, 23–27, 79–81, 410
  guilt and, 241–242
  hidden vs manifest, 410–411, 420
  hostels for children in war and peace and, 23–27
  psychological aspects of juvenile delinquency and, 46, 49–50
  as symptom of illness, 239
  war and, 420
anxiety
  birth trauma and, 201–202, 207, 208, 216, 217, 228
  defined, 208
  leucotomy and, 467, 481
  guilt and, 302, 319
  transitional objects and instinct tensions, 449, 457
  unconscious, 413
'Appetite and Emotional Disorder' (1936), 139*n*2
art
  Milner, Marion, *On Not Being Able to Paint* (1950; review 1951), **483–485**
  psychoanalysis as, 41
asphyxiation, erotic, 215
Astor, Lady, 471
auto-erotism, allo-erotism, and transitional objects, 448, 455, 456, 459, 461

'The Baby as a Going Concern' (1949), **273–276**
'The Baby as a Person' (1949), **285–288**
Bakwin, Ruth Morris, 492
Bartemeier, Leo H., 487
'Basis for Self in Body' (1970), 17
'Battle Neurosis Treated with Leucotomy' (letter to the *British Medical Journal* 1947), **113**

BBC broadcasts
  'The Baby and Its Food (Home Service; 1949), 277
  'The Baby at Feeding Time' (Home Service; 1949), 289
  'Caring for Children and How Babies Develop Their Personalities' (Home Service; 1949), 269
  'Knowing and Learning How to be a Mother (Home Service; 1950), 387
  'The Mind of a Child (Home Service; 1949), 273
  'No Baby can Grow Properly Without Love' (Home Service; 1949), 285
  'The Passing of Excretions' (Home Service; 1949), 281
  'Presenting the World to a Baby' (Home Service; 1949), 293
  'Problems of Management' (Home Service; 1949), 299
  'Symptoms of Illness' (Home Service; 1950), 393
  'Weaning' (Home Service; 1949), 303
Beethoven, Ludwig van, 173
Beveridge, William, Lord, letter to (1946), **37–38**
Bion, W. R., 12, 147*n*i
  'The Imaginary Twin' (1950), 433*n*i
  letter to (1951), **433**
birth memories
  aggression, early roots of, 340
  analytical methodology for, 204
  anxiety and, 201–202, 207, 208, 216, 217, 228
  'Birth Memories, Birth Trauma and Anxiety' (1949), 16, 17, **201–220**, 221*n*i, 225–228, 340
  as break in infant's continuity of being, 212, 215–216, 217–218
  categorization of, 207
  chest, constriction of, 214–215
  clinical examples of, 134, 204–206, 211–213
  erotic asphyxiation and, 215
  as experience versus trauma, 204, 207, 217–218
  Freud on, 201–202, 207, 209, 217, 228
  Greenacre on, 201, 202–203, 207, 217, 220*n*1, 222, 226, 227
  head, emergence of, 213–214
  identification of whole body with penis and, 214
  mother-child relationship and, 215, 227–228
  normal birth experience, 209–213, 216, 226
  'Notes on the Discussion Held on Dr Winnicott's Paper "The Birth Trauma"' (1949), **225–228**
  psychological disorders and, 217–219, 225–227
  Read on, 203–204
  reliving, 226, 250–254
  traumatic births, handling of infants after, 226–227

body, sense of living in, 129, 167, 169–170, 192
Bollas, Christopher, 12
Bonaminio, Vincenzo, 3
Bowlby, John, 385, 400
  Maternal Care and Mental Health (1951), 405*n*2, 437–439
Bowley, Agatha H., *The Psychology of the Unwanted Child* (review; 1947), 149–150
BPAS. *See* British Psychoanalytical Society
Bradley, C., 354, 356
breastfeeding. *See also* weaning
  biting during, 301
  bottle-feeding and, 133, 277–278, 304
  described, 290–291
  first-time management of, 291–292
  maternal knowledge about nutrition and, 388
  methodological approach of DWW to child development and, 6–7
  personhood of baby and, 99, 100
  primary narcissism in, 10–11
  turning away from the breast, 291
Brierley, Marjorie, 121
British Journal of Medical Psychology
  articles by DWW first published in, 23, 123, 245, 265, 363, 483, 487, 489, 491
British Medical Journal
  articles by DWW first published in, 69, 353, 437
  'Battle Neurosis Treated With Leucotomy' (letter 1947), **113**
  'Ethics of Prefrontal Leucotomy' (letter 1951), **467–468**
  'Paddington Green Children's Hospital' (letter 1949), **243–244**
  '"Pathies in a State Service' (letter 1948), **141**
  'Psychology in the Child's Education' (letter 1946), **35–36**
  reviews originally published in, 149, 151, 157, 159, 235, 431, 469, 473
  'Taking Children's Temperatures' (letter 1949), **181–182**
British Medical Student's Journal, 259
British Psychoanalytical Society (BPAS)
  'Birth Memories, Birth Trauma and Anxiety' (1949) presented at, 201, 221*n*i, 222, 225
  candidates for membership, 233–234
  discussion on 'Consultation Technique' (1946), 42*n*i
  'Mind and Its Relation to the Psyche-Soma' (1949) read before, 245
  reparation, importance of recognizing, 121–122
  'Transitional Objects and Transitional Phenomena' first presented to (1951), 435
Britton, Clare. *See* Winnicott, Clare
broken homes. *See* deprivation of home life

Bruch, H., 356
Burlingham, Dorothy, 157

Cassel Hospital, 351
Casteret, N., *My Caves* (1947), 213
castration, as medical treatment, 479
castration anxiety
  brain mutilation and, 478
  childhood sexuality and, 102, 104, 110
  displacements of, 213
  dreams and, 62, 63
  penis envy and, 490
The child, the family, and the outside world (1964), 313, 323, 393, 421n4, 441
'The Child and Sex' (1947), **101–111**
The child and the family (1957), 313, 387, 393
The child and the outside world (1957), 313, 323
Child Care and Protection Act, 423
Child Study Association of America, *Parents' Questions* (review; 1947), 151
Child-Family Digest, 441
'Childhood Psychosis' (1950), **353–356**
Children's Act (1948), 425, 439
'Children's Hostels in War and Peace' (1948), **23–27**
citizenship, home life as basis for, 35
claustrophobia
  infant management and, 135
  potential space, DWW's concept of, 12
clinical observations
  birth memories, 134, 204–206, 211, 212–213
  transitional objects, 448, 451–455
'Close-up of Mother Feeding Baby' (1949), **289–292**
Collected papers: Through paediatrics to psycho-analysis (1958), 59, 117, 201, 245, 333, 447
concern, stage of
  aggression and, 5, 335–336
  in child development, 402–403
continuity of being
  birth memories as break in, 212, 215–216, 217–218
  child development and, 404
  mind and its relationship to psyche-soma, 247, 248, 249, 250, 256
continuity of management, child's need for, 24
controlled projection test, 149
convulsion therapy (electric shock, shock therapy, E.C.T.), 59, 70–71, 72–75
corporal punishment
  hate in the countertransference and, 65
  in hostels, 84, 93n4, 432
  as substitute climax, 105
Cottington, F., 356
countertransference
  anticipation by DWW of later developments in understanding, 3–4
  classification of phenomena of, 60
  'Hate in the Countertransference' (1947), 3–4, 7, 8–9, 15, **59–68**
  interpsychic processes, DWW's account of, 7–9
Creak, E. M., 356
Crichton-Miller, Hugh, 327ni
crime
  expiation and propitiation, value to criminal of, 241–242
  letter to *The Times* (1949) on punishment and crime, **237–238**, 239, 241–242
  penal reform, 357–359
  as psychological illness, 44–45
  'Punishment and Crime: A Psychologist's View' (letter to *the Times*, 1949), **237–238**, 241, 359, 359ni
  WWII and increase in, 410
Criminal Justice Act (1948), 432
'Curtis Report on the Care of Children' (1946); Curtis Committee (Home Office Care of Children Committee), 162, 439, 92n2, 149, 350, 423

Davies, W. H., 'Infancy', 132
day nurseries versus nursery school, 471
delinquent children
  antisocial behaviour and, 46
  child psychosis and, 353
  hostels and prevention of, 26, 47, 81–82
  letter to *The Times* (1949) on punishment and crime, **237–238**
  link to deprivation, 42, 45–47, 95
  'Psychological Aspects of Juvenile Delinquency' (undated; ca. late 1940s), **49–55**
  'Some Psychological Aspects of Juvenile Delinquency' (1946), **43–48**, 322n1
democracy
  developmental growth of child towards, 398
  defined, 408
  different uses for term, 407–408
  education in, 419
  gender, political leadership, and fear of women, 416–417, 421n4
  geographical boundaries, 418–419
  immature identification with authority/society and, 410–411
  innate democratic tendency, analysing, 410–412, 421n2
  machinery of, 409–410
  ordinary good homes fostering, 412–414, 415, 421n3
  parent-child relationship in, 417–418

democracy (*Cont.*)
  proportional representation, 421*n*1
  psychiatric health and, 408–409
  social unrest and memory of dependence, 339*n*iii
  'Some Thoughts on the Meaning of the Word Democracy' (1950), 195*n*1, 197, 199, 405*n*1, **407–421**
  voting and elections, 409, 414–415
  at war, 419–420
dependence, social unrest and memory of, 339*n*iii
depression
  child psychosis and, 353
  deprived children and, 370–371
  electric shock and, 73
  emotional development, depressive position in, 157–158, 335, 402, 457–458
  helping friends with, 424–425
  'Reparation in Respect of Mother's Organized Defence Against Depression' (1948), 12–13, 14–15, **117–122**
  Romeo in *Romeo and Juliet*, latent depressed mood of, 186, 190–191
  weaning delays and, 187–189
deprivation of home life
  assessment of deprivation, 368–371
  classification of broken homes, 368–369
  delinquency and, 43, 47–48
  and depression, 158, 370
  'The Deprived Child and How He Can Be Compensated for Loss of Family Life' (1950), **367–380**
  early history of child, importance of taking, 376–378
  effects on emotional development, 438–439
  foster parents, 373, 375
  hospital, visiting children in, 438, 441–445
  hostels, 373–374
  large institutions, 374, 375–376, 377–378
  non-interference with functioning households, 367–368
  physical care as psychological care, 98
  providing care for deprived children, 371–374
  small homes, 373
  therapeutics and management, 375–376
  transitional objects and, 378–380
  value of stays away from home for older children, 444
Descuret, J. B. Felix, 157
Despert, J. L., 356
Deutsch, Helene, 490
diagnostic interviews with child, 125
discussions (at societal meetings)
  on 'Consultation Technique' at BPAS (1946), 42*n*i

'Notes on the Discussion Held on Dr Winnicott's Paper "The Birth Trauma" (1949), **225–228**
disillusionment, 99–100, 306, 322, 458
'Disorders of Childhood' (1948), **153–155**
displacement, transitional objects and, 456
divorce and child development, 367
Dobinson, C. H., 472
dolls
  Lilly (doll played with by DWW as child), 331
  with sex organs, 183–184
dreams
  of birth experience, 212–213
  healing, 62–63
  'Interpretation of Dreams' (S. Freud), 458, 461
  and reality, 220*n*3, 262, 295, 296, 337
  sexuality and, 105
dropping and throwing away, 287, 304–305
dummies, as transitional objects, 452

E.C.T. (electric shock, shock therapy, convulsion therapy), 59, 70–71, 72–75
education
  of children (*See* school and teaching)
  and democracy, 415, 419, 421
  of parents, 399–401
'Educational Diagnosis' (1946), **29–33**
'Ego Distortion in Terms of True and False Self' (1960), 4, 14
electric shock (shock therapy, convulsion therapy, E.C.T.), 59, 70–71, 72–75
The End of the Digestive Process (1949), **281–284**
'Enuresis: Notes for a Lecture to the Tavistock Children's Department' (ca. 1949), **327–328**
environment
  birth memories and, 204, 210, 211–212
  child's need for environmental stability, 24, 88, 128
  classification of environmental factors, 223, 381
  delinquent children and, 51–53
  'Environmental Needs; the Early Stages; Total Dependence and Essential Independence' (1948), **171–176**, 185
  good-enough environment, 247–248, 369–370
  growth and development resulting from, 397–398
  in hostels, 90–92
  'The Innate Morality of the Baby' (1949), **299–302**
  Klein birthday book and, 223, 229, 381
  primary home experience, concept of, 80–81
  for psychoanalysis, 63–64
  sense of responsibility for, 250
ethics. *See* morality and ethics

Index 519

'Ethics of Prefrontal Leucotomy' (letter to the
   British Medical Journal 1951), **467–468**
euthanasia, 260
evacuation of children, World War II
   antisocial behaviour of, 23–27, 79–81, 410
   development of hostels for, 77–78
Evans, Philip, and Ronald MacKeith,
   Infant Feeding and Feeding Difficulties
   (review 1951), **491–493**
excited state, child management of, 401–403
excretion
   child's reactions to, 395
   disgust and, 395
   The End of the Digestive Process (1949),
      281–284
   'Enuresis: Notes for a Lecture to the Tavistock
      Children's Department' (ca. 1949), **327–328**
   relation to mother, 99. *See also* mother-child
      relationship
external reality. *See* reality

Fabozzi, Paolo, 3, 9, 11
Fain, M., 341, 347*n*1
Fairbairn, W. R. D., 'Endopsychic structure
   considered in terms of object-relationships'
   (1944), 461
Fairhurst, William, 161
The family and individual development
   (1965), 367, 397, 407
fantasies (phantasies)
   aggression and, 165, 311, 402
   asphyxiation as masturbation fantasy, 215
   of birth, 216, 218, 251
   of conflict against parents, 80, 103
   fantasy vs. reality, 296, 337
   fear of domination by fantasy women, 417
   of primitive love impulse, 314, 320
   in psychoanalysis, 121–122
   of re-entry into mother head-first, 214
   sex fantasies, 104–106
   transitional objects and, 458, 459
father-child relationship and sexual
   development in children, 102–104, 105–106
'fathers and mothers' (childhood game), 106,
   307–308, 445
fear
   Ernest Jones on, 490
   leucotomy, associated with, 481
   normal, 396
   of women, 416–417
Federn, Paul
   'Ego Psychology and the Psychoses'
      (1952), 179*n*i
   letter to (1949), **179–180**
feeding. *See also* breastfeeding; weaning
   belching, 278–279

bottle versus breast, 277–278, 304
'Close-up of Mother Feeding Baby' (1949),
   289–292
digestive process, 278–280
The End of the Digestive Process (1949), **281–284**
Evans, Philip, and Ronald MacKeith,
   Infant Feeding and Feeding Difficulties
   (review 1951), **491–493**
institutional versus maternal, 289–292
maternal knowledge about, 388
mother-child relationship and, 309
paediatrics and psychiatry, interplay between,
   125, 130–133
reality, introduction of child to, 296–297
refusal of food and finickiness, 395
spoon game (spatula game), 285–288, 304
'Where the Food Goes' (1949), **277–280**
Field, Joanna, 461
finger-sucking, as transitional object, 452, 454
Fitzgerald, Otho W. S., letter to (1950), **351–352**
Flügel, J. C., 147*n*i
Follett, M. P., *Creative Experience* (1924), 483
foster parents, 373, 375, 426
'The Foundation of Mental Health' (1951), **437–439**
Fremont-Smith, Frank, 487
Freud, Anna
   on aggression, at Royal Society of Medicine
      symposium (1947), 148*n*iii, 333, 473
   'Aggression in Relation to Emotional
      Development: Normal and Pathological'
      (1947), 147*n*i, 148*n*iii
   circle of influence, 474
   The Ego and the Mechanisms of Defence (1937),
      460–461
   Harms, Ernest, ed. *Handbook of Child
      Guidance* (1947; review 1949), 235
   on identification with the aggressor, 347*n*6
   letter to (1948), **147–148**
   on mother-child relationship, 126
   The Psychoanalytic Study of the Child, Volume 2
      (1946; review 1948), **157–158**
   *The Psychoanalytic Study of the Child, Volumes
      3-4 and 5* (1949; review 1951), 461, **473–474**
   reparation, DWW's concept of, 13
Freud, Sigmund
   accomplishments of, 397
   on aggression, 339
   Angst defined by, 208
   Beyond the Pleasure Principle, 208
   on birth trauma and anxiety, 201–202, 207,
      208, 209, 217, 228
   on childhood roots of adult
      psychoneurosis, 123
   on denial, 14
   in Harms, Ernest, ed. *Handbook of Child
      Guidance* (1947; review 1949), 235

Freud, Sigmund (*Cont.*)
  Susan Isaacs and, 161
  Jones, Ernest, *Papers on Psycho-Analysis* (1948; review 1951), 489, 490
  methodological approach of DWW and, 6
  on mother-child relationship, 66
  obsessional neurosis, theory of, 257*n*1
  reparation, DWW's concept of, 13
  Joan Riviere as translator of, 221
  scientific psychology and, 70
  on sexuality in childhood, 102, 103, 397, 490
  James Strachey as translator of, 435
  on transitional objects, 458–459, 460, 461
  on the unconscious, 43, 54
Freud, Sigmund, works
  'Collected Papers' Vol. 3, 459
  The Ego and the Id (1923), 460
  Fliess Letters (1895), 461
  Group Psychology and the Analysis of the Ego (1921), 202, 460
  Instincts and their Vicissitudes (1915), 65
  The Interpretation of Dreams (1900), 458
  'Introductory Lectures on Psychoanalysis' (1916-1917), 459
  Project for a Scientific Psychology, 461*n*i
  'Three Essays on the Theory of Sexuality' (1915), 459
Friedlander, Kate, 126–127
Fry, Margery, *Child Care and the Growth of Love* (1953), 405*n*2
'Further Thoughts on Babies as Persons' (1947), **95–100**

Galeerd, Elizabeth, 157
Gesell, Arnold, 461
Giannakoulas, A., 11
Gillespie, William, 225
Glover, Edward, 121, 167
  letter to (1951), **475**
  The Psychoanalytic Study of the Child, Volume 2 (1946; review, 1948), **157–158**, 475*n*i
  The Psychoanalytic Study of the Child, Volumes 3-4 and 5 (1949; review 1951), 461, **473–474**
Goodenough, Sir William, and Goodenough Report, 243
good-enough mothering/environment, 247–248, 343, 369–370
Green, André, 'The Dead Mother' (1980), 15*n*vi
Greenacre, P., 201, 202–203, 207, 217, 220*n*1, 222, 226, 227
'Growth and Development in Immaturity' (1950), **397–405**
guilt
  antisocial behaviour and, 241–242
  in depressive position, 457

Ernest Jones on, 490
  reparation and, 117
  in stage of concern, 335–336, 402–403
'The Gwrw Tree' (1948), **143–145**

Harms, Ernest, ed. *Handbook of Child Guidance* (1947; review 1949), **235**
Hartmann, H., 341
Haskell, Arnold, 119
hate and hatred
  capacity for, 80, 148, 369
  child's, for foster parents, 375
  DWW's, 38
  feeling in psychiatric discourse and, 3
  'Hate in the Countertransference' (1947), 3–4, 7, 8–9, 15, **59–68**
  Ernest Jones on, 490
  for father, 103
  frustration and, 311
  love, coincidence of hate with, 61, 64
  in mother-child relationship, 66–67
  repressed, 44, 370
  in transference, **59–68**, 70
Hazlehurst, R. S., letter to (1949), **239**
healing dreams, 62–63
Health Visitors, 303
Heimann, Paula, 226, 229, 233
  'On Counter-transference' (1950), 3*n*ii
Henriques, Basil, 431
Henry, Hannah 'Queen', 197, 383
  letter to (1950), **383–384**
Hernandez, M., 11
hidden antisocials, 410–411, 420
Hill, Adrian, *Art Versus Illness* (1948; review, 1949), **265–267**
history-taking. *See* medical histories, taking
Hodge, S. H., letter to (1949), **241–242**
Hoffer, Willie, 461
  The Psychoanalytic Study of the Child, Volume 2 (1946; review, 1948), **157–158**, 461, 475*n*i
  The Psychoanalytic Study of the Child, Volumes 3-4 and 5 (1949; review 1951), 461, **473–474**
holding and picking up babies, 96–97, 168, 209, 388–391
Holloway Gaol, 237
home, value of stays away from, 444
homeopathy, 141
homosexuality, 104, 119, 214
Horney, Karen, 490
hospital, visiting children in. *See* visiting children in hospital
hostels
  administrative development of, 82–83
  antisocial behaviour and, 23–27
  central therapeutic idea of, 88–92

'Children's Hostels in War and Peace'
  (1948), **23–27**
 delinquency, preventing, 26, 47, 81–82
 deprived children, providing care for, 373–374
 development of wartime hostels scheme for
  evacuated children, 77–78
 environment of, 90–92
 for evacuated children with antisocial
  behaviour, 23–27, 79–81
 'Maladjusted Children: Damaging Effect of
  Delay' (letter to the *Times*, 1950), **361–362**
 placement of children in, 25–26, 85–88
 as primary home experience, 80–81
 provision of, 25
 psychiatric teams in, 83–85
 purpose and effectiveness of, 81–82
 'Residential Management as Treatment for
  Difficult Children' (with Clare Britton;
  1947), 27n1, **77–93**
 self-government, problem of, 93n5
 training of staff, 89–90
Human Relations, 27n1, 195, 407
Hussey, B. J., 181
hypochondriacs, 117–122
hypo-manic patients' view of analyst, 60

Ilg, Frances, 461
illegitimacy, 325, 369
Illingworth, R. S., 'Sleep Disturbances in Young
  Children' (1951), 461
'The Impulse to Steal' (1949), **319–322**
'The Infancy of Juliet' (1949), 174n1, **185–193**
infant development
 'Further Thoughts on Babies as Persons'
  (1947), **95–100**
 'Growth and Development in Immaturity'
  (1950), **397–405**
 paediatrics and psychiatry, interaction of, 124,
  128–136
 psychoanalytical re-enactment of, 132–136
'The Innate Morality of the Baby' (1949),
  299–302
inner world of the child, 173, 336–339, 463
'insane', use of word, 92n3
instinct
 'Instincts and Normal Difficulties' (1950),
  393–396
 transitional objects and instinct tensions, 457
Institute of Child Psychology, 183
Institute of Education, University of London, 171
Institute of Public Health and Hygiene, 153
Integration, 6, 14
 aggression and, 335, 340 345
 of the ego, 9, 340
 of the personality, 70, 167, 334–335
 hate and, 65–66

as maturational process, 15–17, 128,
  167–168, 403
 non-integration and, 14
 in *Romeo and Juliet*, 186, 192
intelligence testing and educational
  diagnosis, 30
Interdepartmental Committee on Medical
  Schools, 243n1
intermediate area, 6–7, 16
International Conference on Mental Health (11-
  21 August 1948), 147n1
International Journal of Psychoanalysis, 59, 223,
  447, 460
International Psychoanalytical Association,
  DWW at Seventeenth Congress (1951),
  Amsterdam, 20
introjection and transitional objects, 456
Isaacs, Nathan, 163
Isaacs, Susan, 169, 472
 Childhood and After, 162, 460
 'Children in Institutions' in *Childhood and
  After*, 162
 The Children We Teach, 162
 Intellectual Growth in Young Children (1930), 161
 'The Nursery Years' (1929), 162
 obituary, **161–163**
 Social Development in Young Children (1933), 161

jealousy
 Ernest Jones on, 490
 Ziman, Edmund, *Jealousy in Children* (review
  1951), **469**
Jones, Ernest, 245, 475
 Papers on Psycho-Analysis (1948; review 1951),
  489–490
Josiah H. Macy, Jr. Foundation, 487
*Journal of the Royal Institute of Public Health and
  Hygiene*, 153
Jung, Carl, 54, 122, 235, 463
Juvenile Courts
 hostel committees and, 47
 psychological methods, use of, 44
 Watson, J. A. F., *The Child and the Magistrate*
  (1950, review 1951), **431–432**
juvenile delinquency. *See* delinquent children

Kanner, Leo, 354
Khan, Masud, 12
Klein, Melanie
 on aggression, 335, 338, 347n6
 on depressive position in emotional
  development, 157–158, 335, 457
 environment and, 223, 381, 385
 Glover's critique of, 121, 475
 Harms, Ernest, ed. *Handbook of Child
  Guidance* (1947; review 1949), 235

Klein, Melanie (*Cont.*)
  IJPA birthday festschrift (1952), 223, 229, 231, 365*n*1, 381, 385
  Susan Isaacs and, 162, 163
  normal child behaviour compared to psychosis, by, 13
  on paranoid anxiety, 217
  potential space, DWW's concept of, 12
  and reparation, 13, 14, 121, 402
  scientific psychology and, 70
  on sexual development in girls, 490
  theories of, 5, 12–13
  on transitional objects, 460, 461
Klein, Melanie, works
  'Notes on Some Schizoid Mechanisms' (1946), 4–5, 256*n*12
  The Psycho-Analysis of Children (1932), 460
  'The Psychogenesis of the Manic-Depressive States' (1935), 461
'Knowing and Learning' (1950), **387–391**

The Lancet, 463, 467
leucotomy
  benefits of, 259, 260
  DWW's critique of, 59, 72, 259–263
  'Ethics of Prefrontal Leucotomy' (letter to the *British Medical Journal* 1951), **467–468**
  'Leucotomy' (1949), 59, **259–263**
  'Leucotomy in Psychosomatic Disorders' (letter to *The Lancet* 1951), **465–466**
  'Notes on the General Implications of Leucotomy' (1951), **477–481**
Little, H. M., 356
Little, Margaret, 218
London School of Economics, 423, 477
love
  of DWW for wife Clare, 331
  hate, coincidence with, 61, 64
  in mother-child relationship, 270–271, 274
  primitive love impulse, 340, 394, 457

MacAlpine, I., 246
MacKeith, Ronald, and Philip Evans, *Infant Feeding and Feeding Difficulties* (review 1951), **491–493**
maladjusted children
  'Maladjusted Children: Damaging Effect of Delay' (letter to the *Times*, 1950), **361–362**
  transitional object, lack of, 379
  use of word 'maladjusted', 92
Malleson, Joan, 181–182
'A Man Looks at Motherhood' (1949), **269–271**
'The Manic Defence' (1935), 14
manic-depressive disease, 137
Mannheim, Hermann, 49, 49*n*i
Marty, P., 341, 347*n*1

masturbation, 108–110
  asphyxiation as fantasy of, 215
  compulsive, 109, 459
  sex education in schools and, 324
maturity
  democracy and, 408
  as development process, 397
  health as, 95, 408–409
Maudsley Hospital, 266, 357
McCarthy, Desmond, 174
McMillan, Margaret, 472
Mead, Margaret, 147*n*i
medical histories, taking
  deprived children, 376–378
  paediatrics and psychiatry, interplay between, 124–125, 136–137
Medical Press, 323
medical profession. *See also* nurses
  disorders of childhood, lessons learned from, 153–155
  inter-speciality discussion, 351–352, 487
  mother-child relationship and, 291–292, 310–311
  nationalization of, 37–38, 39, 141
  osteopathy, homeopathy, and other practices not accepted on scientific grounds, 141
  science in medical practice, 69–70
melancholia, 137
mental disability
  educational diagnosis of, 30
  psychosis confused with, 134, 204, 353
mental health
  development of, 126–127, 274
  'The Foundation of Mental Health' (1951), **437–439**
  as maturity, 95
  theory of, 71–72
'Metapsychological and Clinical Aspects of Regression within the Psycho-Analytical Set-Up', 257*n*2
Middle Group, 41
Middlemore, Merell P., *The Nursing Couple* (1941), 124, 130
Mill Hill (former location of Maudsley Hospital), 266
Milner, Marion, *On Not Being Able to Paint* (1950) review (1951), **483–485**
  on transitional objects, 461
mind
  brain and, 260
  as entity, 245
  as function of psyche-soma, 246–247
  head, localization in, 254–256
  'Mind and Its Relation to the Psyche-Soma' (1949), 17, 220*nn*5–6, **245–257**
  reliving birth experience and, 250–254
  theory of, 247–250

Index

Ministry of Health
  Goodenough Report, 243*n*i
  hostels, establishment of, 26, 47, 78, 79, 82, 92*n*1
Moncrieff, A., 181
Money-Kyrle, Roger
  democracy defined by, 408
  letters to (1949), **195, 197, 199, 223, 229, 231**
  letters to (1950), **365, 381, 385**
  letters to (1952), 10
  Psychoanalysis and Politics (1951), 365
  'Some Aspects of State and Character in Germany' (1951), 408*n*i
morality and ethics
  of leucotomy and shock therapy, 465, 467, 478
  'Ethics of Prefrontal Leucotomy' (letter to the *British Medical Journal* 1951), **467–468**
  'The Innate Morality of the Baby' (1949), **299–302**
  of the child, 171, 299–302
  imposition of, 312, 325
mother-child relationship
  aggression and, 5, 165–166, 311–312
  'The Baby as a Going Concern' (1949), **273–276**
  'The Baby as a Person' (1949), **285–288**
  birth memories and, 215, 227–228
  'dead mother', Greene's concept of, 15*n*vi
  development of, 126–127
  enjoyment and pleasure in, 274–275
  excretion, maternal management of, 282–284
  father, existing within structure provided by, 6*n*iii, 273–274
  feeding and, 309
  good-enough mothering, 247–248
  hate and, 66–67
  hypochondria in mothers, 117–122
  illness versus normal behaviour, 393–396
  'The Innate Morality of the Baby' (1949), **299–302**
  'Instincts and Normal Difficulties' (1950), **393–396**
  interpsychic processes, DWW's awareness of, 7–9
  'Knowing and Learning' (1950), **387–391**
  love in, 270–271, 274
  'A Man Looks at Motherhood' (1949), **269–271**
  medical professionals, role of, 291–292, 310–311
  mental health and, 126–128
  methodological approach of DWW to child development and, 6–7
  personhood of baby and, 96–100, 285–288, 308–310
  physical care as psychological care, 98–99
  picking up and holding babies, 96–97, 168, 209, 388–391
  primary maternal preoccupation, 220*n*4
  primary narcissism in, 10–11
  reality, infant contact with, 130–132
  reparation and, 12–15
  sexual development in children and, 102–104, 105–106, 107
  stealing as looking for mother, 46, 314–315, 320, 336*n*ii, 371
  talking to mothers about, 425
  'The World in Small Doses' (1949), **293–297**
  'The Mother's Contribution to Society', 421*n*4
music, as occupation therapy, 266–267

National Association for Mental Health, 147*n*i
National Froebel Foundation Bulletin, 29
National Health Service, 37–38, 39, 141
National Society for the Prevention of Cruelty to Children, 349
Nature, 161
Nazis and Nazism, 35
negative mother transference, 233
'Neglected Children' (letter to the *Times*, 1950), **349–350**
Nemon, Oscar, bust of D. W. Winnicott (1971), *ii*
neurosis
  analyst, neurotic patient's view of, 60
  psychoanalytical environment and, 64
neurosurgery and psychology, 261, 466
New Directions in Psychoanalysis, 223
New Era in Home and School, 43, 95, 441
night terrors, and sexual climax, 105
'Notes on the Discussion Held on Dr Winnicott's Paper "The Birth Trauma"' (1949), **225–228**
'Notes on the General Implications of Leucotomy' (1951), **477–481**
Not-Me, 344–347, 447, 456
nursery school
  day nurseries versus, 471
  'Nursery Schools: A Definition of Functions' (letter to *the Times* 1951), **471–472**
nurses
  breastfeeding opinions of, 291–292
  mother-child relationship and, 291–292, 310–311
  visiting children in hospital and, 438, 441–445

'Obituary: Susan Isaacs' (1948), **161–163**
obsessional neurosis
  analyst, obsessional neurotic's view of, 60
  Freud's theory of, 257*n*1
occupation therapy, 266–267
Oedipus complex, 102–103, 339
Ogden, Thomas, 4
oral erotism, 214, 334
The ordinary devoted mother and her baby (1949), 269, 273, 277, 281, 285, 289, 293, 299, 303
osteopathy, 29, 39, 141, 167

Paddington Green Children's Hospital, 24, 227
  'Paddington Green Children's Hospital' (letter to the *British Medical Journal* 1949), **243–244**
  threat to close, 221–222, 243–244
paediatrics and paediatricians
  and childhood sexuality, 108–109
  childhood psychosis, awareness of, 353
  and psychiatry, 126, 136, 487
  and mental disorders, 71
  out of touch with psychology, 181, 204, 354
  'Paediatrics and Psychiatry' (1948), 13–14, **123–139**
  'Taking Children's Temperatures' (letter to *British Medical Journal*, 1949), **181–182**
pain and transitional objects, 455–456
panic attacks, 12
paranoia and birth memories, 217, 225–227
parents
  Child Study Association of America, *Parents' Questions* (review; 1947), **151**
  democracy, ordinary good homes fostering, 412–414, 415, 421n3
  democracy, parent-child relationship in, 417–418
  disillusionment as job of, 99–100, 306, 322
  education of, 399–401
  foster parents, 373, 375, 380
  medical professionals, what parents need from, 154
  mother-child relationship existing within structure provided by father, 6niii, 273–274
  morality and standards, role of, 299–302
  quarrelling between, 338
Parents' Magazine, 162
part objects, transitional objects as, 456
"Pathies in a State Service' (letter to the *British Medical Journal* 1948), **141**
penal reform, 357–359
penis
  identification of whole body with, 214
  penis envy, 110, 490
Pennington, Lady Sarah, 'Advice to her daughters in 1824', 227
personal management, child's need for, 24
personhood of baby, 96–100, 285–288, 308–310
phantasies. *See* fantasies
physical care as psychological care, 98–99
'Physical Therapy of Mental Disorder' (1947), 59, **69–75**
picking up and holding babies, 96–97, 168, 209, 388–391
play
  dolls with sex organs, letter to manufacturer of, 183–184
  'fathers and mothers' (childhood game), 106, 307–308, 445

hospital experience and, 445
imagination and, 286, 288, 290
sexuality and, 104–106
spoon (spatula) game, 285–288, 304
Playing and Reality (1971), 447
pleasure-pain principle and transitional objects, 455–456
The Possible Significance of the Nurse Scene in *Romeo and Juliet* (1966), 185
potential space
  DWW's semantics of, 11–12
  methodological approach of DWW to child development and, 6–7
The Practitioner, 101
pre-school children. *See also* nursery school
  intensity of feeling in, 294
  reality, introduction of child to, 294–296
  Wolff, Werner, *The Personality of the Preschool Child: The Child's Search for His Self* (1947; review, 1948), **159–160**
primary home experience, 80–81, 86, 92
'Primary Introduction to External Reality: The Early Stages' (1948), **165–170**, 185
'Primary Maternal Preoccupation' (1956), 220n4
'Primitive Emotional Development' (1945), 4, 6, 9, 17, 139n3, 246
primitive love impulse, 340, 394, 457
Princess Louise Hospital for Children, 243
prisoners of war, 226
probation officers, talk on 'Psychological Aspects of Juvenile Delinquency' (undated; ca. late 1940s) given to, **49–55**
'The Problem of Homeless Children' (with Britton), 27n1
projection
  controlled projection test, 149
  projective identification, 5
  transitional objects and, 456
proportional representation, 421n1
psyche-soma
  head, localization of mind in, 254–256
  'Mind and Its Relation to the Psyche-Soma' (1949), 17, 220nn5–6, **245–257**
  mind as function of, 246–247
  reliving birth experience and, 250–254
  theory of mind and, 247–250
psychiatric social workers
  antisocial children in hostels, arranging psychotherapy for, 25
  deprived children, taking histories of, 377–378
psychiatrists
  antisocial children in hostels, arranging psychotherapy for, 24–25, 27n2
  hate in the countertransference and, 59–68
  inter-speciality discussion, 351–352, 487

Index

regression of patient, importance of adapting to, 234
reparation and, 121–122
psychoanalysis
　as an art, 41
　of BPAS candidates, 233–234
　defined, 54
　environment for, 63–64
　infant development, re-enactment of, 132–136
　interpsychic processes, DWW's awareness of, 7–9
　potential space in, 12
　repressed memories, regaining, 101–102
The Psychoanalytic Study of the Child (ed. Anna Freud, W. Hoffer, and E. Glover)
　Volume 2 (1946; review, 1948), **157–158**, 461, 475ni
　Volumes 3–4 and 5 (1949; review 1951), 461, **473–474**
'Psychological Aspects of Juvenile Delinquency' (undated; ca. late 1940s), **49–55**
psychology
　scientific, 70
　study of, 423–427
'Psychology in the Child's Education' (letter to *British Medical Journal* 1946), **35–36**
'Psychoses and Child Care', 248
psychosis
　analyst, psychotic patient's view of, 60
　'Childhood Psychosis' (1950), **353–356**
　countertransference, DWW's understanding of, and, 4
　hate in the countertransference and, 59–68
　mental disability confused with, 134, 204, 353
　methodological approach of DWW to, 6–7
　normal child behaviour compared, 13–14, 125–126
　psychoanalytical environment and, 64
　regressions, psychotic, 125
psychosomatic disorders
　birth memories and, 217
　'Leucotomy in Psychosomatic Disorders' (letter to *The Lancet* 1951), **465–466**
　in paediatrics, 139
　purpose of, 255–256
　sexual development in children and, 108
punishment. *See also* corporal punishment
　expiation and propitiation, value to criminal of, 241–242
　letter to *The Times* (1949) on punishment and crime, **237–238**, 239, 241–242
　penal reform, 357–359
　'Punishment and Crime: A Psychologist's View' (letter to *the Times*, 1949), **237–238**, 241, 359, 359ni
　as substitute climax, 105

quiet states and transitional objects, 457

radio, as occupation therapy, 267
rage, in infants and young children, 394, 396
Rank, O., *Trauma of Birth* (1929), 212, 213
Rapaport, J., 356
Raven, John C., 149
Read, Grantly Dick, 203–204
reality, infant introduction to
　child development and, 403–404
　environmental needs and, 172
　paediatrics and psychiatry, interaction of, 128–132, 135–136, 137–139
　'Primary Introduction to External Reality: The Early Stages' (1948), **165–170**, 185
　in *Romeo and Juliet*, 192
　'The World in Small Doses' (1949), **293–297**
refugees, 226
regression
　analyst needing to adapt to, 234
　in childhood schizophrenia, 134
　psychotic, 125
　theory of mind and, 247, 251
remand homes, 51, 52
reparation
　in child development, 402
　DWW's understanding of, 12–15
　'Reparation in Respect of Mother's Organized Defence Against Depression' (1948), 12–13, 14–15, **117–122**
repressed unconscious, 101–102, 208
'Residential Management as Treatment for Difficult Children' (with Clare Britton; 1947), 27n1, **77–93**. *See also* hostels
responsibility, reliability, and child growth and development, 398–399
reviews
　Bowley, Agatha H., *The Psychology of the Unwanted Child* (1947; review 1948), **149–150**
　Child Study Association of America, *Parents' Questions* (1947; review 1948), **151**
　Evans, Philip, and Ronald MacKeith, *Infant Feeding and Feeding Difficulties* (1951), **491–493**
　Freud, A., Hoffer, W., Glover, E., eds., *The Psychoanalytic Study of the Child, Volume 2* (1946, review 1948), **157–158**, 475ni
　Freud, A., Hoffer, W., Glover, E., eds., *The Psychoanalytic Study of the Child, Volumes 3–4 and 5* (1949; review 1951), **473–474**
　Harms, Ernest, ed. *Handbook of Child Guidance* (1947; review 1949), **235**
　Hill, Adrian, *Art Versus Illness* (1948; review 1949), **265–267**
　Jones, Ernest, *Papers on Psycho-Analysis* (1948, review 1951), **489–490**

reviews (*Cont.*)
    Milner, Marion, *On Not Being Able to Paint* (1950; review 1951), **483–485**
    Senn, M. J. (Ed.), *Problems of Infancy and Childhood. Transactions of the Third Conference* (1949; review 1951), **487**
    Stein, Leopold, *The Infancy of Speech and the Speech of Infancy* (1949; review 1950), **363–364**
    Watson, J. A. F., *The Child and the Magistrate* (1950; review 1951), **431–432**
    Wickes, Frances G., *The Inner World of Man: With Psychological Drawings and Paintings* (1950; review 1951), **463**
    Wolff, Werner, *The Personality of the Preschool Child: The Child's Search for His Self* (1947; review 1948), **159–160**
    Ziman, Edmund, *Jealousy in Children* (1951), **469**
Rickman, John, 147*n*i
Riviere, Joan, 233*n*i, 341, 460, 490
    letters to (1949), **221–222, 233–234**
Robertson, James, 400
    Going to Hospital with Mother (film), 405*n*2
    A Two-year-old goes to Hospital (film), 405*n*2
    Young Children in Hospital (1958), 405*n*2
'Rockabye Baby', 67
Rodman, F. Robert, 234*n*ii
Romeo and Juliet (Shakespeare), 174, 185–193
Rosenberg, Dr, 228
Royal Society of Medicine, 148, 333
ruthlessness
    stage of ruth, 335, 339, 402
    ruthless love, 66
    of primitive impulses, 311, 457
    'pre-ruth', 5, 335, 340

St Mary's Hospital Paddington Green, 222, 243–244. *See also* Paddington Green Children's Hospital
Sandy, J. R., 141
Sargant, William, 113, 465
    'The Mechanism of Conversion', 467
schizoid states
    child psychosis and, 353
    countertransference, DWW's understanding of, and, 4
    management of, 137
schizophrenia
    birth memories and, 212–213
    in childhood, 353, 354
    infant development and, 125, 128, 134, 135, 137
    reality, relationship to, 172–173
Schmideberg, Melitta, 179
school and teaching
    continuity of teachers at a school, 175

'Educational Diagnosis' (1946), **29–33**
management of children in, 169
'Primary Introduction to External Reality: The Early Stages' (1948), **165–170**, 185
'Psychology in the Child's Education' (letter to *British Medical Journal*, 1946), **35–36**
reality, introduction of child to, 295
relationship between teachers and children, 176
'Sex Education in Schools' (1949), **323–326**
Schorstein, Joseph, 467
science
    human nature, scientific inquiry into, 404
    in medical practice, 69–70
scientific psychology, 70
Scott, P. D., letter to (1950), **357–359**
Scott, W. C. M., 245, 253, 255
    on environmental factors, 228
    on pregnant mothers, 227
Sechehaye, M. A., 347*n*2
Senn, M. J. (Ed.), *Problems of Infancy and Childhood. Transactions of the Third Conference* (1949; review 1951), **487**
sexuality
    adult sexual disorders and childhood development, 104, 106–107, 111
    aggression and eroticism, 344–347
    anal erotism, 108, 110, 181
    in boys, 102–103, 109–110
    'The Child and Sex' (1947), **101–111**
    contact with reality and, 137
    dolls with sex organs, letter to manufacturer of, 183–184
    'fathers and mothers' (childhood game), 106, 307
    Freud on childhood sexuality, 102, 103, 397, 490
    genital excitement, onset of, 110
    in girls, 103–104, 107, 110, 490
    homosexuality, 104, 119, 214
    Juliet's falling over in presence of nurse's husband in *Romeo and Juliet*, 187, 189, 193
    male genitalia, value placed on, 109–111
    maternal knowledge and handling of, 395
    oral erotism, 214, 334
    play and, 104–106
    psychosomatic disorders and, 108
    'Sex Education in Schools' (1949), **323–326**
    transitional objects, auto-erotism, and allo-erotism, 448, 455, 456, 459, 461
    urinary erotism, 110
Shakespeare, William
    feuds, external and internal, 185–187
    Hamlet, 174, 426

'The Infancy of Juliet' (1949), 174*n*i, **185–193**
inner world of, 173
Romeo and Juliet, 174, 185–193
Sharpe, Ella Freeman, letter to (1946), **41**
shell shock, 113, 327*n*i
Shelley, Percy Bysshe, 492
Shenley Hospital, St Albans, 351
shock therapy (electric shock, convulsion therapy, E.C.T.), 59, 70–71, 72–75
siblings
  differences between, 313
  holding younger siblings, 388–389
  maternal role taken on by, 398
  transitional objects, different uses of, 451–455
social unrest and memory of dependence, 339*n*iii
society's unconscious reactions to insanity, 75
'Some Psychological Aspects of Juvenile Delinquency' (1946), **43–48**, 322*n*1
'Some Thoughts on the Meaning of the Word Democracy' (1950), 195*n*i, 197, 199, 405*n*1, **407–421**
speech and speaking
  Stein, Leopold, *The Infancy of Speech and the Speech of Infancy* (1949; review 1950), **363–364**
Spence, James, 130, 139*n*1
Spitz, René A., 157–158, 473–474, 492
  'Autoerotism' (1949), 461
  'Relevancy of Direct Infant Observation' (1950), 461
spoon game, 285–288, 304
stealing
  as belief in something good, 52, 55
  child's lack of understanding of, 239, 242, 319–320
  as delinquency and antisocial behaviour, 46, 52–53, 55, 79, 239, 241–242
  'The Impulse to Steal' (1949), **319–322**
  psychological significance of, 46, 242, 314–315, 320, 336*n*ii, 371, 451
  sexual desire and, 107
  'Stealing and Telling Lies' (1949), **313–317**
Steele, G. D. F., 467
Stein, Leopold, *The Infancy of Speech and the Speech of Infancy* (1949; review 1950), **363–364**
Stewart, C. M., 113
Stone, Marjorie, letter to (1949), **183–184**
Strachey, James, letter to (1951), **435–436**
'String' (1960/1965), 447
Stungo, E., 35, 36
subjective object, 6–7
suicide
  child psychosis and, 353
  erotic asphyxiation versus, 215
  inner world, child's management of, 338
  as murder, 333
  right to commit, 468
Sutherland, Miriam, 161
symbolism of transitional objects, 456

'Taking Children's Temperatures' (letter to the *British Medical Journal* 1949), **181–182**
tantrums, 396
Tavistock Clinic, 327, 438
Taylor, Alice (later Winnicott; first wife), 195*n*ii, 197*n*i, 383–384
temperature, taking, 181–182
theft. *See* stealing
theory of mind, 247–250
thumb-sucking, as transitional object, 452, 454
The Times
  'Maladjusted Children: Damaging Effect of Delay' (letter 1950), **361–362**
  on nationalization of medical profession (DWW letter 1946), **39**
  on nationalization of medical profession (J. R. Sandy letter 1948), 141
  'Neglected Children' (letter 1950), **349–350**
  'Nursery Schools: A Definition of Functions' (letter 1951), **471–472**
  'Punishment and Crime: A Psychologist's View' (letter 1949), **237–238**, 239, 241, 359, 359*n*i
Tod, Robert, 327
toilet training, 282–283
total happenings, 287–288
training
  of children, 299
  of hostel staff, 89–90
transference, 233. *See also* countertransference
transitional objects
  abnormalities associated with, 450–451
  aggression, correlation with DWW's conception of, 9–10
  auto-erotism and allo-erotism, 448, 455, 456, 459, 461
  characteristics of, 450
  clinical descriptions, 448, 451–455
  defined, 448
  depressive position and, 457–458
  deprivation of home life and, 378–380
  DWW's theory of, 448–451
  infant development and, 405
  instinct tensions and quiet states, 457
  introjection and projection, 456
  Klein's birthday book, possible article for, 381
  literature review, 458–461
  methodological approach of DWW to child development and, 6–7
  normal sequence of, 448–450
  primary narcissism and, 10–11

transitional objects (*Cont.*)
  psychology of stealing and, 451
  theoretical approach to, 455–458
  'Transitional Objects and Transitional Phenomena' (presentation notes, 1951), 435, **447–461**
  'Transitional Objects and Transitional Phenomena' (published 1953/1958/1971), 447
transitional space
  aggression, correlation with DWW's conception of, 9–10
  primary narcissism and, 11
twins
  adult psychiatric issues stemming from infant treatment of, 133–134, 175
  Bion, 'The Imaginary Twin' (1950), 433ni
  birth memories of, 214
  transitional objects and, 452

the unconscious
  delinquent children and, 43–44, 54
  Freud on importance of, 43, 54
  infancy and childhood, adult memory of, 101
  repressed unconscious, 101–102, 208
  society's unconscious reactions to insanity, 75
unconsciousness (physical), 210–211
United Nations programme for the welfare of homeless children, 438
United States, DWW on, 352, 418
urinary erotism, 108
'The Use of an Object' (1968), 4, 18

van Gogh, Vincent, 138
visiting children in hospital
  foundations of mental health and, 438
  'Visiting Children in Hospital' (1952), **441–445**

war, democracy at, 419–420
Watson, J. A. F., *The Child and the Magistrate* (1950, review 1951), **431–432**
weaning
  good feeding experience and, 303–306
  of Juliet in *Romeo and Juliet*, 187–189
  transitional objects and, 451, 452, 453
  'Weaning' (1949), **303–306**
Welfare Centres, 273
'Where the Food Goes' (1949), **277–280**
Whitehead, A. N., 121
WHO (World Health Organization), Expert Committee on Mental Health, 437–439
Wickes, Frances G.
  chapter in Harms, Ernest, ed. *Handbook of Child Guidance* (1947; review 1949), 235

The Inner World of Man: With Psychological Drawings and Paintings (1950; review 1951), **463**
Wilson, Dr, 227
Winnicott, Alice (née Taylor; first wife), 195$n$ii, 197ni, 383–384
Winnicott, Clare (née Britton; second wife)
  letter to (1950), **331**
  occupation therapy, use of, 266
  'The Problem of Homeless Children' (with Winnicott), 27n1
  'Residential Management as Treatment for Difficult Children' (with Winnicott; 1947), 27n1, **77–93**
Winnicott, Donald Woods (DWW)
  1946, 23–55
  1947, 59–113
  1948, 117–176
  1949, 179–328
  1950, 331–427
  1951, 431–493
  chronology, 495–501
  heart condition, 221$n$ii, 383
  images of, ii, 20
  interpsychic processes, awareness of, 7–9
  methodological approach to psychosis in children, 6–7
  separation from first wife, 195$n$ii, 197ni
Wolff, Werner, *The Personality of the Preschool Child: The Child's Search for His Self* (1947; review, 1948), **159–160**
women, fear of, 416–417, 421n4
Wordsworth, W., *Ode: Intimations of Immortality* (1807), 100ni
World Health Organization (WHO), Expert Committee on Mental Health, 437–439
'The World in Small Doses' (1949), **293–297**
World War I, shell shock in, 327ni
World War II. *See also* evacuation of children
  bombings and air raids, 454
  effect on antisocial behaviour and crime, 410
  prisoners of war and refugees, 226
  Tavistock Clinic and, 327ni
Wulff, M., 'Fetishism and Object Choice in Early Childhood' (1946), 458

'Yes, but How Do We Know It's True?' (1950), **423–427**
Young Children (1949), 307
'Young Children and Other People' (1949), **307–312**
Ziman, Edmund, *Jealousy in Children* (review 1951), **469**